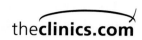

OTOLARYNGOLOGIC CLINICS OF NORTH AMERICA

Advances in Oculo-facial Surgery

GUEST EDITOR
Stephen L. Bosniak, MD

October 2005 • Volume 38 • Number 5

SAUNDERS

An Imprint of Elsevier, Inc.
PHILADELPHIA   LONDON   TORONTO   MONTREAL   SYDNEY   TOKYO

W.B. SAUNDERS COMPANY
A Division of Elsevier Inc.

1600 John F. Kennedy Boulevard, Suite 1800, Philadelphia, PA 19103–2899

http://www.theclinics.com

THE OTOLARYNGOLOGIC CLINICS	**Volume 38, Number 5**
OF NORTH AMERICA	**ISSN 0030–6665**
October 2005	**ISBN 1-4160-2864-1**
Editor: Molly Jay	

Reprints. For copies of 100 or more, of articles in this publication, please contact the Commercial Reprints Department, Elsevier Inc., 360 Park Avenue South, New York, New York 10010-1710. Tel. (212) 633-3813; Fax: (212) 462-1935; email: reprints@elsevier.com

The ideas and opinions expressed in *The Otolaryngologic Clinics of North America* do not necessarily reflect those of the Publisher. The Publisher does not assume any responsibility for any injury and/or damage to persons or property arising out of or related to any use of the material contained in this periodical. The reader is advised to check the appropriate medical literature and the product information currently provided by the manufacturer of each drug to be administered to verify the dosage, the method and duration of administration, or contraindications. It is the responsibility of the treating physician or other health care professional, relying on independent experience and knowledge of the patient, to determine drug dosages and the best treatment for the patient. Mention of any product in this issue should not be construed as endorsement by the contributors, editors, or the Publisher of the product or manufacturers' claims.

The Otolaryngologic Clinics of North America (ISSN 0030–6665) is published bimonthly by W.B. Saunders Company. Corporate and editorial offices: Elsevier, Inc., 1600 John F. Kennedy Boulevard, Suite 1800, Philadelphia, PA 19103-2899. Accounting and circulation offices: 6277 Sea Harbor Drive, Orlando, FL 32887–4800. Periodicals postage paid at Orlando, FL 32862, and additional mailing offices. Subscription price is $199.00 per year (US individuals), $350.00 per year (US institutions), $100.00 per year (US student/resident), $269.00 per year (Canadian individuals), $430.00 per year (Canadian institutions), $280.00 per year (international individuals), $430.00 per year (international institutions), $140.00 per year (international & Canadian student/resident). Foreign air speed delivery is included in all *Clinics'* subscription prices. All prices are subject to change without notice. POSTMASTER: Send address changes to *The Otolaryngologic Clinics of North America*, W.B. Saunders Company, Periodicals Fulfillment, Orlando, FL 32887–4800. **Customer Service: 1-800-654-2452 (US). From outside the US, call 407-345-4000.**

The Otolaryngologic Clinics of North America is also published in Spanish by McGraw-Hill Interamericana Editores S.A., P.O. Box 5-237, 06500 Mexico D.F., Mexico.

The Otolaryngologic Clinics of North America is covered in *Index Medicus, Current Contents/Clinical Medicine, Excerpta Medica, BIOSIS, Science Citation Index,* and *ISI/BIOMED.*

Printed in the United States of America.

GUEST EDITOR

STEPHEN L. BOSNIAK, MD, Attending Surgeon, Manhattan Eye, Ear and Throat Hospital; and Private Practice, New York, New York

CONTRIBUTORS

ERIC B. BAYLIN, MD, Clinical Instructor of Ophthalmology and Oculoplastics, Department of Ophthalmology, William Beaumont Hospital, Royal Oak; and Consultants in Ophthalmic and Facial Plastic Surgery, Southfield, Michigan

STEPHEN L. BOSNIAK, MD, Attending Surgeon, Manhattan Eye, Ear and Throat Hospital; and Private Practice, New York, New York

CYNTHIA A. BOXRUD, MD, FACS, Assistant Clinical Professor, Department of Ophthalmology, Division of Ophthalmic Plastic and Reconstructive Surgery, Jules Stein Eye Institute, University of California-Los Angeles, Los Angeles, California

CAT NGUYEN BURKAT, MD, Assistant Professor, Oculoplastics Service, Department of Ophthalmology and Visual Sciences, University of Wisconsin-Madison, Madison, Wisconsin

MARIAN CANTISANO-ZILKHA, MD, Center for Clinical Studies, Oftalmoclinica Botafogo; and Private Practice, Rio de Janeiro, Brazil

DAMON B. CHANDLER, MD, Clinical Instructor in Ophthalmology and Fellow, Oculoplastic and Orbital Surgery, Scheie Eye Institute, University of Pennsylvania, Philadelphia, Pennsylvania

TACIANA DE OLIVEIRA DAL'FORNO, MD, Dermatologist; and Fellow in Training, Federal University of Rio Grande do Sul, Porto Alegre, Brazil

BRENDA C. EDMONSON, MD, Clinical Assistant Professor, Hahnemann University, Philadelphia; and Private Practice, Warrington, Pennsylvania

IRA ELIASOPH, MD, FACS, Associate Clinical Professor of Ophthalmology, Mount Sinai School of Medicine, New York; Associate Attending Ophthalmic Surgeon, Mount Sinai Hospital, New York; Chief of Oculoplastic Surgery, Veterans Hospital, Bronx; Chief of Oculoplastic Surgery, Emeritus, Beth Israel Hospital, New York; Chief of Ophthalmology, Jewish Home and Hospital, Bronx; and Associate Attending Ophthalmic Surgeon, Manhattan Eye, Ear, and Throat Hospital, Manhattan, New York

ROBERTA E. GAUSAS, MD, Assistant Professor of Ophthalmology and Director, Oculoplastic and Orbital Surgical Service, Scheie Eye Institute, University of Pennsylvania, Philadelphia, Pennsylvania

JEFFREY P. GILBARD, MD, Clinical Assistant Professor, Department of Ophthalmology, Harvard Medical School, Boston; and Founder, CEO, and Chief Scientific Officer, Advanced Vision Research, Woburn, Massachusetts

GEOFFREY J. GLADSTONE, MD, FAACS, Clinical Professor of Ophthalmology, Michigan State University School of Medicine, East Lansing; Assistant Clinical Professor of Ophthalmology and Otolaryngology, Wayne State University School of Medicine, Detroit; Co-Director, Oculoplastic Surgery, Department of Ophthalmology, William Beaumont Hospital, Royal Oak; and Consultants in Ophthalmic and Facial Plastic Surgery, Southfield, Michigan

IOANNIS P. GLAVAS, MD, Department of Ophthalmology, New York University Medical School, Manhattan Eye, Ear and Throat Hospital, New York, New York

DORIS MARIA HEXSEL, MD, Dermatologist; and Coordinator, Cosmetic Dermatology Department, Brazilian Society of Dermatology, Brazil

JONATHAN A. HOENIG, MD, Assistant Clinical Professor, Jules Stein Eye Institute, University of California-Los Angeles Medical Center, Los Angeles; and Private Practice, Encino, California

BRADLEY N. LEMKE, MD, Lemke Facial Surgery, Madison, Wisconsin

JANET M. NEIGEL, MD, FACS, Private Practice, West Orange, New Jersey

T.G. PAIKIDZE, MD, TOTALCharm, Clinic of Plastic and Aesthetic Surgery, Moscow, Russia

BHUPENDRA C.K. PATEL, MD, FRCS, FRC OPHTH, Professor, Division of Facial Plastic Reconstructive and Cosmetic Surgery, John Moran Eye Center, University of Utah, Salt Lake City, Utah

RANDAL T. PHAM, MD, Clinical Assistant Professor, Division of Ophthalmic Plastic & Reconstructive Surgery, Department of Ophthalmology, Stanford University, Stanford; and Medical Director, Aesthetic & Refractive Surgery Medical Center, San Jose, California

DEBORA ZECHMEISTER DO PRADO, PHARM, Pharmacist; and Research and Scientific Development Assistant, Doris Hexsel Dermatologic Clinic, Porto Alegre, Brazil

JOHN G. ROSE JR, MD, Oculofacial and Facial Cosmetic Surgery, Davis Duehr Dean, Madison, Wisconsin; and Oculoplastics Service, Department of Ophthalmology and Visual Sciences, University of Wisconsin-Madison, Madison, Wisconsin

STUART R. SEIFF, MD, FACS, Michal D. Vilensky Professor or Ophthalmology and Director, Department of Ophthalmic Plastic and Reconstructive Surgery, University of California San Francisco; and Chief, Department of Ophthalmology, San Francisco General Hospital, San Francisco, California

MARCIO SERRA, MD, Dermatologist; and Study Group on Lipodystrophy, Brazilian Health Ministry–Sexually Transmitted Diseases Department, Rio de Janeiro, Brazil

G.M. SULAMANIDZE, MD, TOTALCharm, Clinic of Plastic and Aesthetic Surgery, Moscow, Russia

M.A. SULAMANIDZE, MD, TOTALCharm, Clinic of Plastic and Aesthetic Surgery, Moscow, Russia

ALLAN E. WULC, MD, FACS, Clinical Associate Professor, University of Pennsylvania, Philadelphia; Private Practice, Warrington, Pennsylvania

LISA A. ZDINAK, MD, Fellow, Bosniak + Zilkha, New York, New York

ORIN M. ZWICK, MD, Department of Ophthalmic Plastic and Reconstructive Surgery, University of California San Francisco, San Francisco, California

CONTENTS

most recently, glabelar lines. This article discusses the development of the use of botulinum toxin, with focus on its benefits in treating facial dystonia and upper facial rhytidosis.

Current Techniques of Entropion and Ectropion Correction

903

Ira Eliasoph

The entities of entropion and ectropion have some important common factors in their genesis. Preoperative examination requires similar careful assessment and planning. The need for surgery must first be established, and the changes in the anatomy must be evaluated. Prior local trauma or surgery, conjunctival or skin changes, septal shortening, weakness of muscles, retractor thinning or dehiscence, orbicularis muscle shift, and, most importantly, the status of the lateral canthal tendon must all be considered. In performing any eyelid surgery, entropion or ectropion should not be produced, and preventive techniques must be incorporated into such undertakings. Anesthetic injections should be subcutaneous and only as deep as needed. The amount injected should not be excessive, because distortion or stretching can occur. Dealing with orbital fat should never involve any pulling, which can shear off a deep orbital vessel with serious consequences. Immediate and adequate measures for intraorbital bleeding should be familiar to the surgeon and instituted without delay. Restoration of lid anatomy with precise surgical methods yields improved lid function, comfort, and cosmesis.

Ptosis Evaluation and Management

921

Brenda C. Edmonson and Allan E. Wulc

Drooping of the upper eyelids is one of the most common complaints in oculoplastic practice. This anatomic and morphologic state is termed ptosis, from the Greek "to fall." This article discusses some of the more common types of ptosis and provides an introduction to the evaluation and management of the ptosis patient. Complications of ptosis surgery and recent innovations in ptosis surgery are discussed.

Comprehensive Management of Eyebrow and Forehead Ptosis

947

Jonathan A. Hoenig

The inferior displacement of the eyebrows results in apparent redundancy of the upper eyelid skin and hooding in the multicontoured areas of the medial and lateral canthal regions. Patients often present to the aesthetic surgeon complaining of dermatochalasis and request blepharoplasty. The re-establishment of the structural integrity of the eyebrow is fundamental to achieving an aesthetically acceptable surgical result for cosmetic and functional periocular surgery.

peripheral blood suppressor/cytotoxic T8+ lymphocytes, and a depressed T4/T8 ratio. Environmental and genetic factors, such as HLA-DR histocompatibility loci, may play a role in developing thyroid orbitopathy, although a specific cause has not yet been undetermined. Both cellular and humoral immune mechanisms contribute to the disorder.

five sessions of phosphatidylcholine injections in facial areas of localized fat, with a minimum interval of 3 to 4 weeks between applications. Clinical evaluations and photographic assessments were performed before and after injections. The degree of patient satisfaction with the results was assessed by means of a telephone questionnaire performed 3 years after treatment. Ninety percent of the sample reported a reduction of localized fat deposits on the face and neck. Of these, 50% reported a marked reduction, 33.3% reported a moderate reduction, and 16.6% reported a discreet reduction. Eighty percent reported a persistent improvement 3 years after the treatment sessions. All the HIV-positive patients reported a marked and persistent improvement. All members of the sample reported pain and presented with erythema, edema, itching, and bruises in the treated areas. No systemic side effect was reported. Phosphatidylcholine can be used successfully in small areas of localized fat on the face. It is a minimally invasive procedure with few and reversible side effects.

FORTHCOMING ISSUES

RECENT ISSUES

The Clinics are now available online!

Access your subscription at
www.theclinics.com

Otolaryngol Clin N Am
38 (2005) xiii

OTOLARYNGOLOGIC
CLINICS
OF NORTH AMERICA

Preface

Advances in Oculo-facial Surgery

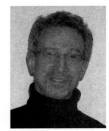

Stephen L. Bosniak, MD
Guest Editor

In the past two decades, new techniques, anatomic considerations, and an ever-expanding menu of noninvasive therapies have revolutionized the science and art of oculo-facial surgery. When used in combination, these techniques function well and have enhanced effects.

This issue of the *Otolaryngologic Clinics of North America* will address the most current understanding of eyelid and peri-orbital anatomy, approaches to patients in need of oculo-facial reconstruction or rejuvenation, recognition and treatment of patients with dry eyes, and the state-of-the-art of botulinum toxin injections for the management of blepharospasm as an adjunct or alternative to surgery and as the foundation of a noninvasive therapeutic regimen.

The oculo-facial surgeon's cosmetic approaches to the forehead, eyebrows, and eyelids are treated in great detail. The latest surgical techniques for the management of eyelid, lacrimal, and thyroid-related deformities—entropion and ptosis correction, upper and lower eyelid reconstruction, dacryostenosis, and thyroid ophthalmopathy—are also presented in this issue.

It is a privilege to share our perspectives and insights. We acknowledge this opportunity as a milestone in cross- and multidisciplinary cooperation that will ultimately enhance our profession and benefit our patients.

Stephen L. Bosniak, MD
135 East 74th Street
New York, NY 10021, USA

E-mail address: sbosniak@mindspring.com

ELSEVIER
SAUNDERS

Otolaryngol Clin N Am
38 (2005) 825–856

OTOLARYNGOLOGIC
CLINICS
OF NORTH AMERICA

Anatomy of the Orbit and Its Related Structures

Cat Nguyen Burkat, MD[a],*, Bradley N. Lemke, MD[b]

[a]Oculoplastics Service, Department of Ophthalmology and Visual Sciences,
F4/336-3220 Clinical Science Center, 600 Highland Avenue,
University of Wisconsin-Madison, Madison, WI 53792, USA
[b]Lemke Facial Surgery, Madison, WI, USA

A comprehensive knowledge of orbital and periorbital anatomy is necessary to understand disorders in these regions and to apply medical and surgical management appropriately and safely.

The configuration of the bony orbit resembles a four-sided pyramid that becomes three-sided near the apex, with a volume of approximately 30 cm³. The adult orbital rim measures, on average, 40 mm horizontally and 35 mm vertically, with the widest dimension of the orbit 1 cm behind the anterior orbital rim. The medial walls are roughly parallel and are 25 mm apart in adults. The length of the medial orbital wall from the anterior lacrimal crest is 45 to 50 mm, whereas the lateral wall from the rim to the superior orbital fissure measures 40 mm [1,2]. The lateral orbital walls are angled 90° from each other. The lateral orbital rim is approximately at the level of the equator of the globe. The globe has an average volume of 6.5 cm³ and has a shape formed by two spheres, the cornea and the sclera, with radius of curvatures equal to 8 and 12 mm, respectively [2]. Globes in the average adult and newborn infant measure 24 mm and 16.4 mm, respectively, in the anteroposterior dimension.

Osteology

Whitnall [2] described the orbital rim as a spiral with its two ends overlapping medially on either side of the lacrimal sac fossa (Fig. 1). The inferior orbital rim is comprised of the maxillary bone medially and the zygomatic bone laterally. The zygomatic bone forms the lateral orbital rim,

---

* Corresponding author.
E-mail address: catburkat@yahoo.com (C.N. Burkat).

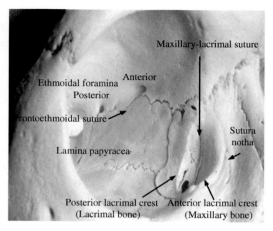

Fig. 1. Bony anatomy of the lacrimal sac fossa and medial orbital wall, right orbit. The anterior and posterior lacrimal crests are formed by the maxillary and lacrimal bones, respectively.

and the frontal bone forms superior orbital rim. In most skulls, the superior rim is indented by a supraorbital notch at the junction of its medial one third and lateral two thirds, where the supraorbital nerve and artery pass to supply the forehead. In approximately 25% of skulls, a foramen within the frontal bone is present, rather than a notch [3,4]. Large studies by Webster [5] and Miller [6] found that 46% to 49% of skulls had bilateral supraorbital notches, 26% to 28% had bilateral supraorbital foramina, and 25% had a notch and a foramen on the other side. The supraorbital landmark is generally located 27 mm from the midline of the face, with a range of 15 to 38 mm [5–9]. The average vertical distance of the supraorbital foramen from the orbital rim is 1.6 mm, although it may vary from 1 to 19 mm [5,10]. Beer [10] found that a single supraorbital exit site was found in 84% of orbits, and more than one notch or foramen exited a single orbit in 14%. Multiple bony landmarks were also previously classified by Kimura [11].

Studies have been unable to identify consistently a supratrochlear notch or foramen as seen with the supraorbital nerve. In general, the mean distance of the supratrochlear nerve from the midline is 16 to 17 mm [6,9,12]. In contrast, Webster [5] found that supratrochlear notches were found in 97% of skulls, with 1% having bilateral foramina.

The medial orbital rim is formed anteriorly by the frontal process of the maxillary bone rising to meet the maxillary process of the frontal bone. The lacrimal sac fossa is a depression in the inferomedial orbital rim, formed by the maxillary and lacrimal bones (Fig. 1). It is bordered by the anterior lacrimal crest of the maxillary bone and the posterior lacrimal crest of the lacrimal bone. The fossa is approximately 16 mm high, 4 to 9 mm wide, and 2 mm deep [2,13]. The fossa is widest at its base, where it is confluent with the opening of the nasolacrimal canal. The lower nasolacrimal fossa and the nasolacrimal canal are narrower in females, which may contribute to the female predominance of nasolacrimal obstruction [14].

The nasolacrimal duct is 3 to 4 mm in diameter and courses in an inferolateral and slightly posterior direction toward the inferior turbinate. The duct has an interosseous length of 12 mm and terminates as a 5-mm extension within the inferior meatus. All the walls of the canal, except the medial wall, are formed by the maxillary bone. The medial wall of the bony canal is formed by the lateral nasal wall inferiorly and the descending process of the lacrimal bone superiorly [15]. On the frontal process of the maxilla, just anterior to the lacrimal sac fossa, a fine groove, the sutura notha, or sutura longitudinalis imperfecta of Weber, runs parallel to the anterior lacrimal crest (Fig. 1) [2]. Small branches of the infraorbital artery pass through this groove to supply the bone and nasal mucosa. The presence of these branches should be anticipated during lacrimal surgery to avoid bleeding.

The orbital walls, consisting of seven bones, are embryologically derived from neural crest cells. Ossification of the orbital walls is completed by birth except at the orbital apex. Although the lesser wing of the sphenoid is initially cartilaginous, the other orbital bones develop by intramembranous ossification. The frontal bone forms most of the orbital roof, except the posterior 1.5 cm, which is formed by the lesser wing of the sphenoid bone as the roof tapers into the anterior clinoid process. The optic foramen is located in the lesser wing of the sphenoid, through which the optic nerve enters the orbit at a 45° angle from the midline. The lacrimal gland fossa is located in the lateral orbital roof, and the trochlear fossa is located in the anteromedial orbital roof.

The medial orbital wall is formed, from anterior to posterior, by the frontal process of the maxilla, the lacrimal bone, the ethmoid bone, and the lesser wing of the sphenoid bone. The thinnest portion of the medial wall is the lamina papyracea, which covers the ethmoid sinuses medially. Infectious, inflammatory, or neoplastic processes of the ethmoid sinuses commonly extend through the lamina papyracea to cause orbital cellulitis and proptosis. The ethmoid bullae appear as a honeycomb pattern medial to the ethmoid bone. The medial wall becomes thicker posteriorly at the body of the sphenoid and anteriorly at the posterior lacrimal crest of the lacrimal bone.

The frontoethmoidal suture marks the approximate level of the ethmoid sinus roof, so dissection superior to this suture may expose the cranial cavity. The anterior and posterior ethmoidal foramina conveying branches of the ophthalmic artery and the nasociliary nerve are located at the frontoethmoidal suture 24 mm and 36 mm posterior to the anterior lacrimal crest, respectively (Fig. 2) [16].

A vertical suture running centrally between the anterior and posterior lacrimal crests represents the anastomosis of the maxillary bone to the lacrimal bone (Fig. 1). A suture located more posteriorly within the fossa

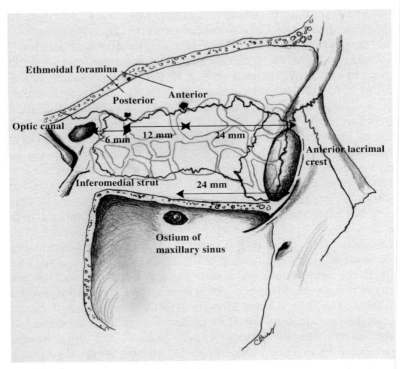

Fig. 2. Anteroposterior distances of the foramina from the anterior lacrimal crest. The ostium of the maxillary sinus lies approximately in a vertical line to the anterior ethmoidal foramen.

indicates predominance of the maxillary bone, whereas a more anteriorly placed suture indicates predominance of the lacrimal bone. The lacrimal bone at the lacrimal sac fossa has a mean thickness of 106 μm, which allows it to be easily penetrated during dacryocystorhinostomy surgery [17]. In contrast, the thicker bone of a maxillary bone dominant fossa renders creation of the osteotomy more difficult.

The floor, the shortest of the orbital walls, is bordered laterally by the inferior orbital fissure and medially by the maxilloethmoidal strut. The orbital plate of the maxillary bone comprises nearly the entire floor with small contributions from the palatine bone posteriorly and from the zygoma anterolaterally. The posterior infraorbital groove becomes a canal anteriorly as the nerve and artery pass through to exit the infraorbital foramen. With facial bone growth, the foramen migrates 6 to 10 mm below the orbital rim. The floor medial to the infraorbital nerve is thinner because of the underlying maxillary sinus expansion.

The lateral orbital wall is formed mainly by the greater wing of the sphenoid, with contributions anteriorly by the zygoma and the lateral angular (zygomatic) process of the frontal bone. The recurrent meningeal branch of the middle meningeal artery may be seen coursing through a foramen along the suture between the frontal and sphenoid bones. This artery anastomoses the external carotid circulation with the internal carotid system through the lacrimal branch of the ophthalmic artery. Approximately 4 to 5 mm behind the lateral orbital rim and 1 cm inferior to the frontozygomatic suture is the lateral orbital tubercle of Whitnall [18]. The lateral canthal tendon, the lateral rectus check ligament, the lateral horn of the levator aponeurosis, the suspensory ligament of the lower lid (Lockwood's ligament), the orbital septum, and the lacrimal gland fascia attach at Whitnall's tubercle.

The frontal process of the zygomatic bone and the zygomatic process of the frontal bone are thick and protect the globe from lateral trauma. Behind this facial buttress area, the posterior zygomatic bone and the orbital plate of the greater wing of the sphenoid are thinner, making the zygomaticosphenoid suture a convenient breaking point for bone removal during lateral orbitotomy. The zygomaticofacial and the zygomaticotemporal nerves and vessels course through canals within the lateral orbital wall to terminate in the cheek and temporalis region, respectively. Posteriorly, the lateral wall thickens and meets the temporal bone, which forms the lateral wall of the cranial cavity. In a lateral orbitotomy, only 12 to 13 mm may separate the posterior aspect of the osteotomy from the middle cranial fossa. In women, however, this distance may be 5 to 6 mm shorter [19].

The superior orbital fissure is a transverse notch between the greater and lesser wings of the sphenoid bone that descends medially (Fig. 3). The superior portion is usually narrower where the lacrimal, frontal, and trochlear nerves pass outside the annulus of Zinn. The structures passing through the superior orbital fissure within the annulus of Zinn include the

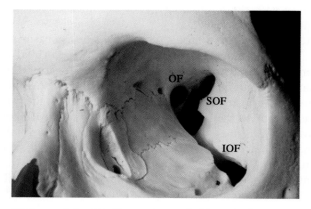

Fig. 3. Bony orbital apex, left orbit. The narrow vertical bony optic strut separates the optic foramen from the superior orbital fissure. OF, optic foramen; IOF, inferior orbital fissure; SOF, superior orbital fissure.

superior and inferior divisions of the oculomotor nerve, the abducens nerve, and the nasociliary branch of the ophthalmic trigeminal nerve. The majority of the orbital venous drainage exits the superior orbital fissure to drain into the cavernous sinus.

Medial to the superior orbital fissure is the optic foramen within the lesser wing of the sphenoid, which conveys the optic nerve and the ophthalmic artery (Fig. 3). The optic foramen and canal are separated from the superior orbital fissure by the bony optic strut, the inferior root of sphenoid bone that joins the body of the sphenoid to its lesser wing. In adults, the optic canal is 8 to 10 mm long and 5 to 7 mm wide, and the optic foramen is 6.5 mm in diameter. The optic canal attains adult dimensions by age 3 years and is symmetric in most persons; therefore, a foramen that is 1 mm or more larger than the contralateral foramen is considered abnormal.

The inferior orbital fissure lies between the lateral orbital wall and orbital floor and measures approximately 20 mm in length. The maxillary division of the trigeminal nerve, the zygomatic nerve, branches from the sphenopalatine ganglion, and branches of the inferior ophthalmic vein leading to the pterygoid plexus travel through the fissure. The inferior orbital fissure extends more anteriorly than the superior orbital fissure, ending about 20 mm from the orbital rim. The maxillary trigeminal nerve and the terminal branch of the internal maxillary artery enter the infraorbital groove and canal to become the infraorbital nerve and artery that exit the infraorbital foramen to supply to lower eyelid, cheek, upper lip, and upper anterior gingiva.

Nasal and paranasal sinuses

The bones forming the orbital floor, roof, and medial wall are pneumatized by air sinuses arising from the primitive nasal cavities. Because they retain communication with the nasal cavity, they are lined by a continuation of the nasal mucous membrane [2].

The maxillary sinus is the largest paranasal sinus, measuring 15 cm^3 in volume [2]. The roof of the maxillary sinus forms the orbital floor, which declines from the medial wall to lateral wall at an angle of approximately 30°. The maxillary sinus drains into the hiatus semilunaris within the middle meatus through an ostium located near the level of the orbital floor, immediately inferior to the middle portion of the maxilloethmoidal orbital strut. The ostium measures, on average, 24 mm from the orbital rim, which is approximately in a vertical line to the anterior ethmoidal foramen in the medial orbital wall (Fig. 2) [20].

The frontal sinus usually is not evident radiologically until about the sixth year of life and continues to expand until early adulthood. It may be larger in males and drains into the middle meatus through the frontonasal duct. The sphenoid sinus also continues to grow until adulthood, with varying degrees of pneumatization, and drains into the sphenoethmoid recess under the superior turbinate. When the sphenoid body is fully pneumatized, only sinus mucoperiosteum, a thin layer of bone, and periosteum separate the respiratory tract from the overlying internal carotid artery, the cavernous sinus, and branches of the trigeminal nerve.

The ethmoid sinuses are the first to develop, reaching adult configuration at as early as 12 years of age [21]. Ethmoid bullae may pneumatize the orbital plate of the frontal bone and even develop as frontal sinuses. Frequently, the ethmoid sinuses extend past the suture of the ethmoid bone and into the lacrimal and maxillary bones of the lacrimal sac fossa (Figs. 1, 2) [22,23]. The ethmoid sinuses are shaped like a rectangular box slightly wider posteriorly where they articulate with the sphenoid sinus. The ethmoid sinuses are comprised of three main groups—the anterior, middle, and posterior ethmoidal air cells. The anterior and middle ethmoidal air cells drain into the middle meatus; the posterior air cells drain into the superior meatus of the nasal cavity.

The orbital roof slopes down medially, and this slope continues at the frontoethmoidal suture to become the roof of the ethmoid sinus, or fovea ethmoidalis. The ethmoid roof continues to slope inferiorly and medially to overlie the nasal cavity as the cribriform plate. The crista galli bisects the cribriform plate on its superior aspect. Directly inferior, the vertical nasal plate, or vomer, is located. Because of this sloping, which is most prominent over the anterior ethmoidal air cells, it is important to know the individual anatomy before surgery to avoid inadvertent entry into the cranial cavity, cerebrospinal fluid leak, or more severe intracranial injury [24].

It is important to understand the anatomic relationship of the anterior ethmoidal air cells to the lacrimal sac fossa to avoid confusion between the ethmoid and nasal cavities during creation of a dacryocystorhinostomy ostium. Past studies have demonstrated an intimate relationship between the anterior ethmoidal air cells, or agger nasi cells, and the lacrimal sac fossa [21–23,25–27]. These agger nasi bullae may pneumatize the lacrimal bone and rarely extend into the frontal process of the maxillary bone.

In 1911, Whitnall [22] described the relationship of the anterior ethmoidal air cells directly medial to the lacrimal sac fossa in 86% of skulls [22]. In 32% of skulls, the air cells extended anteriorly to the vertical maxillary–lacrimal suture, and in an additional 54% the air cells extended even farther to the anterior lacrimal crest. Similarly, on orbital CT scans, Blaylock [23] found that, the anterior ethmoid cells extended anterior to the posterior lacrimal crest in 93% of orbits; in 40% the cells extended anterior to the maxillary–lacrimal bone suture and entered the frontal process of the maxilla [23]. In only 7% of orbits was the nasal cavity directly adjacent to the entire lacrimal sac fossa. Typically, the anterior extension of the ethmoid cells was adjacent to the superior half of the lacrimal sac fossa, with the inferior half of the fossa directly next to the middle meatus [21–23,25,27,28].

The bony nose is formed by the frontonasal process during embryology. The nasal septum bisects the nasal cavity and is comprised of the bony perpendicular plate of the ethmoid and vomer, a cartilaginous anterior triangle, and an inferior membranous columella that divides the nares anteriorly. Laterally, the nasal wall has three or more horizontal ridges termed turbinates, with a corresponding meatus below each (Fig. 4). During the sixth week of embryologic development, before cartilage forms in the walls of the primitive nasal cavities, linear outgrowths of the lining epithelium occur on the sides and roof of each nasal side. Each outgrowing gutter becomes a meatus; the ridges left behind form the turbinates [2,29].

The inferior turbinate is the largest and arises from the medial wall of the maxillary sinus. The smaller and more posterior middle, superior, and supreme turbinates are derived from the ethmoid bone. The supreme turbinate may be found in up to 65% of patients. The middle turbinate originates posteriorly from the roof of the nose at the cribriform plate and arises anteriorly from the medial wall of the maxillary sinus. The lacrimal sac fossa is located just anterior and lateral to the anterior tip of the middle turbinate (Fig. 5).

Within the middle meatus lies a curvilinear gutter, the hiatus semilunaris, into which the ostium of the maxillary sinus drains. It is bordered inferiorly by the uncinate process bony ridge and superiorly by the bulla ethmoidalis prominence, which represents the most anterior ethmoidal air cells (Fig. 6) [30]. The middle meatus receives the drainage of the ethmoid (anterior and middle), frontal, and maxillary sinuses. The frontonasal duct drains the frontal sinus into the anterosuperior portion of the hiatus semilunaris. The posterior ethmoid air cells drain into the superior meatus, along with the sphenoid sinus.

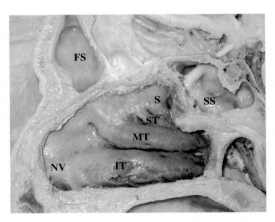

Fig. 4. Endonasal sagittal view. Each nasal turbinate has a corresponding meatal space located immediately below. FS, frontal sinus; IT, inferior turbinate; MT, middle turbinate; NV, nasal vestibule; S, supreme turbinate; SS, sphenoid sinus; ST, superior turbinate.

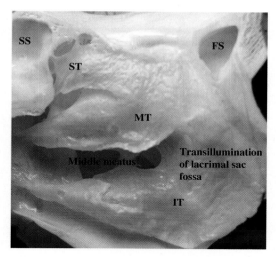

Fig. 5. Endonasal site of a dacryocystorhinostomy ostium. Transillumination through the lacrimal sac fossa demonstrates its location at the anterior tip of the middle turbinate. FS, frontal sinus; IT, inferior turbinate; MT, middle turbinate; SS, sphenoid sinus; ST, superior turbinate.

Orbital soft tissues

Orbital septum

The orbital septum is the anterior soft tissue boundary of the orbit (Fig. 7). It acts as a physical barrier against pathogens and contributes to the normal posterior position of the orbital fat pads. It is a thin, multilayered sheet of fibrous tissue derived from the mesodermal layer of the embryonic eyelid. The septum is covered anteriorly by a thin layer of preseptal orbicularis oculi muscle and skin and originates from the superior and inferior orbital rims at a thick, white fibrous line, the arcus marginalis. Medially, the septum covers the posterior aspect of Horner's muscle as it inserts along the inferior posterior lacrimal crest. Laterally, the orbital septum fuses with the lateral canthal tendon to attach to the lateral orbital rim [31].

The superior orbital septum does not insert onto tarsus because of the intervening levator aponeurosis. Instead, it inserts onto the aponeurosis approximately 10 mm above the upper eyelid margin or 2 to 5 mm above the superior tarsal border [31]. In the lower eyelid, the septum inserts onto the inferior border of tarsus after joining with the inferior retractors 4 to 5 mm below the tarsus (Fig. 8). In contrast, in Asian eyelids, the orbital septum fuses to the levator aponeurosis at a level below the superior tarsus, which allows preaponeurotic fat to prolapse inferior and anterior to tarsus; in the lower eyelid, it may fuse directly to the inferior tarsal border rather than joining with the retractors. An absent or lower eyelid crease in Asian eyelids

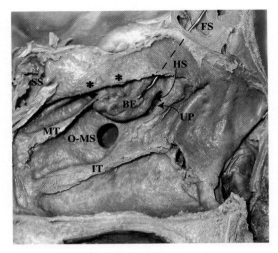

Fig. 6. Endonasal view of lateral nasal wall with turbinates removed. BE, bulla ethmoidalis; FS, frontal sinus; HS, hiatus semilunaris; IT, inferior turbinate; MT, middle turbinate; O-MS, ostium of maxillary sinus; SS, sphenoid sinus; UP, uncinate process; *, ethmoid ostia.

may result from this orbital fat prolapse and other subcutaneous fat that inhibit levator fibers from inserting into the subdermal skin [32]. Loose areolar tissue, termed the suborbicularis fascia, lies immediately anterior to the septum [33] and shares the same plane as the eyebrow retro-orbicularis oculi fat and malar fat pads further from the eyelid margins.

Periorbita

The periorbita is the periosteal lining of the orbital walls. The periorbita is firmly attached at the suture lines, the foramina, the fissures, the arcus

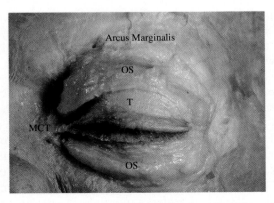

Fig. 7. Anterior view of orbital septum (OS) overlying the orbital fat pads, left orbit. The orbital septum arises from a thick, white fibrous band, the arcus marginalis, along the entire orbital rim. MCT, medial canthal tendon; T, tarsus.

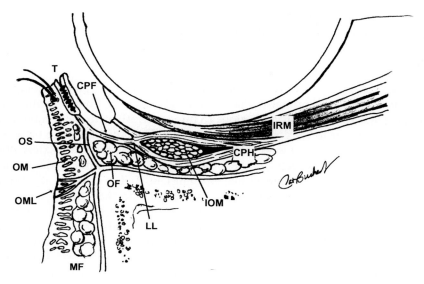

Fig. 8. Normal lower eyelid anatomy in cross-section. CPF, capsulopalpebral fascia; CPH, capsulopalpebral head; IOM, inferior oblique muscle; IRM, inferior rectus muscle; LL, Lockwood's ligament; MF, malar fat; OF, orbital fat; OM, orbicularis oculi muscle; OML, orbitomalar ligament; OS, orbital septum; T, tarsus.

marginalis, and the posterior lacrimal crest. Elsewhere, it is loosely adherent to the bone and is a potential space for accumulation of blood, pus, or tumor growth; it also provides a convenient plane of dissection for the surgeon. Posteriorly, the periorbita is continuous with the optic nerve sheath where the dura is fused to the optic canal. Likewise, the superior orbital fissure is surrounded by thickened periorbita, which is also continuous with intracranial dura. Anteriorly, the periorbita is continuous with the orbital septum at the arcus marginalis. Inferomedially, the periorbita lines the lacrimal fossa, and an extension termed the lacrimal fascia covers the lateral aspect of the lacrimal sac. The periorbita is extensively vascularized with interconnections between its bone and soft tissue sides; therefore, the periosteum does not serve as a vascular barrier [34]. It may, however, restrain subperiosteal hematomas and temporally provide resistance to the spread of infections and tumors from the surrounding sinuses and bones into the orbit.

Kikkawa [35] described the orbitomalar ligament as a distinct bony attachment originating from the periosteum of the inferior orbital rim and fanning out in a lamellar fashion through the orbicularis oculi overlying the inferior orbital rim to insert into the malar dermis (Fig. 8). The orbitomalar ligament continues along the entire inferior orbital rim with its lateral component firmly attaching the superficial musculoaponeurotic system to the lateral orbital rim. Attenuation and loss of elastic fibers with age result in descent of the infraorbital cutaneous insertion of the orbitomalar ligament and upper midfacial ptosis.

Orbital fascia

Extensive work by Koornneef [36] has shown a highly complex organization of the orbital fascia. Tenon's capsule is a fibrous membrane that extends from the posterior globe to fuse anteriorly with the conjunctiva slightly posterior to the corneoscleral junction. The potential space between the adherent Tenon's fascia and the globe is Tenon's space. Externally, Tenon's capsule connects to the network of fibrous septa dividing the lobules of orbital fat. Tunnel-like openings in Tenon's fascia allow the extraocular muscles to pass from the orbital fat into the Tenon's space to insert onto the sclera. A muscular fascia sheathes each extraocular muscle and extends between them. Each muscle sheath sends extensions to the orbital walls. Anteriorly, the extensions are especially prominent and are called check ligaments. The lateral rectus check ligament is the strongest and inserts primarily on Whitnall's lateral orbital tubercle with lesser extensions to the lateral conjunctival fornix and lateral orbital septum. The medial rectus check ligament mainly inserts behind the posterior lacrimal crest [37].

Orbital fat

The orbital fat provides a resilient cushion to support the globe and other orbital structures. In the upper eyelid, the orbital fat is located anterior to the levator palpebrae superioris complex and posterior to the orbital septum. The central preaponeurotic fat pad and smaller medial fat pad are separated by the trochlea and superior oblique tendon (Fig. 9). The medial fat pad is more fibrous and whiter in color. The infratrochlear nerve and medial palpebral artery branch of the ophthalmic artery course through the medial fat pad. In the lower eyelid, there are three clinical orbital fat pads [38]. The lateral and central fat pads are separated by the arcuate expansion fascial attachments of the inferior oblique muscle that pass to the inferolateral orbital floor. The central and medial fat pads are separated by the inferior oblique muscle, which may be inadvertently injured during fat removal for blepharoplasty (Fig. 10). In Asians, the lower eyelid orbital fat may protrude anterior to the inferior orbital rim and more superior toward the inferior tarsus because of differences in orbital septum insertion with the capsulopalpebral fascia [39].

Extraocular muscles

Except for the inferior oblique, all the extraocular muscles arise from the orbital apex. The four rectus muscles originate from the thick, fibrous annulus of Zinn, which surrounds the optic foramen at the orbital apex and divides the superior orbital fissure into intraconal and extraconal spaces.

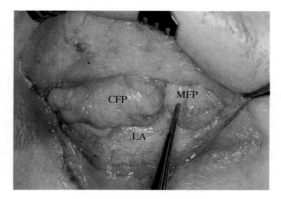

Fig. 9. The whiter medial fat pad (MFP) and central preaponeurotic fat pad (CFP) lie anterior to the levator aponeurosis (LA) of the right upper eyelid.

The levator palpebrae superioris and superior oblique muscles arise more superomedially on the lesser wing of the sphenoid. Passing through the annulus of Zinn are the oculomotor nerve divisions, the optic, nasociliary, and abducens nerves, and the ophthalmic artery. Passing through the superior orbital fissure outside the annulus are the trochlear, lacrimal, frontal nerves, and the superior ophthalmic vein.

The four rectus muscles course through the orbital fat and define the muscle cone. The muscles pass through openings in Tenon's fascia to insert on the anterior portion of the globe in a configuration called the spiral of Tilleaux, with the medial rectus inserting nearest at 5.5 mm posterior to the limbus. The medial and inferior recti and inferior oblique muscles are innervated by the inferior division of the oculomotor nerve; the superior rectus and levator palpebrae superioris muscles are innervated by the

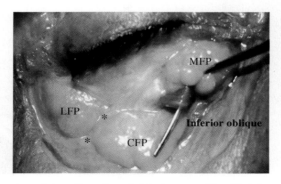

Fig. 10. Anterior view of deep dissection of right lower eyelid orbital fat pads. The inferior oblique muscle divides the medial from the central fat, and the arcuate expansion fascia (asterisks) of the inferior oblique muscle divides the central from the lateral fat pads. CFP, central fat pad; LFP, lateral fat pad; MFP, medial fat pad.

superior oculomotor division; the superior oblique muscle is innervated by the trochlear nerve; and the lateral rectus muscle is innervated by the abducens nerve. The innervation enters each muscle on its ocular surface at the junction of the posterior third with the anterior two thirds of the muscle.

Fibrous septa from the inferior rectus muscle radiate to the inferior periorbita, suggesting that incarceration of this tissue, without muscle entrapment in a floor fracture, may cause restricted extraocular motility. The inferior oblique muscle arises from a shallow depression in the orbital plate of the maxilla at the anteromedial orbital floor, just lateral to the lacrimal excretory fossa, and courses posterolaterally underneath the inferior rectus muscle. The fascia of the inferior rectus muscle divides to encircle the inferior oblique muscle, and their conjoined fascia just anterior to the inferior oblique forms the suspensory ligament of Lockwood before continuing as the capsulopalpebral fascia and lower lid retractor complex (Figs. 8, 11).

The superior oblique muscle arises from the superomedial annulus of Zinn and courses anteriorly along the superomedial orbital wall. Between the superior oblique and medial rectus muscles are the ethmoidal branches of the nasociliary nerve and ophthalmic artery. The superior oblique muscle becomes tendinous just before it passes through the trochlea. The tendon then makes a 54° angle to continue posterolaterally underneath the superior rectus to insert on the globe [37]. The superior oblique muscle depresses, intorts, and abducts the eye.

The trochlea is located in a shallow fossa in the anteromedial orbital roof, 5 to 10 mm posterior to the orbital rim. Crescent-shaped rings of cartilage suspended from the periorbita support the reflected tendon [40,41]. The periorbita to which the trochlea is attached can be carefully elevated from the bone by the surgeon and replaced if needed, although injury to the

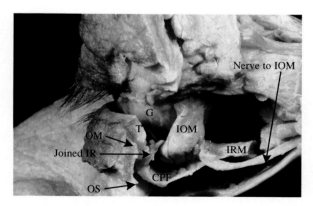

Fig. 11. Parasagittal view of a left lower eyelid anatomic dissection of the inferior retractor complex. CPF, capsulopalpebral fascia; G, globe; IOM, inferior oblique muscle; IR, joined inferior retractors at Lockwood's ligament; IRM, inferior rectus muscle; OM, orbicularis oculi muscle; OS, orbital septum; T, tarsus.

tissues surrounding the trochlea can cause scarring and possible superior oblique restriction or Brown's syndrome.

Blood supply for the extraocular muscles is from the medial and lateral muscular branches of the ophthalmic artery, the lacrimal artery, and the infraorbital artery. Except for the lateral rectus, each muscle receives two anterior ciliary arteries that communicate with the major arteriole circle of the ciliary body. The lateral rectus is supplied by a single vessel derived from the lacrimal artery [42].

Orbital nerves

Entering the orbit are the optic (cranial nerve II), oculomotor (cranial nerve III), trochlear (cranial nerve IV), abducens (cranial nerve VI), first and second divisions of the trigeminal (cranial nerve V), sympathetic, and parasympathetic nerves.

As a peripheral nerve tract of the central nervous system, the optic nerve has supporting neuroglial cells and is surrounded by cerebrospinal fluid within dural layers. The optic nerve axons arise from the ganglion cell layer of the retina to form the optic nerve, which is cushioned by retrobulbar intraconal fat lobules. The intraorbital optic nerve measures 25 mm, on average, betweer the back of the globe and the optic foramen, but the distance between these structures is only 18 mm. This 7 mm of slack in the optic nerve results in a gentle curve with a convexity directed inferotemporally in the orbit. This degree of slack in the nerve allows freedom of eye movement and affords a margin of safety in proptotic states. The dural sheath covering the optic nerve thickens near the optic foramen, where it becomes continuous with the posterior periorbita.

The oculomotor nerve divides into a superior and inferior division within the anterior cavernous sinus, several millimeters posterior to the annulus of Zinn. The superior division innervates the superior rectus on its inferior surface before terminating in the overlying levator palpebrae superioris muscle. The inferior branch of the oculomotor nerve innervates the medial and inferior rectus muscles (Fig. 12). A large, terminal branch runs along the lateral inferior rectus muscle before terminating in the inferior oblique muscle. This inferior oblique branch also supplies a parasympathetic branch to the ciliary ganglion, eventually innervating the ciliary body and iris sphincter.

The ophthalmic and maxillary divisions of the sensory trigeminal nerve course through the orbit. The ophthalmic division enters the orbit through the superior orbital fissure as three branches: the lacrimal, frontal, and nasociliary nerves. The lacrimal nerve passes through the extraconal superior orbital fissure and joins the lacrimal artery to reach the posterior lacrimal gland, where it divides into superior and inferior branches. The superior branch of the lacrimal nerve supplies the gland, conjunctiva, and the lateral upper eyelid. The inferior branch anastomoses with the zygomaticotemporal branch of the maxillary trigeminal nerve where it

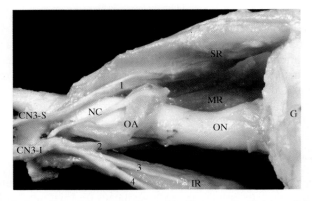

Fig. 12. Lateral view of the right retrobulbar orbit. The superior division of the oculomotor nerve (CN3-S) supplies a branch (1) to the superior rectus and levator palpebrae superioris muscles, whereas the inferior division of the oculomotor nerve (CN3-I) supplies branches to the medial rectus (2), inferior rectus (3), and inferior oblique muscles (4). The nasociliary branch of the ophthalmic trigeminal nerve (NC) and the ophthalmic artery (OA) cross over the optic nerve (ON) from lateral to medial to subsequently course the medial orbit. G, globe; IR, inferior rectus; MR, medial rectus; SR, superior rectus muscle.

picks up parasympathetic secretory fibers to the gland. The frontal branch of the ophthalmic trigeminal nerve divides anteriorly in the orbit to form the supratrochlear and larger supraorbital nerves that supply sensation to the medial canthus, upper eyelid, brow, and forehead (Fig. 13).

The nasociliary branch of the ophthalmic trigeminal nerve is the only branch to enter the orbit through the annulus of Zinn. It passes from lateral to medial over the optic nerve with the ophthalmic artery to course between the superior oblique and medial rectus muscles (Fig. 13). The nasociliary nerve gives off branches to the ciliary ganglion, the globe, and the anterior and posterior ethmoidal nerves that supply the nasal mucosa. The terminal infratrochlear branch supplies the tip of the nose and may be involved in herpes zoster ophthalmicus, known as Hutchinson's sign.

The maxillary division of the trigeminal nerve exits the foramen rotundum and crosses the pterygopalatine fossa to enter the inferior orbital fissure. The maxillary trigeminal nerve gives off the infraorbital nerve which enters the infraorbital groove approximately 3 cm posterior to the orbital rim, traverses the infraorbital canal, and exits from the infraorbital foramen. Sphenopalatine and posterior superior alveolar branches of the maxillary trigeminal nerve provide sensation to the nasal mucosa, gingiva, teeth, and upper lip; middle and anterior superior alveolar branches arise from within the infraorbital canal. The zygomatic branch of the maxillary trigeminal nerve enters the inferior orbital fissure and divides into the zygomaticotemporal and zygomaticofacial nerves, with the former carrying parasympathetic secretory fibers from the sphenopalatine ganglion to the lacrimal gland.

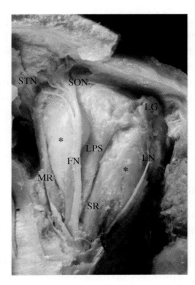

Fig. 13. Superior view of right orbit. Course of the ophthalmic division of the trigeminal nerve in the orbit. FN, frontal nerve; LG, lacrimal gland; LN, lacrimal nerve; LPS, levator palpebrae superioris muscle and aponeurosis; MR, medial rectus muscle; SON, supraorbital nerve; SR, superior rectus muscle; STN, supratrochlear nerve.

The sympathetic nerve supply to the orbit controls pupillary dilatation, function of the smooth tarsal muscles of the eyelids, and vasoconstriction. Lyon [43] found that the sympathetic nerves entered through the superior orbital fissure rather than the optic foramen [2,43]. The exact pathway of the sympathetic fibers to and through the orbit is not clearly defined, however.

The parasympathetic innervation to the lacrimal gland is discussed in the section on the lacrimal gland. The parasympathetic nerves to the globe reach the ciliary ganglion by a branch from the inferior oblique nerve, synapse in the ganglion, and pass to the globe through multiple short posterior ciliary nerves. The ciliary ganglion is located 15 mm posterior to the globe and is frequently adherent to the lateral aspect of the optic nerve [44].

Orbital vessels

The orbital arteries are primarily branches of the ophthalmic artery with small contributions from the internal maxillary artery. The internal and external carotid systems have several areas of anastomoses for collateral circulation.

The ophthalmic artery is the first large branch off the internal carotid artery just as it emerges from the cavernous sinus. The optic nerve within its canal is supplied by pial branches of the ophthalmic artery. The ophthalmic artery exits the optic foramen on the inferolateral aspect of the nerve and crosses over the optic nerve in up to 90% of orbits to course medially (Fig. 12) [45]. Approximately 10 mm posterior to the globe, the ophthalmic artery provides the central retinal artery branch, which enters the ventral surface of the optic nerve. Other branches include the lacrimal, supraorbital, ethmoidal, long posterior ciliary arteries, and the muscular arteries that supply the extraocular muscles. The terminal ophthalmic artery exits the medial orbit as the supratrochlear, dorsal nasal, and medial palpebral arteries. Significant variability exists regarding the order in which the ophthalmic artery gives rise to its branches.

Orbital lymphatic drainage

Traditionally thought to be devoid of any lymphatic vessels or lymph nodes, the orbital lymphatic drainage has been the subject of many animal studies [46–48].

Studies by Sherman [49] and Gausas [50] distinguished orbital lymphatic channels from blood capillaries histochemically by light microscopy using a 5'-nucleotidase and alkaline phosphatase double-staining method. Lymphatics were not identified in the extraocular muscles or orbital fat. Cook [51,52] used this same technique and found both a superficial preorbicularis muscle lymphatic plexus and a deep pretarsal (postorbicularis muscle) plexus that were not interconnected in the upper and lower eyelids. Lymphoscintigraphy demonstrated lymphatic drainage of the medial and central lower eyelid along the facial vein to the submandibular lymph nodes, whereas the entire upper eyelid, medial canthus, and lateral lower eyelid drained into the preauricular lymph nodes. The central upper eyelid also had dual drainage into the submandibular nodes [52]. In contrast, the lymphatic drainage of the medial upper eyelid and medial canthus traditionally was thought to drain into the submandibular rather than the preauricular lymph nodes (Fig. 14) [46].

Eyelid structures

The pertinent elements of the eyelid anatomy from anterior to posterior are the skin, orbicularis oculi muscle, orbital septum, orbital fat, inferior oblique muscle, levator complex (levator palpebrae superioris muscle and aponeurosis), canthal tendons, inferior retractors, Müller's muscle, tarsus, and conjunctiva. Several of these have been discussed previously.

Anterior lamella

The eyelid skin is extremely thin and contains very little or no fat. The orbicularis oculi muscle runs in concentric sheets around the eyelids and can be divided regionally into pretarsal, preseptal, and orbital portions,

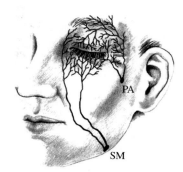

Fig. 14. Traditional schematic for lymphatic drainage of the eyelids. PA, preauricular lymph nodes; SM, submandibular lymph nodes.

corresponding to the structure they overly. Sebaceous glands of Zeis that empty into hair follicles and eccrine sweat glands of Moll are found near the eyelid margin. The orbicularis oculi muscle of Riolan marks the posterior limit of the anterior lamella, known as the gray line (Fig. 15).

Tarsus

The tarsal plate and conjunctiva comprise the posterior lamella, separated from the anterior lamella by the gray line. The tarsus measures 8 to 11 mm in height in the upper eyelid and 4 mm in the lower eyelid. The tarsus is composed of dense connective tissue approximately 1 mm in thickness that gives the eyelid its structure. It extends, on average, 28 mm in length from the lateral canthus to the punctum medially. The tarsus contains the meibomian glands that secrete the sebaceous layer of the tear film; the meibomian gland orifices are visible in a line posterior to the gray line. The palpebral conjunctiva is tightly adherent to the posterior tarsus and continues superiorly or inferiorly to the fornix where it is reflected onto the globe as the bulbar conjunctiva. Accessory lacrimal glands of Krause and Wolfring are located in the conjunctival fornices and along the superior tarsal border, respectively [53–55].

Levator complex

The levator palpebrae superioris muscle and aponeurosis comprise the levator complex. The levator palpebrae superioris muscle arises from the lesser wing of the sphenoid superior to the annulus of Zinn. The supraorbital artery, frontal nerve, and the trochlear nerve pass superior to the levator muscle. The muscular portion of the levator is approximately 40 mm in length, in contrast to its aponeurosis, which measures 14 to 20 mm to the terminal attachments on the anterior inferior tarsus (Fig. 16) [56]. Superiorly, a transverse fibrous condensation termed the superior transverse ligament, or

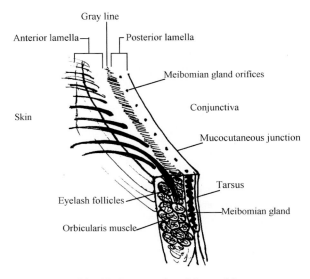

Fig. 15. Topography of the eyelid.

Whitnall's ligament, attaches the widening levator muscle to the superior orbit [57]. Whitnall's ligament is a thick condensation of elastic fibers of the anterior sheath of the levator, located superior to the transition from levator muscle to aponeurosis. Although its function is not entirely clear, it has been suggested that Whitnall's ligament acts as a suspensory ligament for the upper lid as well as a fulcrum for the levator muscle to change vector force from an anterior–posterior direction to a superior–inferior direction [58]. The ligament terminates medially in the fascia surrounding the trochlea. Laterally, Whitnall's ligament forms septa through the lacrimal gland before

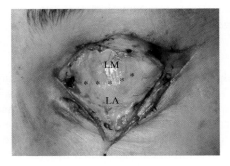

Fig. 16. Left upper eyelid. The asterisks demarcate the musculo-aponeurotic junction between the levator palpebrae superioris muscle (LM) and its fibrous levator aponeurosis (LA).

attaching to the inner lateral orbital wall, up to 10 mm superior to the lateral orbital tubercle of Whitnall. Attenuation of the levator aponeurosis with age or disorders of the levator muscle may lead to upper eyelid ptosis.

A light and electron microscopic study by Stasior [59] showed that the levator complex forms an intricate insertion into the upper eyelid. As the levator aponeurosis approaches the mid-tarsal level, approximately two thirds of the aponeurotic elastic fibers radiate away from the tarsus to fuse into the pretarsal orbicularis oculi muscle bundles and dermis to create the eyelid crease. The remaining one third of the aponeurotic elastic fibers insert onto the anterior surface of the inferior tarsus. Stasior suggested that this complex elastic fiber network degenerates with age, rather than the aponeurosis itself.

As the levator aponeurosis descends toward the tarsus, it expands into a broad, fibrous sheath to insert onto the orbital rims as medial and lateral horns. The lateral horn is a strong, fibrous band incompletely dividing the lacrimal gland into two lobes and continuing inferiorly to insert onto the lateral canthal tendon and the lateral orbital tubercle (Fig. 17). The medial horn, in contrast, is thin and filmy as it passes over the reflected superior oblique tendon to insert onto the medial canthal tendon and posterior lacrimal crest. The lateral horn of the levator complex should not be confused with the superior transverse ligament (Whitnall's ligament) located superiorly.

Lateral and medial canthal tendons

The lateral canthal tendon is formed by fibrous extensions of the upper and lower eyelid tarsal plates and pretarsal orbicularis muscles that unite into a common tendon 1 mm thick and 3 mm wide [60]. As the lateral

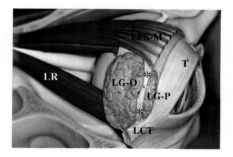

Fig. 17. Superolateral oblique view of the right orbit. The levator palpebrae superioris muscle transitions into the levator aponeurosis, which has been mostly excised to demonstrate the palpebral lobe of the lacrimal gland located posterior to the lateral horn of the levator aponeurosis (asterisks). LCT, lateral canthal tendon; LG-O, orbital lobe of lacrimal gland; LG-P, palpebral lobe of lacrimal gland; LPS-M, levator palpebrae superioris muscle; LR, lateral rectus; T, tarsus.

canthal tendon approaches the orbital rim, it widens to 6 to 7 mm as the lateral horn of the levator aponeurosis, the check ligament of the lateral rectus muscle, and Lockwood's ligament fuse with it before its bony insertion into the lateral orbital tubercle of Whitnall, 5 mm inside the orbital rim. Knowledge of lateral canthal tendon anatomy is important when reconstructing the lateral canthal angle and securing it to intact or elevated periosteum inside the orbital rim to simulate the normal anatomic insertion [60–62].

The medial canthal tendon is comprised of an anterior and posterior limb. The superficial heads of the pretarsal orbicularis oculi muscle surround the lacrimal canaliculi and, together with fibrous extensions of the tarsal plates, form the anterior limb of the medial canthal tendon, which inserts onto the upper anterior lacrimal crest. The deep heads of the pretarsal orbicularis oculi muscle fuse near the common canaliculus to form Horner's muscle, which forms the posterior limb that inserts onto the posterior lacrimal crest. Therefore, the anterior and posterior limbs of the medial canthal tendon envelop the superior half of the lacrimal sac (Fig. 18A, B). Medial canthal tendon laxity should be addressed before lateral canthal tightening to avoid pulling the punctum laterally away from the tear lake [63].

Inferior retractors

The inferior retractors in the lower eyelid are analogous to the levator aponeurosis of the upper eyelid. The inferior retractor complex is comprised of aponeurotic expansions of the inferior rectus muscle that form the capsulopalpebral head. This layer divides around the inferior oblique muscle and fuses into Lockwood's suspensory ligament anterior to the inferior oblique muscle [64,65]. The capsulopalpebral fascia connects Lockwood's suspensory ligament to the inferior fornix, to the inferior border of the tarsus, and to the preseptal orbicularis muscle and skin at the level of the eyelid crease (Figs. 8, 11) [65]. Lockwood's suspensory ligament may help support the globe in the absence of an intact orbital floor. The inferior retractor complex also contains diffusely distributed adrenergic smooth muscle fibers of the inferior tarsal muscle, which is not as distinct a layer as Müller's muscle.

Müller's muscle

The smooth superior tarsal muscle (Müller's muscle) arises from the undersurface of the striated levator palpebrae superioris muscle, approximately 15 mm above the superior tarsal border. It is firmly attached to the levator muscle only at its origin and may be easily separated from the

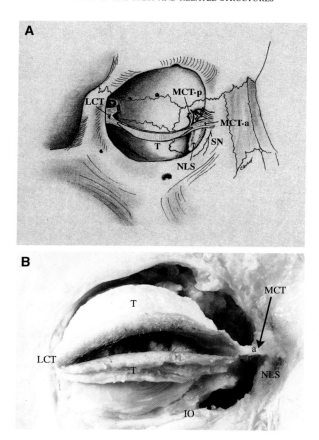

Fig. 18. Relationship of the right medial canthal tendon to the nasolacrimal sac. (*A*) Diagrammatic illustration. (*B*) Anatomic dissection. The thick anterior limb of the medial canthal tendon wraps along the anterior upper half of the lacrimal sac to insert onto the anterior lacrimal crest. The thin posterior limb passes behind the sac to insert onto the posterior lacrimal crest. The upper eyelid tarsus is much greater in height than the lower eyelid tarsus. IO, inferior oblique muscle origin; LCT, lateral canthal tendon; MCT-a, medial canthal tendon, anterior limb; MCT-p, medial canthal tendon, posterior limb; NLS, nasolacrimal sac; SN, sutura notha; T, tarsus.

levator aponeurosis to form the subaponeurotic space [53]. Müller's muscle inserts onto the superior tarsus, where the peripheral arterial arcade courses along the superior tarsal border in the plane between Müller's muscle and the overlying levator aponeurosis. The analogous inferior tarsal muscle of the lower eyelid is less well developed and is found posterior to the inferior retractors. Sympathetic denervation, as in Horner's syndrome, results in approximately 2 mm of upper eyelid ptosis and may manifest as lower eyelid elevation or "reverse ptosis." The exact sympathetic nerve course to these smooth muscles is unknown [66].

The lacrimal system

Lacrimal gland and accessory glands

The main lacrimal gland is located in the superotemporal orbit in a shallow lacrimal fossa of the frontal bone. The gland is composed of numerous secretory acinar units that drain into progressively larger tubules and ducts. The gland measures 20 mm by 12 mm by 5 mm and is divided incompletely by the lateral horn of the levator aponeurosis into a larger orbital lobe and a lesser palpebral lobe below (Fig. 17) [54,67]. The orbital lobe lies posterior to the orbital septum and preaponeurotic fat and anterior to the levator aponeurosis [54]. A prolapsed orbital lobe should not be confused with the preaponeurotic orbital fat pad (Fig. 19). The palpebral lobe is located posterior to the levator aponeurosis in the subaponeurotic space and anterior to the conjunctiva and may be visible through conjunctiva with eyelid eversion. Two to six secretory ducts from the orbital lobe pass through the palpebral lobe or along its fibrous capsule, joining with ducts from the palpebral lobe to form 6 to 12 tubules that empty into the superolateral conjunctival fornix 4 to 5 mm above the tarsus [1,53]. Damage to the palpebral lobe may therefore block drainage of the entire lacrimal gland.

Approximately 20 to 40 accessory lacrimal glands of Krause are located in the superior conjunctival fornix, and half that number are located in the lower eyelid. Fewer but larger accessory glands of Wolfring are found along the superior tarsal border of the upper eyelid and the inferior tarsal border of the lower eyelid [54,55].

The innervation of the lacrimal gland is derived from cranial nerves V and VII, as well as from the sympathetic nerves of the superior cervical ganglion [68]. The lacrimal branch of the ophthalmic division of the

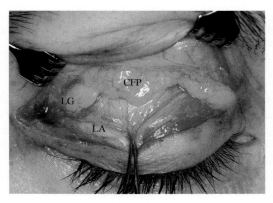

Fig. 19. Right upper eyelid. A prolapsed lacrimal gland (LG) should not be mistaken for the central preaponeurotic fat pad (CFP). Both overlie the white levator aponeurosis (LA).

trigeminal nerve carries sensory stimuli from the lacrimal gland. The lacrimal gland receives arterial supply from the lacrimal artery, with contributions from the recurrent meningeal artery and a branch of the infraorbital artery. The venous drainage follows approximately the intra-orbital course of the artery and drains into the superior ophthalmic vein.

Parasympathetic secretomotor fibers originate in the lacrimal nucleus of the pons and exit the pons–medullary junction between cranial nerves VI and VIII. These fibers travel a long course within the nervus intermedius, the greater superficial petrosal nerve, the deep petrosal nerve, and the vidian nerve finally to synapse in the pterygopalatine ganglion [1]. The deep petrosal nerve also carries sympathetic fibers from the internal carotid plexus. Postganglionic parasympathetic fibers leave the pterygopalatine ganglion through the pterygopalatine nerves to innervate the lacrimal gland [69,70]. Some parasympathetic fibers join the zygomatic nerve branch of the maxillary trigeminal nerve and enter the orbit through the inferior orbital fissure. The zygomatic nerve may enter the posterior lacrimal gland either alone or in combination with the lacrimal nerve [54]. In 2004, however, Ruskell [71] found that parasympathetic fibers travel along a branch of the middle meningeal artery through the superior orbital fissure before joining the ophthalmic or lacrimal artery to supply the lacrimal gland, rather than passing to the gland through the zygomatic and lacrimal nerves.

Sympathetic nerves arrive with the lacrimal artery of the ophthalmic artery and along with parasympathetic nerves in the zygomatic nerve. The zygomatic branch of the maxillary trigeminal nerve gives off the lacrimal branch before dividing into zygomaticotemporal and zygomaticofacial branches. This sympathetic lacrimal branch anastomoses with the sensory lacrimal nerve of the ophthalmic trigeminal nerve or enters the posterolateral gland independently.

Lacrimal drainage system

The lacrimal excretory system begins at a 0.3-mm opening on each medial eyelid termed the punctum [2,53]. The maxilla grows more rapidly than the frontal bone during embryologic development, and the lateral migration pulls the inferior canaliculus laterally, causing the lower eyelid punctum to be located slightly lateral to the upper eyelid punctum [29]. The puncta are directed posteriorly to appose the tear lake. The punctal opening widens into the ampulla, which is 2 mm in height and perpendicular to the eyelid margin, before making a sharp turn into the canaliculi. The canaliculi measure 0.5 to 1.0 mm in diameter and course parallel to the eyelid margins. The superior canaliculus is 8 mm in length; the inferior canaliculus is 10 mm (Fig. 20).

In more than 90% of individuals, the superior and inferior canaliculi merge into a common canaliculus before entering the nasolacrimal sac [53,72]. A study using digital subtraction dacryocystograms demonstrated

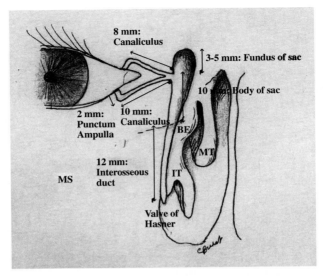

Fig. 20. Approximate dimensions of the lacrimal excretory system. BE, bulla ethmoidalis; IT, inferior turbinate; MS, maxillary sinus; MT, middle turbinate.

a common canaliculus in 94% of individuals. The upper and lower canaliculi joined at the wall of the lacrimal sac without a common canaliculus in 4%, and only 2% of systems had completely separate drainage of the upper and lower canaliculi into the lacrimal sac [73]. The opening of the common canaliculus into the lacrimal sac is known as the common internal punctum.

The functional valve between the common canaliculus and the lacrimal sac has traditionally been attributed to the valve of Rosenmuller, although some studies have been unable to document this structure [74]. Tucker demonstrated that the angulation within the canalicular system (the canaliculi bend at the canaliculus–common canaliculus junction at an angle of 118° and then enter the lacrimal sac at an acute angle of 58°) may contribute to a valvelike effect that prevents retrograde flow from the lacrimal sac [75]. Other mucosal folds have been reported within the lacrimal drainage system, such as the valve of Krause, located between the sac and duct, and the valve of Hasner (plica lacrimalis) that is present at the opening of the duct into the inferior meatus [76]. An imperforate Hasner's valve frequently persists in newborns, resulting in congenital nasolacrimal obstruction [77,78].

The lacrimal drainage system is lined by stratified squamous epithelium in the canaliculi and by nonciliated columnar epithelium in the nasolacrimal sac and duct that contains goblet cells as it approaches the nasal cavity. The total nasolacrimal sac measures 12 to 15 mm vertically and 4 to 8 mm anteroposteriorly and may be slightly larger in males (Figs. 20, 21) [16]. The fundus of the sac extends 3 to 5 mm above the medial canthal tendon, and

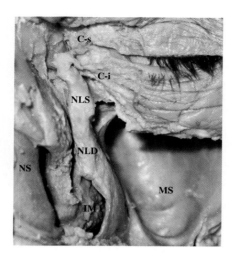

Fig. 21. Anatomic dissection of the lacrimal drainage system within the bony wall between the nasal cavity and maxillary sinus. The nasolacrimal duct drains into the inferior meatus. C-i, inferior canaliculus; C-s, superior canaliculus; IM, inferior meatus; MS, maxillary sinus; NLD, nasolacrimal duct; NLS, nasolacrimal sac; NS, nasal septum.

the body of the sac is 10 mm in height [53]. The sac rests in the lacrimal sac fossa with its medial aspect tightly adherent to the periorbital lining of the fossa. The lower nasolacrimal fossa and the duct are narrower in females, which may account for the female predominance of nasolacrimal obstruction [14]. The nasolacrimal duct then travels inferolaterally and slightly posteriorly in its bony course to the inferior turbinate for an interosseous distance of 12 mm. The nasolacrimal duct ostium within the inferior meatus is located 25 to 30 mm posterior to the lateral margin of the anterior nares [2]. The long axis of the duct and canal forms an angle of 15° to 25° posterior to the frontal plane, or in a line connecting the medial commissure to the first molar tooth [2]. The mean height of the lacrimal sac is 8.8 mm above the middle turbinate insertion on the lateral nasal wall and 4.1 mm inferior to it [79].

The canaliculi are encased in superficial pretarsal orbicularis oculi muscle that contributes to the lacrimal pump mechanism [53,80–85]. The lacrimal sac is wrapped in the lacrimal fascia, which refers to the periorbital lining that splits at the posterior lacrimal crest into one layer that lines the fossa and another layer that encases the lateral sac to reach the anterior lacrimal crest. Additionally, the lacrimal sac is enveloped by the thick anterior and thin posterior limbs of the medial canthal tendon. The thicker anterior limb wraps along the anterior upper half of the lacrimal sac before inserting onto the anterior lacrimal crest, and a very thin posterior limb passes behind the sac to insert onto the posterior lacrimal crest (Fig. 18). The deep portion of the

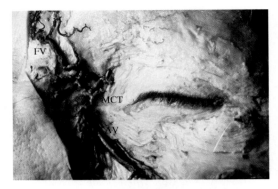

Fig. 22. The angular vein (AV, blue) and artery (red) are located approximately 5 mm medial to the anterior lacrimal crest. FV, frontal vein; MCT, medial canthal tendon.

pretarsal orbicularis muscle important in lacrimal outflow (Horner-Duverney muscle, tensor tarsi, or pars lacrimalis) passes posterior to the lacrimal sac and posterior limb of the medial canthal tendon and inserts onto the upper posterior lacrimal crest [2,53,86]. The anterior cranial fossa is in close proximity to the medial canthal tendon. A study of coronal maxillofacial CT scans found the mean vertical dimension between the medial canthal tendon to the level of the cribriform plate to be 17 mm ± 4 mm [87]. The oblique distance between the common internal punctum and the most anterior aspect of the cribiform plate is 25 ± 3 mm [88].

The angular artery branch of the facial artery runs along the line of the nasojugal skinfold with the angular vein and passes superficial to the medial canthal tendon. The vessels are located approximately 5 mm anteromedial to the anterior lacrimal crest; their presence should be anticipated to avoid bleeding (Fig. 22) [2].

References

[1] Lemke BN, Lucarelli MJ. Anatomy of ocular adnexa and orbit. In: Smith BC, editor. Ophthalmic plastic and reconstructive surgery. 2nd edition. St. Louis (MO): CV Mosby; 1997. p. 3–78.
[2] Whitnall SE. The anatomy of the human orbit and accessory organs of vision. New York: Oxford University Press; 1932. p. 1–252.
[3] Williams PL, Bannister LH, Berry MM, et al, editors. Gray's anatomy. 38th edition. New York: Churchill-Livingstone; 1995. p. 550–5.
[4] Hollinshead WH, Rosse C. Textbook of anatomy. 4th edition. Philadelphia: Harper & Row; 1985. p. 890.
[5] Webster RC, Gaunt JM, Hamdan US, et al. Supraorbital and supratrochlear notches and foramina: anatomical variations and surgical relevance. Laryngoscope 1986;96:311–5.

[6] Miller TA, Rudkin G, Honig M, et al. Lateral subcutaneous brow lift and interbrow muscle resection: clinical experience and anatomic studies. Plast Reconstr Surg 2000;105: 1120–7.

[7] Lorenc ZP, Ivy EM, Aston SJ. Neurosensory preservation in endoscopic forehead plasty. Aesthetic Plast Surg 1995;19:411–3.

[8] Park JI, Hoagland TM, Park MS. Anatomy of the corrugator supercilii muscle. Arch Facial Plast Surg 2003;5:412–5.

[9] Burkat CN, Lucarelli MJ, Lemke BN. Comprehensive glabellar anatomy for the cosmetic surgeon. American Journal of Cosmetic Surgery 2005; in press.

[10] Beer GM, Putz R, Mager K, et al. Variations of the exit of the supraorbital nerve: an anatomic study. Plast Reconstr Surg 1998;102:334–41.

[11] Kimura K. Foramina and notches on the supraorbital margin in some racial groups. Acta Anatomica Nipponica 1977;52:203–9.

[12] Shumrick KA, Smith TL. The anatomic basis for the design of forehead flaps in nasal reconstruction. Arch Otolaryngol Head Neck Surg 1992;118:373–9.

[13] Bailey JH. Surgical anatomy of the lacrimal sac. Am J Ophthalmol 1923;6:665–71.

[14] Groessl SA, Sires BS, Lemke BN. An anatomical basis for primary acquired nasolacrimal duct obstruction. Arch Ophthalmol 1997;115:71–4.

[15] Whitnall SE. The naso-lacrimal canal: the extent to which it is formed by the maxilla, and the influence of this upon its caliber. Ophthalmoscope 1912;10:557–8.

[16] Lemke BN, Della Rocca R. Surgery of the eyelids and orbit: an anatomical approach. East Norwalk (CT): Appleton & Lange; 1990.

[17] Hartikainen J, Aho HJ, Seppa H, et al. Lacrimal bone thickness at the lacrimal sac fossa. Ophthalmic Surg Lasers 1996;27:679–84.

[18] Whitnall SE. On a tubercle on the malar bone, and on the lateral attachments of the tarsal plates. J Anat Physiol 1911;45:426.

[19] Simonton JT, Garber PF, Ahl N. In margins of safety in lateral orbitotomy. Arch Ophthalmol 1977;95:1229.

[20] Kim JW, Goldberg RA, Shorr N. The inferomedial orbital strut. Ophthal Plast Reconstr Surg 2002;18:355–64.

[21] Mattox DE, Delaney RG. Anatomy of the ethmoid sinus. Otolaryngol Clin North Am 1985; 18:3–42.

[22] Whitnall SE. The relations of the lacrimal fossa to the ethmoidal cells. Ophthalmic Review 1911;30:321–5.

[23] Blaylock WK, Moore CA, Linberg JV. Anterior ethmoid anatomy facilitates dacryocysto-rhinostomy. Arch Ophthalmol 1990;108:1774–7.

[24] McCormick CD, Bearden WH, Hunts JH, et al. Cerebral vasospasm and ischemia after orbital decompression for Graves ophthalmopathy. Ophthal Plast Reconstr Surg 2004;20: 347–51.

[25] Mosher HP. The surgical anatomy of the ethmoid labyrinth. Ann Otol Rhinol Laryngol 1929;38:869–901.

[26] Bagatella R, Guiado C. The ethmoid labyrinth: an anatomical and radiological study. Acta Otolaryngol (Stockh) 1983;403(Suppl):1–19.

[27] Terrier F, Weber W, Ruefennacht D, et al. Anatomy of the ethmoid: CT, endoscopic and macroscopic. Am J Radiol 1985;144:493–500.

[28] Masala W, Perugini S, Salvolini U, et al. Multiplanar reconstructions in the study of ethmoid anatomy. Neuroradiology 1989;31:151–5.

[29] Hurwitz JJ. Embryology of the lacrimal drainage system. In: Hurwitz JJ, editor. The lacrimal system. Philadelphia: Lippincott-Raven; 1996. p. 9–13.

[30] Bridger MWM, Van Nostrand AWP. The nose and paranasal sinuses-applied surgical anatomy. J Otolaryngol 1978;(Suppl 6):1–33.

[31] Meyer DR, Linberg JV, Wobig JL, et al. Anatomy of the orbital septum and associated eyelid connective tissues. Ophthal Plast Reconstr Surg 1991;7:104.

[32] Jeong S, Lemke BN, Dortzbach RK, et al. The Asian upper eyelid. Arch Ophthalmol 1999;
     117:907.
[33] Putterman AM, Urist MJ. Surgical anatomy of the orbital septum. Ann Ophthalmol 1974;6:
     290.
[34] Lang J. The vascularization of the periorbita [abstract]. Gegenbaurs Morphol Jahrb 1975;
     121:174.
[35] Kikkawa DO, Lemke BN, Dortzbach RK. Relations of the superficial musculoaponeurotic
     system to the orbit and characterization of the orbitomalar ligament. Ophthal Plast Reconstr
     Surg 1966;12:77.
[36] Koornneef L. Spatial aspects of orbital musculo-fibrous tissue in man: a new anatomical and
     histological approach. Amsterdam: Swets en Zeitlinger; 1977.
[37] Fink WH. An anatomical study of the check mechanism of the vertical muscles of the eyes.
     Am J Ophthalmol 1957;44:800.
[38] Castanares S. Blepharoplasty for herniated intraorbital fat: anatomical basis for a new
     approach. Plast Reconstr Surg 1951;8:46.
[39] Carter SR, Chang J, Aguilar GL, et al. Involutional entropion and ectropion of the Asian
     lower eyelid. Ophthal Plast Reconstr Surg 2000;16:45.
[40] Helveston EM, Merriam WW, Ellis FD, et al. The trochlea: a study of the anatomy and
     physiology. Ophthalmology 1982;89:124.
[41] Sacks JG. The shape of the trochlea. Arch Ophthalmol 1984;102:932.
[42] Hayreh SS, Scott WE. Fluorescein iris angiography: I. Normal pattern. II. Disturbances in
     iris circulation following strabismus operation on various recti. Arch Ophthalmol 1978;96:
     1383.
[43] Lyon DB, Lemke BN, Wallow IH, et al. Sympathetic nerve anatomy in the cavernous sinus
     and retrobulbar orbit of the cynomolgus monkey. Ophthalmic Plast Reconstr Surg 1992;8:1.
[44] Simreich Z, Nathan H. The ciliary ganglion in man (anatomical observations). Anat Anz
     1981;150:287.
[45] Bergen MP. A literature review of the vascular system in the human orbit. Acta Morphol
     Neerl Scand 1981;19:273.
[46] Duke-Elder S, Wybar KC. The anatomy of the visual system. In: Duke-Elder S, editor.
     System of ophthalmology, vol. 2. New York: Kimpton; 1961. p. 551.
[47] Jakobiec FA, McLean I, Font RL. Clinico-pathologic characteristics of orbital lymphoid
     hyperplasia. Ophthalmology 1979;86:948.
[48] McGetrick JJ, Wilson DG, Dortzbach RK, et al. A search for lymphatic drainage of the
     monkey orbit. Arch Ophthalmol 1989;107:255.
[49] Sherman DD, Gonnering RS, Wallow IHL, et al. Identification of orbital lymphatics:
     enzyme histochemical light microscopic and electron microscopic studies. Ophthalmic Plast
     Reconstr Surg 1993;9:153.
[50] Gausas RE, Gonnering RS, Lemke BN, et al. Identification of human orbital lymphatics.
     Ophthalmic Plast Reconstr Surg 1999;15:252.
[51] Cook BE Jr, Lucarelli MJ, Lemke BN, et al. Eyelid lymphatics I: histochemical comparisons
     between the monkey and human. Ophthalmic Plast Reconstr Surg 2002;18:18.
[52] Cook BE Jr, Lucarelli MJ, Lemke BN, et al. Eyelid lymphatics II: a search for drainage
     patterns in the monkey and correlations with human lymphatics. Ophthalmic Plast Reconstr
     Surg 2002;18:99.
[53] Jones LT. An anatomical approach to problems of the eyelids and lacrimal apparatus. Arch
     Ophthalmol 1961;66:111–24.
[54] Dutton JJ. The lacrimal systems. In: Dutton J, editor. Atlas of clinical and surgical orbital
     anatomy. Philadelphia: WB Saunders; 1994. p. 140–2.
[55] Seifert P, Spitznas M, Koch F, et al. Light and electron microscopic morphology of accessory
     lacrimal glands. Adv Exp Med Biol 1994;350:19–23.
[56] Anderson RL, Beard C. The levator aponeurosis attachments and their clinical significance.
     Arch Ophthalmol 1977;95:1437.

[57] Whitnall SE. On a ligament acting as a check to the action of the levator palpebrae superioris muscle. J Anat Phys 1910;14:131.

[58] Anderson RL, Dixon RS. The role of Whitnall's ligament in ptosis surgery. Arch Ophthalmol 1979;97:705.

[59] Stasior GO, Lemke BN, Wallow IH, et al. Levator aponeurosis elastic fiber network. Ophthal Plast Reconstr Surg 1993;9:1.

[60] Tarbet KJ, Lemke BN. Small-incision periosteal flap canthopexy: aesthetic applications. Am J of Cosmetic Surg 2001;18:21.

[61] Lemke BN, Cook BE Jr, Lucarelli MJ. Canthus-sparing ectropion repair. Ophthal Plast Reconstr Surg 2001;17:161.

[62] Lemke BN, Khwarg SI. Adjuvant lateral canthal advancement in the surgical management of exophthalmic eyelid retraction. Arch Ophthalmol 1999;117:274.

[63] Burkat CN, Lemke BN, Rosenberg PN, et al. Anatomic considerations in cosmetic blepharoplasty of the lower eyelid: an oculoplastic perspective. American Journal of Cosmetic Surgery 2004;21:29–36.

[64] Lockwood CB. The anatomy of the muscles, ligaments, and fascia of the orbit, including an account of the capsule of tenon, the check ligaments of recti, and of the suspensory ligament of the eye. J Anat Physiol 1886;20:1.

[65] Hawes MJ, Dortzbach RK. The microscopic anatomy of the lower eyelid retractors. Arch Ophthalmol 1982;100:1313.

[66] Collin JRO, Beard C, Wood I. Terminal course of nerve supply to Müller's muscle in the rhesus monkey and its clinical significance. Am J Ophthalmol 1979;87:234.

[67] Morton AD, Elner VM, Lemke BN, et al. Lateral extensions of the Müller muscle. Arch Ophthalmol 1996;114:1486–8.

[68] Walcott B. Anatomy and innervation of the human lacrimal gland. In: Albert DM, Jakobiec F, Robinson N, editors. Principles and practice of ophthalmology: basic sciences. Philadelphia: WB Saunders; 1994. p. 454–8.

[69] Ruskell GL. The distribution of autonomic post-ganglionic nerve fibers to the lacrimal gland in monkeys. J Anat 1971;109:229–42.

[70] Ruskell GL. The orbital branches of the pterygopalatine ganglion and their relationship with internal carotid nerve branches in primates. J Anat 1970;106:323–39.

[71] Ruskell GL. Distribution of pterygopalatine ganglion efferents to the lacrimal gland in man. Exp Eye Res 2004;78:329–35.

[72] Lemke BN. Lacrimal anatomy. Adv Ophthalmic Plast Reconstr Surg 1984;3:11–23.

[73] Yazici B, Yazici Z. Frequency of the common canaliculus: a radiological study. Arch Ophthalmol 2000;118:1381–5.

[74] Schaeffer JP. The genesis and development of the nasolacrimal passages in man. Am J Anat 1912;13:1–23.

[75] Tucker NA, Tucker SM, Linberg JV. The anatomy of the common canaliculus. Arch Ophthalmol 1996;114:1231–4.

[76] Aubaret E. Les replis valvulaires des canalicules et du conduit lacrymo-nasal, au point de vue anatomique et physiologique [The valves of the lacrymo-nasal passages]. Arch d'Ophthal 1908;28:211–36 [in French].

[77] Petersen RA, Robb RM. The natural course of congenital obstruction of the nasolacrimal duct. J Pediatr Ophthalmol Strabismus 1978;15:246–50.

[78] Yuen SJ, Oley C, Sullivan TJ. Lacrimal outflow dysgenesis. Ophthalmology 2004;111: 1782–90.

[79] Wormald PJ, Kew J, Van Hasselt A. Intranasal anatomy of the nasolacrimal sac in endoscopic dacryocystorhinostomy. Otolaryngol Head Neck Surg 2000;123:307–10.

[80] Ploman K, Engel A, Knutsson F. Experimental studies of lacrimal passageways. Acta Ophthalmol (Copenh) 1928;6:55–90.

[81] Rosengren B. On lacrimal drainage. Ophthalmologica 1972;164:409–21.

[82] Maurice DM. The dynamics and drainage of tears. Int Ophthalmol Clin 1973;13: 103–16.

[83] Doane MG. Blinking and the mechanics of the lacrimal drainage system. Ophthalmol 1981; 88:844–51.

[84] Becker BB. Tricompartment model of the lacrimal pump mechanism. Ophthalmol 1992;99: 1139–45.

[85] Thale A, Paulsen F, Rochels R, et al. Functional anatomy of the human efferent tear ducts: a new theory of tear outflow mechanism. Graefes Arch Clin Exp Ophthalmol 1998;236: 674–8.

[86] Ahl NC, Hill JD. Horner's muscle and the lacrimal system. Arch Ophthalmol 1982;100: 488–93.

[87] McCann DP, Lucarelli MJ. Radiologic analysis of the ethmoid bone-cribriform plate spatial relationship [abstract 2281]. Invest Ophthalmol Vis Sci 1998;39(Suppl):498.

[88] Botek AA, Goldberg RA. Margins of safety in dacryocystorhinostomy. Ophthalmic Surg 1993;24:320–2.

ELSEVIER
SAUNDERS

Otolaryngol Clin N Am
38 (2005) 857–869

OTOLARYNGOLOGIC
CLINICS
OF NORTH AMERICA

Patient Evaluation

Lisa A. Zdinak, MD

Bosniak + Zilkha, 135 East 74th Street, New York, NY 10021, USA

The initial clinical encounter between the cosmetic surgeon and a patient considering facial rejuvenation is a time of information gathering for the patient and the surgeon. During the consultation, the physician should attempt to understand the patient's motivations for surgery and expectations regarding the surgical outcome. Once rapport has been established, preoperative photographs and measurements are taken and used to delineate which of the features can be successfully surgically altered in accordance with the patient's desires. The general risks of surgery are explained as well as risks specific to the proposed interventions. The surgical plan is devised with the patient, and questions regarding preoperative preparations and the expected clinical course are discussed. A second consultation may be needed to allow the patient and surgeon to scrutinize the details of proposed interventions further as well as to facilitate the development of an uninhibited mode of communication.

Patient selection

One of the most important things for the surgeon to ascertain during the initial clinical encounter with the patient is the motivation for cosmetic surgery. Some patients may have specific complaints about their appearance and a definitive idea of what results they desire, whereas others may be passively vague and seek significant input from the surgeon. It is the surgeon's responsibility to determine which of the objectionable physical parameters can be surgically altered and to convey this information to the patient in language that he or she can understand. The surgeon must be able to translate the patient's subjective complaint into an objective physical finding. Several illustrative tools, such as old photographs, photographs taken during the initial patient encounter, mirrors, and computer-generated

E-mail address: lisazdinak@aol.com

images that demonstrate proposed postsurgical improvements, can help the patient to relate the desired surgical outcome objectively to the surgeon. In turn, the surgeon can use these same tools to convey what physical parameters can be successfully altered in accordance with the patient's desires. Patients with specific complaints and a clear idea of surgical limitations are ideal candidates for cosmetic surgery. Patients who do not involve themselves in the decision-making process may not be happy with the surgical outcome [1].

Patient preparation

The patient must understand that cosmetic surgery done well is not designed to effect a lifestyle change. The patient should expect to look more alert, less weary, and not necessarily younger. Patients must be informed of the potential pitfalls of the surgery—at least the generalized possibilities of bleeding, infection, and scarring. Potential complications specific to blepharoplasty, including abnormalities of lid level and contour, lid closure dysfunction, and tear film deficiencies, should also be discussed. The patient should anticipate a transient superficial numbness of the upper eyelid secondary to resection of the subcutaneous fascia and its sensory nerve endings, but it can be expected to resolve within 6 to 8 weeks after surgery. Lower lid anesthesia does not occur with the transconjunctival approach. Asian patients should understand that cosmetic blepharoplasty may occidentalize their appearance if a high lid crease incision is made. Darker skinned patients must accept the remote possibility of postoperative postinflammatory dyspigmentation. Patients with darkly pigmented skin may not be ideal candidates for skin resurfacing, and preoperative test laser applications may be required. Patients who smoke, have had phenol peels, or have taken isotretinoin during the preceding year may not be candidates for laser facial rejuvenation. It is essential for patients to avoid aspirin, aspirin-containing compounds, and cigarette smoking for at least 2 weeks before surgery. During the preoperative months, reducing the quantity of cigarettes smoked or eliminating them entirely can facilitate wound healing and decrease postoperative edema. Anticoagulant therapy should be discontinued 2 weeks before surgery so as to avoid coagulopathies during surgery. Monoamine oxidase (MAO) inhibitors should also be discontinued so as to avoid complicating interactions at the time of surgery. Preoperative discussions with patients should include familiarizing them with the normal landmarks of the postoperative recovery period. Patients must also be aware of the variability in healing among individuals and that the healing process may take longer on one side of the face than on the other. No matter how benign the surgeon views a patient's recovery, he or she should not forget that most patients have not undergone the intended procedure before and have not seen what a cosmetic surgery patient looks like in the early preoperative days. It is helpful to tell patients that they are not going to look good for the first week after surgery.

Preoperative medical evaluation

Patients' safety should be a prime consideration of the surgeon. Not every operation demands a full laboratory workup. The obvious necessity of establishing patients' cardiopulmonary stability, general health, and blood clotting status is supplemented by the need to discover any systemic ailments that may directly affect the final surgical outcome (Table 1). Chronically boggy upper and lower lids may be the result of thyroid dysfunction, renal disease, or congestive heart failure. Prolapsed orbital fat or ptotic lacrimal glands may be the result of hyperactive thyroid disease. Resection of lid tissue in these patients is unpredictable until the underlying medical condition is stabilized. Young female patients in their 20s and 30s with a history of episodic eyelid swelling may have true blepharochalasis. These patients should be informed that additional procedures may be required in the future as a result of continued episodes of their disease. Acquired inferior scleral show may be related to hyperthyroid lid retraction or retrobulbar tumor. Preoperative ophthalmic examination is essential to document visual acuity, peripheral visual field loss, intraocular pressure, tear film stability, baseline tear function, strength of lid closure, lagophthalmos, and symmetry of palpebral apertures. The preexistence of

Table 1
Preoperative workup

Current photographs
    Full face, both eyes together, each eye separately (front and side views). Appropriate lighting and positioning are essential. For proper orientation, the base of the nose should be on the same horizontal plane as the tragus. Any head or chin depression or elevation will mask the true palpebral aperture.
Old photographs
    To establish the longevity of palpebral aperture asymmetry
    Complete blood cell count in patients over 40 years or with history of anemia. Prothrombin time, partial thromboplastin time, and platelet count in patients with history of easy bruising or bleeding disorder.
    Electrolytes and SMA 12 in patients over 60 years or with history of hypertension.
    Triiodothyronine (T_3) and thyroxine (T_4) if any doubt about thyroid status; if surgeon's index of suspicion for thyroid dysfunction is marked, a more complete endocrinologic workup is indicated.
    Electrocardiogram on every patient over 60 years
    Chest x-ray if there is any history of pulmonary disease

---

dry eyes, lid lag, or lagophthalmos has a bearing on the extent of lid resection proposed by the surgeon.

Preoperative measurements and observations

Photographic documentation should include current photographs of the full face, both eyes together, and each eye separately (front and side views). Appropriate lighting and head position are essential. The base of the nose should be on the same plane as the tragus to prevent chin depression or elevation that could mask the true palpebral aperture. Old photographs are helpful in documenting the duration of palpebral aperture asymmetry. The idealized eyelid and palpebral aperture parameters are compared with the involutionally changed periocular structures in Table 2.

Vertical palpebral aperture

Measuring the distance between the upper and lower lid margins reveals the presence of a true ptosis. The average vertical palpebral aperture is 10 mm, with the upper lid margin 1 to 2 mm below the superior limbus and the

Table 2
Normal periocular anatomic relationships and contrasting involutional changes

	Normal/idealized	Involutional changes
Brow	At or above superior orbital rim	Below level of superior orbital rim
	Gentle arch highest at junction of temporal one-third and nasal two-thirds	Flattened arch
Superior sulcus	Flat	Excessively deep (fat atrophy) Excessively full (skin redundancy)
Vertical palpebral aperture	10 mm	Decreased (ptosis) Increased (inferior scleral show or upper lid retraction)
Upper lid crease	8–10 mm above lashes	Elevated (levator aponeurotic disinsertion) Obliterated (redundant lid fold)
Upper lid fold	Mild draping over crease	Excessive (obliterating crease) Retracted into superior sulcus (levator disinsertion)
Horizontal palpebral aperture	34 mm	Narrowed with canthal tendon laxity
Lateral canthal angle	Acute	Rounded with canthal tendon laxity or dehiscence
Lower lid margin	At or above inferior limbus	Inferior scleral show
Punctal position	Not visible; in lacrimal lake	Vertically directed or everted

lower lid margin at the level of the inferior limbus. The brow should be held at its normal position at the superior orbital rim during measurement.

Horizontal palpebral aperture

The average horizontal palpebral aperture is 30 to 34 mm. Laxity or dehiscence of the medial or lateral canthal tendons causes narrowing of the horizontal palpebral aperture. Lower lid ectropion without canthal tendon laxity causes gross distortion of the lower lid margin but may not shorten the horizontal distance between the canthal angles.

Inferior scleral show

The idealized lower lid rests at the level of the inferior limbus. Inferior scleral show is the distance from the inferior limbus to the lower lid margin. It may occur normally as an anatomic variant (eg, high myopia, shallow orbits, hypoplastic inferior orbital rim), as the result of an underlying pathologic process (eg, hyperthyroid lid retraction, retrobulbar tumor), or as the result of acquired changes from lid margin or canthal tendon laxity. Rarely is a transcutaneous approach to the lower lid indicated. In the case of patients with preexisting scleral show, a transcutaneous approach to lower lid blepharoplasty is contraindicated because of the introduction of variable lower lid retraction caused by the subciliary incision. Lower lid laser resurfacing of the pretarsal skin should also be avoided in patients with preexisting scleral show. Horizontal resection of lax lower lids should be avoided in the presence of inferior scleral show. These patients require superiorly directed support with recession of lower lid retractors and canthal tendon placation.

Superior sulcus

Inferior to the brow, the superior sulcus is tucked under the superior orbital rim. In young patients, the superior sulcus is a flat or concave surface. When evaluating the superior sulcus, the surgeon should make particular note of prolapsed fat pockets, redundant skin, and the presence of ptosis. Patients with prolapsed superior fat pockets have a shallower superior sulcus with a convex contour. Elderly patients with orbital fat atrophy have hollow deep superior sulci. The deep superior sulcus may be accentuated by levator aponeurotic disinsertions with lid crease retraction. A prominent hyperostic superior orbital rim with secondary anterior displacement of the soft tissue of the brow casts the superior sulcus and upper lid into deep shadow. Prominent superior orbital rims can be thinned by resecting the brow fat pocket and orbicularis muscle overlying the superior orbital rim. In extreme cases, however, burring down the orbital rim may be considered. Heavy ptotic brows cause secondary upper lid fold redundancy or temporal hooding. Recontouring the superior sulcus is often the primary objective of blepharoplasty. Although still amenable to cosmetic surgery, the male superior sulcus should not be recontoured to the same extent as the female brow-sulcus complex. The deep smooth female superior sulcus exhibits a high arched lid crease and a delicate lid fold. This is in direct contrast to the male superior sulcus, which is full, with a flat contour and a low flat lid fold with minimal central arching. Patients with ptosis and levator aponeurotic disinsertions may have deep flat superior sulci. They might find their ptosis objectionable but like their superior sulcus contours. Repair of the levator aponeurosis without resection of excess lid skin may correct the lid level and palpebral aperture asymmetry but produce a redundant lid fold that abuts the upper lid lashes. Patients who had smooth upper lid contours before surgery may have prominent convexities and draping of the fold after reapproximation of a dehisced levator aponeurosis. Ptosis repair without appropriate myocutaneous resection and fat contouring in these patients corrects their ptosis but changes their superior sulcus contour, usually to their dissatisfaction.

Brows

The idealized female brow lies above the level of the superior orbital rim, with a gentle arch reaching its peak at the junction of the nasal two thirds and the temporal one third (on-line with the temporal limbus). The brow contour can be altered by plucking or other methods of hair removal and is usually left at its fullest nasally as far medial as the medial orbital rim and tapered temporally to overlie the superior orbital rim. The male brow is thicker and less well defined, with minimal to no arch. Although it may be tempting for the surgeon to elevate the male brow to deepen the superior sulcus, this should be approached with caution, because a flat superior sulcus is more in keeping with the traditionally accepted male physiognomy. Temporal brow ptosis with secondary hooding of the upper lid can be corrected with direct temporal brow resection or internal suspension and forehead laser resurfacing.

Suborbicularis brow fat pocket

Patients with heavy upper lids, a full superior sulcus, and an upper lid crease obscured by a thick upper lid fold require sculpting of the suborbicularis brow fat pocket. Resecting preaponeurotic fat alone does not yield a well-defined superior sulcus in these patients.

Lateral canthal angle

In non-Asian patients, the lateral canthus is slightly superior to the medial canthus. In general, the lateral canthal angle is more acute than the medial canthal angle. There is a prominently sharp angle at the outer canthus. Any rounding or inferior displacement of the lateral canthus is cosmetically significant. Bilaterally rounded lateral canthi should alert the surgeon that previous cosmetic surgery may have been performed.

Lid surface contour irregularities

Lid irregularities secondary to prolapsed orbital fat displacing orbicularis muscle and skin are dome shaped and smooth. Not all smooth dome-shaped upper lid convexities are prolapsed orbital fat, however. Frontoethmoidal mucoceles often occur as dome-shaped masses in the medial superior sulcus, which can look like a medial fat pocket in some instances. They are firm, usually noncompressible, and contiguous with the orbital rims medially and superiorly, however. Dermoid or epidermoid cysts of the zygomaticofrontal or nasofrontal sutures may appear as an ill-defined temporal or nasal upper lid fullness mimicking a temporal or nasal fat pocket. These also tend to be firm and noncompressible. Tumors of the orbital lobe of the lacrimal gland may appear as temporal lid masses. They may be firm, noncompressible, adherent to the orbital rim, and associated with ptosis or proptosis. Gentle pressure on the globe exaggerating the prominence of the masses in their characteristic locations is the hallmark of prolapsed fat. Each fat pad may yield a discrete mass (two in the upper lid and three in the lower lid). Pressure on the globe via the upper lid accentuates the inferior pockets. Qualitative and quantitative assessment of these inferior fat pockets is facilitated by observing them in all fields of gaze. Inferior pockets are accentuated with supraduction. Abduction accentuates the nasal pocket, and adduction accentuates the temporal pocket. Pressure applied inferiorly accentuates the superior pockets. Preoperative drawings delineating these fat pockets are useful during surgery when subcutaneous infiltration of the lids and the patient's supine position cause a coalescing of the lid surface contours. Care must be taken in demarcating the nasal fat pocket because it often lies medial to the nasal border of the upper lid incision and may not be fully exposed during dissection. The skin-muscle flap can be retracted to expose these medial fat pockets effectively and avoid the need for enlarging the initial incision. Of most direct relevance to cosmetic blepharoplasty is the ptotic palpebral lobe of the lacrimal gland. It appears as a soft, compressible, movable mass in the temporal portion of the upper lid, where a distinct temporal fat pocket does not exist. It can be rolled between the examiner's fingers, and it may be unilateral or bilateral. For an acceptable cosmetic result after blepharoplasty in these patients, a resuspension or carbon dioxide laser contraction of the lacrimal gland is indicated.

Hypertrophic orbicularis muscle

Hypertrophic orbicularis muscle can be recognized as a transverse ridge or band on the anterior tarsal surface that is accentuated by smiling.

Inferior orbital rim

The inferior orbital rim should be palpated in patients considering lower lid blepharoplasty. Prolapsed fat and redundant folds may be part of a malar bag and not amenable to standard lower lid approaches. Mild malar cutaneous redundancy may be effectively treated with laser skin resurfacing. More prominent malar deformities require direct resection and secondary resurfacing. Facial skin lying within the boundaries of the orbital rims is thinner than facial skin lying distal to the orbital rims and must be treated differently. Tear-trough deformities may be the result of a hypoplastic or flat inferior orbital rim and may require malar augmentation. Concave deformities of the inferior orbit can be softened by fat pedicle flap transposition, microlipoinjection, or malar and tear-trough implants.

Lid margin and punctal malpositions

The idealized lower lid rests at the level of the inferior limbus. Involutional entropion and ectropion of the lower lid can be corrected concurrently with lower lid blepharoplasty. The punctum is normally not visible without retracting the lower lid. Punctal eversion exists if the punctum can be seen without touching the lid and poses an added consideration during operative planning. Lower lid skin resection or pretarsal laser skin resurfacing can accentuate preexisting punctual eversion, leading to epiphora and an unhappy patient.

Canthal tendon laxity

Lid margin laxity is determined by grasping the lid and pulling it away from the globe. If it can be retracted 6 mm or more from the globe, it is deemed to be lax (distraction test). Lateral canthal tendon laxity can be determined if nasal traction on the lid brings the lateral canthal angle closer to the temporal limbus. A subtle rounding of the lateral canthal angle or mild S-shaped deformity of the lower lid with a slightly increased vertical palpebral aperture temporally is indicative of lateral canthal tendon laxity. In the absence of frank medial ectropion or punctual eversion, a lax medial canthal tendon may be discovered with the application of lateral traction to the lower lid margin. In the presence of a lax medial canthal tendon, this maneuver displaces the inferior punctum temporally toward the nasal limbus. To avoid shortening of the horizontal palpebral aperture, the medial canthal tendon must be plicated before horizontal shortening of the lower lid is performed by wedge resection. Lower lid laxity left unaddressed during blepharoplasty may predispose the lid to postoperative eversion or retraction of the lid margin. Canthal tendon laxity must be repaired before horizontal shortening of the lid margin to avoid horizontal palpebral fissure distortion. Any lower lid margin laxity must be addressed before lower lid resurfacing is performed.

Malar festoons

Malar festoons are excessive redundancies of lower lid skin and orbicularis muscle that cascades below the inferior orbital rim. These deformities have been most difficult to correct in the past using standard blepharoplasty techniques. Historically, a subciliary lower lid blepharoplasty incision with extensive subcutaneous undermining beyond the inferior orbital rim characteristically leaves a postoperative pocket of subcutaneous edema and residual redundancy over the malar eminence. Extensive undermining of a skin-muscle flap with periosteal anchoring at the lateral palpebral raphe and internal suspension of malar suborbicularis fat to the inferior orbital rim has been described to eliminate the festoons. A rhytidectomy with subcutaneous musculoaponeurotic system (SMAS) plication supplies additional superiorly directed support to the lid-cheek complex. Carbon dioxide laser resurfacing of the malar festoon can significantly reduce mild to moderate deformities. Residual malar festoons are corrected with direct resection, but this leaves the patient with an uncamouflaged scar that has to be resurfaced with the carbon dioxide laser in most instances.

Special considerations in blepharoplasty: male, Asian, and African-American patients

Men can be excellent candidates for cosmetic blepharoplasty, but the patient and the surgeon must be aware of differences in anatomy, technique, and postoperative course from female patients. Men are often less tolerant of postoperative discomfort. Their incisions remain indurated and erythematous for a longer time, and their eyelids may also remain swollen longer. The low flat contour of the male brow parallels a lid fold that is full and generously draped over the lid crease. Aggressive sculpting of the male superior sulcus and overresecting of the male lid fold are inappropriate. Frequently, upper lid dermatochalasis and septal weakness in men are accompanied by brow ptosis, which can be medial, central, or lateral. Often, transblepharoplasty internal brow suspension may be all that is necessary.

Asian patients are particularly attentive to the height, depth, length, and symmetry of their lid crease-fold complexes. They are specific and exact about their desires and expectations. There are three areas of potential concern: the lid crease-fold complex, the epicanthal folds, and the angle and width of the horizontal palpebral fissure aperture. Of paramount importance is the lid crease-fold complex. The double eyelid exists when the lid crease is 6 mm or more above the lid margin. When it is less than 4 mm above the margin, it may be perceived as a single eyelid. There are profound ethnic variations among Chinese, Japanese, Korean, and Filipino patients. Patients must understand that any myocutaneous resection of the upper lid may occidentalize their eyelids. Some patients may specifically desire occidentalization of their lids, others may want a double eyelid without changing their ethnic character, and some may simply complain of lid heaviness and request removal of redundant tissue only. Epicanthus tarsalis is the most characteristic fold in northern Chinese and Korean patients. There is a defined lid crease laterally but none nasally. Epicanthus tarsalis can be altered via V-Y plasty. Epicanthus supraciliaris traverses the medial canthus from the eyebrow to the lacrimal sac. Epicanthus palpebralis extends from the nasal pretarsal area to the area of the anterior lacrimal crest. Epicanthus palpebralis and supraciliaris with upper and lower lid components can be modified with double opposing Z-plasties or upper and lower V-Y plasties. Because Asian patients may have a greater propensity for hypertrophic scarring, medial canthal fold revision should be approached with great caution and only by the most experienced surgeons. Skin resurfacing in Asian patients must also be approached with the understanding that there may be a transient postoperative mottled pigmentation that may necessitate the use of bleaching agents and alpha-hydroxy acid peels once the inflammatory phase of healing has subsided.

Persons of African descent have variations in periocular anatomy that deserve special attention during preoperative evaluation, including shallow orbits with prolapsed lacrimal glands, lower lid inferior scleral show, and malar hypoplasia. Typically, upper lid blepharoplasty in dark-skinned patients requires more aggressive lipocontouring, sculpting of the brow fat pocket, and repositioning of a prolapsed lacrimal gland. The shallow orbit and relative malar hypoplasia should alert the surgeon that more aggressive lipocontouring is needed to obtain the desired lower lid contour. Because the globe often sits anterior to the lateral orbital rim, plicating the lateral canthal tendon may not elevate the lower lid margin and, in fact, may draw the lid margin lower. The most acceptable alternative is to perform a transconjunctival blepharoplasty and leave the lid margin where it is. Because of the thinness of the upper lid skin, the possibility of upper lid colloids or hypertrophic scarring is rare. The thin eyelid skin becomes thicker facial skin at the lateral orbital rim; therefore, temporal extensions of the lid incisions beyond the lateral orbital rim are to be avoided. A history of keloid formation on the face or body is not a contraindication to upper lid blepharoplasty. Direct brow elevations should be discouraged in patients with a history of keloid formation.

Classification of skin types and levels of photodamage

Cutaneous aging is a dynamic process influenced by chronologic and environmental factors. Excessive exposure to sunlight-ultraviolet (UV) light is the main cause of chronic photoaging and photodamaged skin. Clinical abnormalities of actinic-damaged skin include dryness, actinic keratosis, irregular pigmentation, elastosis, and a decrease in elasticity accompanied by an increase in wrinkling. Proper evaluation of the skin and its ability to tan or brown from UV exposure is helpful in determining how patients may respond to laser treatment or chemical peeling. Fitzpatrick's classification table can be useful in this analysis (Table 3). Patients with skin types I to III do not generally develop postinflammatory dyspigmentation and are ideal candidates for laser resurfacing. Patients with skin types IV to VI have a greater chance of developing postinflammatory hyperpigmentation, whereas patients with skin types V and VI are often at risk for irregular hypopigmentation from skin resurfacing. Although Fitzpatrick's classification is helpful in predicting the risk of dyschromia after laser skin resurfacing, Glogau's classification of photodamage is helpful in determining the efficacy of different treatments for certain skin types (Table 4). Because there is no single ideal classification system that establishes the appropriate therapy, these are helpful when combined with the surgeon's clinical experience. The introduction of facial rejuvenation techniques with the carbon dioxide laser has significantly expanded the therapeutic options for patients. The intensity of the treatment is modified by the thickness of the skin and the degree of actinic damage. The more severe the actinic changes are, the more dramatic is the result. Rhytid ablation is more prominent, and the lifting effect is more significant. Patients who have previously undergone rhytidectomy but have residual rhytidosis respond well to laser resurfacing performed at least 3 to 6 months after the initial procedure.

Devising the surgical plan

Procedures can be performed singly or in combination with others. Patients may want to see how they are going to look after blepharoplasty before deciding whether they want additional facial surgery. In tailoring a procedure to suit patients, the surgeon can use a variety of techniques. Several procedural principles should be kept in mind. Resecting or resurfacing the upper eye skin without first elevating or supporting the eyebrow is ineffective if there is associated brow ptosis. If the levator aponeurosis is disinserted, as evidenced by an elevated lid crease-fold complex and a deep superior sulcus with normal levator excursions, it must

Table 3
Fitzpatrick's classification table

Skin phototype	Skin color	Characteristics
I	White	Always burns, never tans
II	White	Always burns, tans minimally
III	White	Rarely burns, tans gradually and uniformly
IV	Light brown	Rarely burns, tans more than average
V	Brown	Rarely burns, tans profusely
VI	Dark brown or black	Never burns, deep tan

Table 4
Glogau's classification

Damage	Description	Characteristics
Type 1 (mild)	No wrinkles	Early photoaging: mild pigmentary changes; no keratosis; minimal wrinkles Patient age 20s or 30s: minimal or no makeup; minimal acne scarring
Type 2 (moderate)	Wrinkles in motion	Early to moderate photoaging: early senile lentigines visible Patient age late 30s–40s: some foundation worn; mild acne scarring
Type 3 (advanced)	Wrinkles at rest	Advanced photoaging: obvious dyschromia; telangiectasis; visible keratosis; wrinkles visible at rest Patient age 50s or older: heavier foundation always worn; acne scarring that makeup does not cover
Type 4 (severe)	Only wrinkles	Severe photoaging: yellow-gray skin color; history of skin malignancies; wrinkles all over, no normal skin Patient age 60s or 70s: makeup cannot be worn (it cakes and racks); severe acne scarring

be advanced and repaired during the upper lid blepharoplasty before lipocontouring and myocutaneous resection are performed. Before the lower lid can be resurfaced, laxity of the lid margin and lateral canthal tendon must be corrected. The angle of the lateral canthus and the apposition of the lid margin to the globe must also be restored before the lower lid anterior lamella is treated. Surface irregularities and residual static rhytids after blepharoplasty and browplasty can largely be ablated with laser resurfacing. Full-face carbon dioxide laser resurfacing is conveniently and effectively performed concomitantly with upper and lower lid blepharoplasty, lateral canthoplasty, levator aponeurotic advancement, and internal brow suspension. The dynamic rhytids of the forehead, glabella, and lateral periorbital areas can be addressed with injections of botulinum toxin type A purified neurotoxin complex, followed by carbon dioxide laser resurfacing. Botulinum toxin type A purified neurotoxin complex injection 1 week before the resurfacing or at the conclusion of the resurfacing enhances cosmetic improvement for dynamic rhytids. The erbium:yttrium-aluminum-garnet (Er:YAG) laser yields less penetration than the carbon dioxide laser, causing less thermal damage. This translates into a shorter duration of post-resurfacing erythema and a shorter recovery time. It also means that more passes of laser applications are necessary, however, and this treatment does not work on deep wrinkles or extensive photodamage. Any residual dynamic rhytids and surface depressions can be addressed with volume augmentation and chemodenervation [2]. These include inferior and superior sulcus deformities, glabellar furrows, deeper crow's feet, and laugh lines. The problem of generalized facial laxity should be anticipated before surgery, and a rhytidectomy or full-face resurfacing should be recommended and performed at the time of the blepharoplasty. Radiosurgical removal of benign facial and eyelid lesions using a fine-wire radiosurgical electrode (Ellman International, Hewlett, NY) is a convenient technique for removing flat or elevated lesions of the face and eyelids. Other possible techniques that the surgeon can offer the patient at the time of consultation include treatment of facial lesions and vascular, telangiectatic, and pigmented lesions using the argon laser, tunable dye laser, or intense pulsed light (IPL). Laser hair removal before full-face resurfacing laser hair removal is particularly useful in men because they are not able to shave for the next 3 to 4 weeks.

Summary

Careful planning and establishing a good rapport between the physician and patient are critical to the success of any cosmetic surgeon's practice. Honest communication in an unhurried environment that is geared toward patient comfort yields the most gratifying results for all concerned.

Reference

[1] Bosniak SL, Cantisano-Zilkha M. Cosmetic blepharoplasty and facial rejuvenation. 2nd edition. New York: Lippincott-Raven; 1999.
[2] Bosniak SL, Cantisano-Zilkha M. Minimally invasive techniques of oculofacial rejuvenation. 1st edition. New York: Thieme Medical Publishers; 2005.

ELSEVIER
SAUNDERS

Otolaryngol Clin N Am
38 (2005) 871–885

OTOLARYNGOLOGIC
CLINICS
OF NORTH AMERICA

The Diagnosis and Management of Dry Eyes

Jeffrey P. Gilbard, MD[a,b,*]

[a]*Department of Ophthalmology, Harvard Medical School, Boston, MA, USA*
[b]*Advanced Vision Research, 12 Alfred Street, Suite 200, Woburn, MA 01801, USA*

Dry eye is a condition characterized by symptoms of sandy/gritty irritation, dryness, or burning caused by the ocular surface disease that results from any condition or circumstance that decreases tear secretion or increases tear film evaporation resulting in a loss of water from the tear film sufficient to increase tear film osmolarity.

Dry eye is a common condition that, based on population-based studies, has been estimated to affect between 7.8% and 14% of adults, with the prevalence increasing with age. Women are affected about twice as frequently as men [1–3].

The ability to diagnose and treat dry eye has improved dramatically during the last decade as the understanding of disease mechanisms and pathology has improved. Therefore, the ability to screen patients for dry eye before ophthalmic plastic procedures has improved, and the ability to manage and treat dry eye postoperatively has improved as well.

Anatomy and physiology of the tear film

The anatomy of the tear film really begins with the ocular surface, because a healthy tear film depends upon a healthy ocular surface, and a healthy ocular surface depends upon a healthy tear film. The tear film, therefore, can be considered to have four layers: the ocular surface, the mucous layer, the aqueous layer, and the lipid layer. Together they lubricate, nourish, and protect the ocular surface.

* Advanced Vision Research, 12 Alfred Street, Suite 200, Woburn, MA 01801.
E-mail address: jgilbard@theratears.com

Advanced Vision Research manufactures and distributes TheraTears brand products for dry eye disorders and distributes PanOptx DryEyeWear.

The ocular surface

The normal ocular surface contains numerous features that make it eminently wettable. Ocular surface epithelia are densely packed with microplicae and microvilli covered on their surface by glycoproteins [4]. These physical "ridges" and their glycoprotein covering provide two ways for the mucous layer of the tear film to attach to the ocular surface, creating a very effective glycocalyx. This glycocalyx forms the foundation for the mucous layer.

The mucous layer

The mucous layer is produced by the conjunctival goblet cells that produce gel-forming mucus. Mucus has high lubricity, and the first major function of the goblet cells and the mucus they produce is to provide lubrication for the ocular surface.

The second major function of the mucous layer is to contribute to the defenses of the ocular surface. The mucous layer exists on the ocular surface as a structureless continuum, in granules arraigned in clusters or sheets and as fine strands forming networks. Foreign particles stick to this mucus; with blinking, the clusters, sheets, and strands collapse and move toward the medial canthus where the trapped debris is expelled from the eye [5]. The efficacy of this defense system is enhanced by the nervous innervation of the goblet cells [6]. Goblet cells discharge their mucus in response to pain, increase in tear film osmolarity, and alteration in tear film electrolyte balance, increasing the quantity of mucus available to protect the surface in the face of these threats.

The aqueous layer and lacrimal gland secretion

The aqueous layer of the tear film lies on top of the mucous layer, and its water and electrolyte mixture keeps the mucous layer hydrated. The aqueous tears are produced by the main lacrimal gland that lies deep to the superotemporal fornix and is divided into an orbital and palpebral portion by the levator aponeurosis. The much smaller, accessory glands of Kraus and Wolfring lie mainly in the superotemporal and, to a lesser extent, in the infratemporal fornices. From these glands, the freshly secreted tears first flow to the superotemporal marginal tear strips and then distribute throughout the superior and inferior marginal tear strips [7]. The tears remain in the marginal tear strips until the blink spreads the tears over the surface of the eye [8].

The main and accessory lacrimal glands act in unison, and secretion from these glands is regulated both centrally and peripherally. A large portion of tear secretion is dependent on the sensory reflex arc [9]. Just as irritating the eye increases tear production, anesthetizing the eye surface with a drop of topical anesthetic decreases aqueous tear secretion by 78% [10]. Intact corneal sensation drives tear production and contributes to the physical defense of the ocular surface. Basal tear production from the lacrimal glands is thought to be driven peripherally by serum-borne neurohumoral factors such as vasoactive intestinal peptide that stimulate the lacrimal gland secretory cells directly [11].

Normal tear film osmolarity averages 302 ± 6 (SD) mOsm/L [12]. Tear film osmolarity is lowest upon eye opening [13] and, with the increased evaporation associated with eye opening, increases somewhat as the day progresses [14]. Decreases in tear production also increase tear film osmolarity, because the osmolarity of the lacrimal gland fluid itself increases with decreased rates of lacrimal gland secretion [15].

The aqueous tear supply can be thought of as the "clear blood supply" of the ocular surface, protecting it and nourishing it by providing oxygen by direct absorption from the air and electrolytes from the lacrimal gland fluid. The electrolyte balance of the tears differs from that of serum or aqueous humor. Because of the blood–tear and aqueous tear barriers, the tear supply maintains a unique electrolyte milieu at the ocular surface.

The lipid layer

The lipid or oil layer covers the aqueous layer and is produced by the meibomian glands that lie in the tarsal plates and open onto the lid margin just posterior to the eyelashes. The oil layer coats the tear film and retards evaporation as well as reducing tear film surface tension which holds the tear film "tight" to the eye surface. With loss of the lipid layer, tear film evaporation increases fourfold [16].

The pathogenesis of dry eye disorders

The pathogenesis of dry eye involves several processes. First, in dry eye, the tear film loses water, and tear film osmolarity increases. This increase in tear film osmolarity causes an osmotic dehydration of the eye surface and the symptoms of dry eye. Validated symptom questionnaires have shown that in dry eye symptoms get worse as the day goes on [17], and Farris and co-workers [14] have shown that tear film osmolarity increases as the day goes on. Second, the ocular surface pathology shows an osmotic dehydration of the ocular surface, with water moving across the ocular surface epithelium increasing epithelial desquamation. Ocular surface disease develops first and is most severe in the nasal bulbar conjunctiva in the exposure zone—the area of the ocular surface most remote from the freshly secreted, relatively dilute lacrimal gland fluid [18,19]. Third, biochemically on the ocular surface, glycogen decreases in the cornea as glucose is consumed to power the membrane ion pumps needed to maintain cell volume in the face of a hypertonic tear film [20]. Fourth, elevated tear film osmolarity promotes the increased expression of inflammatory cytokines on the ocular surface described in dry eye [21]. Fifth, surface disease, specifically the decrease in corneal glycogen and the decrease in conjunctival goblet cell density seen in dry eye, is proportional to the degree of elevation in tear film osmolarity and the duration of that increase [22]. The decrease in glycogen is significant, because glycogen is the energy source for the sliding step of corneal wound healing. The decrease in conjunctival goblet cell density is important because goblet cells produce the mucus that acts as the natural lubricant for the ocular surface.

Pathways to dry eye

In approaching the patient with dry eye, it is important to know how patients can develop dry eye (Fig. 1).

Decreased tear secretion

Tear production may decrease because of lacrimal gland disease or decreased corneal sensation. Most cases of dry eye caused by lacrimal gland disease are secondary to inflammatory lacrimal gland disease or Sjögren's syndrome. Sjögren's syndrome may be seen either with or without rheumatoid arthritis. As discussed, decreased corneal sensation decreases tear production. There are a multitude of reasons for decreased corneal sensation, including diabetes, long-term hard contact lens wearing, herpes zoster, laser-assisted intrastromal keratomileusis (LASIK) eye surgery [23], or any surgery that interrupts corneal nerves.

Increased tear film evaporation

Tear film evaporation is directly proportional to the distance between the upper lid and lower lid [24]. Eighty-seven percent of normal persons have

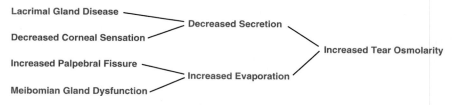

Fig. 1. Decreased tear secretion or increased tear film evaporation increase tear film osmolarity causing the progressive ocular surface changes observed in dry eye disease. (*Modified from* Albert DM, Jakobiec FA, editors. Principles and practice of ophthalmology. Philadelphia: W.B. Saunders Company; 1994. p. 260.)

a palpebral fissure width of 10 mm or less, and most of these have palpebral fissure widths of 9 mm or less [25]. Large palpebral fissure width can be hereditary or may be caused by lid surgery or thyroid eye disease. In patients with thyroid eye disease, palpebral fissure width measurements correlate with elevated tear film osmolarity as well as with dry eye surface disease [26].

The inflammation in the meibomian glands central to meibomitis results first in stenosis and then in closure of the meibomian gland orifices (Fig. 2). Deficiency and then loss of the tear film lipid layer leads to increasing water loss from the tear film, progressively higher tear film osmolarity, and symptomatic dry eye.

Diagnosing dry eye

The history

Although much emphasis has been placed on the use of diagnostic tests to diagnose dry eye, the most helpful diagnostic tool available today in diagnosing dry eye is the history. A classic dry eye history has high sensitivity and specificity and is helpful in separating dry eye from other causes of chronic eye irritation. The following seven questions will extract the information needed:

1. Character: What does the irritation feel like? Is it a sand/-gritty feeling, burning, foreign body sensation, or increased "awareness" of the eyes? Do the eyes itch?
2. Location: Where is the irritation located? Is it on the surface of the eye, in the eye, on the lid margin, or on the skin?
3. Diurnal variation: Are the symptoms worse at any particular time of day? Are they worse on awakening or late in the day? Are there two symptom peaks during the day—one upon awakening and a second late in the day?
4. Onset: Did the symptoms start suddenly, or did they develop gradually? Are the symptoms episodic or continuous?
5. Duration: How long have the symptoms been present?

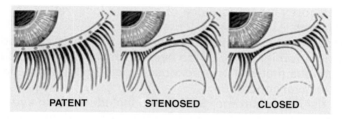

PATENT   STENOSED   CLOSED

Fig. 2. Natural history of meibomitis. Meibomian gland inflammation leads first to stenosis and then to closure of the meibomian gland orifice. (*From* Gilbard JP. Human tear film electrolyte concentrations in health and dry-eye disease. Int Ophthalmol Clin 1994;34:28; with permission.)

Box 1. What causes chronic eye irritation?*

Causes other than dry eye and meibomitis may explain
a patient's chronic eye irritation. Consider these other
possible causes and their symptoms:

Anterior blepharitis: Patients have crusting and irritation at the
base of lashes without diurnal variation. Onset is insidious.

Medicamentosa: Patients complain of burning and irritation
without diurnal variation. Symptoms are equivalent
throughout the day because overuse of topical medications
promotes damage. Suspect this condition in all patients who
use traditional artificial tears more than four times a day.
Patients generally have a history of escalating tear use.

Lacrimal drainage obstruction: Patients often have symptoms of
tearing with actual and demonstrable tear overflow. Patients
with meibomian gland dysfunction may feel like their eyes
are tearing, but these patients have frank epiphora.

Allergic conjunctivitis: The primary symptom for this condition is
itchy eyes. Patients' eyes may also exhibit increased mucus
production. Onset of this condition is commonly seasonal, and
it may be associated with hay fever, asthma and eczema.

Nocturnal lagophthalmos: Patients' eyes may burn upon
awakening. Patients frequently have a history of lid surgery
or thyroid eye disease.

Superior limbic keratoconjunctivitis: Symptoms include burning
and irritation without diurnal variation. Abrupt onset and
remissions characterize this condition. Patients often have
a history of thyroid dysfunction.

Superficial punctate keratitis (Thygenson's keratitis): Patients
with superficial punctate keratitis experience insidious onset
of photophobia, eye irritation, and decreased vision. The
condition is episodic and recurring.

Dry eyelid skin: Patients complain of "dry eyes." This condition
underscores the importance of accurate localization of
symptoms.

Tarsal foreign body: Patients experience a chronic sensation of
having a foreign body in the eye. This sensation results from
exogenous material or an exposed meibomian gland–derived
conjunctival concretion.

Mucus fishing syndrome: Symptoms include chronic eye
irritation and increased mucus production. Patients who reach
into their conjunctival cul-de-sac to remove mucus strands

caused by conjunctival trauma initiate the condition. A vicious cycle can develop.

Blepharospasm: Patients may complain that their eyes feel "tired." Careful questioning reveals that patients are experiencing an involuntary closure of the eyes rather than eye irritation. Driving, reading, and exposure to sunlight worsen symptoms.

Nonspecific ocular irritation: Normal eyes are responding to an abnormal environment. Eye irritation in response to smoke is a typical example.

Normal eyes with hypochondriasis: This condition is uncommon. A careful history that fails to mesh with the examination can provide the first clue to its presence.

---

* Reprinted by permission from www.dryeyeinfo.org.

---

6. Aggravating factors: Is there anything that makes the symptoms worse—wind, smoke, low humidity (ie, airplane cabins), reading, watching television, wearing contact lenses, or artificial tears?
7. Alleviating factors: Is there anything that makes the symptoms better—hot compresses, eye closure, high humidity, or artificial tears?

Patients with dry eye complain of sandy/gritty irritation, dryness, or a burning sensation in the eyes that worsen as the day goes on. Early in the disease they may complain simply of an increased "awareness" of the eyes that worsens as the day goes on. Symptoms worsen as the day goes on because tear film osmolarity increases as the day goes on. The symptoms start gradually over a period of weeks or months. Dry eyes are more sensitive to environmental irritants and to conditions of low humidity such as airplane cabins. Eye closure provides relief, as do conditions of high humidity.

Care must be taken to differentiate the symptoms of dry eye from those of meibomitis. Patients with meibomitis also complain of chronic sandy/gritty irritation, dryness, and burning in their eyes, and the symptoms are also insidious in onset, but in patients with meibomitis the symptoms are worse in the morning. Meibomitis is a condition characterized by inflammation of the meibomian glands in the eyelids. Symptoms are worse in the morning because tear flow decreases at night, and the inflamed eyelids are up against the cornea all night, releasing inflammatory mediators that cause the symptoms upon eye opening. With eye opening, tear flow increases, the lids open, pulling away from the cornea, and patient's symptoms quickly improve.

A third group of patients experiences two symptom peaks—one in the morning on eye opening, and a second that develops late in the day. These patients typically have meibomitis, which causes the symptoms from inflammation upon awakening in the morning, and meibomian gland dysfunction from the meibomitis, which causes symptoms from dryness late in the day. Meibomian gland dysfunction is caused by inflammatory damage to the meibomian glands and results in deficiency of the lipid layer of the tear film, which in turn results in both increased tear film evaporation and increased tear film osmolarity [27–29].

Many other conditions cause chronic eye irritation and, without a careful history, could be confused with dry eye. They are summarized in Box 1.

Examining the patient

A careful history should establish, at least, a very good differential diagnosis and, in many cases, a diagnosis that will be confirmed by examination. The examination is particularly helpful in determining why the patient has dry eye.

First, look at the facial skin. Look for facial telangiectasias and ask about central facial flushing. Central facial flushing is diagnostic for acne rosacea, and facial telangiectasias are highly suggestive. Next, measure the width of the palpebral fissure by having the patient look directly into your contralateral eye and holding a millimeter-scale rule vertically relatively close to the patient's lids. The greater the palpebral fissure width, the less meibomian gland dysfunction or decrease in tear production needed to create symptoms. Next, swing the slit-lamp biomicroscope into position and stage any meibomian gland dysfunction by determining if the meibomian gland orifices are patent, stenosed, or closed (Fig. 2). Press gently on the lid margin just below the lash line and determine if the orifices are stenosed or closed; then assess the thickness and clarity (clear, cloudy, opaque/white, opaque/yellow) of the oils. Look for any oil interference patterns on the surface of the tear film. At this point in the examination, you will know if large palpebral widths or meibomian gland dysfunction contributes to the patient's symptoms.

Next, wet a fluorescein strip with a drop of sterile irrigating solution. Shake the excess water off the strip, pull the patient's lower lid down, paint the strip across the inferior tarsal conjunctiva of both eyes, and have the patient blink. Shine the cobalt blue light on the tear film and look. In normal patients and in patients with early dry eye, the tear film fluoresces, shining a bright yellow. As a dry eye begins to lose tear volume, the nasal inferior marginal tear strip loses its fluorescence. Normally the tear film rapidly follows the raising of the upper lid after a blink, snapping up as the lid rises. In early dry eye, this tear film movement slows, and the film takes on a more viscous appearance. As the dry eye loses more tear volume, the entire tear film loses its fluorescence. Also, as eyes become drier, they develop floating debris in the tear film consisting of desquamated epithelial cells and dehydrated mucus. As surface disease becomes more advanced, dark spots reflective of corneal epithelial cell desquamation develop rapidly in the fluorescein film. On the eye surface, these dark spots have the appearance of cells without the surface specializations and glycoproteins necessary for binding the mucous layer.

In patients with meibomian gland dysfunction, the tear film takes on a more watery appearance. With the loss of the lipid layer, the tears splash around more with each blink.

Next, observe whether the ocular surface picked up any of the fluorescein dye. In early dry eye, there will be no staining. The nasal bulbar conjunctiva in the exposure zone stains first, followed by the temporal conjunctiva in the exposure zone and the inferior cornea. In pure dry eye (with no other concomitant diagnoses), the conjunctiva always stains more than the cornea. The most common staining pattern in meibomitis and the pattern seen in mild meibomitis is no stain at all. As the level of inflammation increases, staining of the superior and inferior bulbar conjunctiva is seen where the lid margins lie with eyes open. As the level of inflammation increases, the staining spills over and includes the cornea and conjunctiva in the exposure zones. In these patients, however, cornea and conjunctival staining are roughly equivalent. Typically, there will be some increased injection of the bulbar conjunctiva in these patients and a papillary reaction of the tarsal conjunctiva that can be observed on flipping the upper lid.

Two other functional points should be checked on examination when appropriate. The first is corneal sensation. When indicated by history, a cotton wisp can be used to test corneal sensation. The second is the functional closure of the lid. Check for lagophthalmos by having the patient gently close the lids; look for a space between the upper and lower lids. In patients who are symptomatic from lagophthalmos, a well-demarcated band of staining runs across the conjunctiva and cornea inferiorly and on a horizontal incline. These patients also typically have abnormal incomplete blinks with their eyes open.

At this point in the examination, you have determined if the patient has decreased tear production based on decreased tear volume, whether there is decreased corneal sensation, whether there are large palpebral fissure widths, and whether there is meibomian gland dysfunction. In other words, you know whether the patient has dry eye and, if so, why the patient has dry eye.

Treating dry eye

The most important goal in treating dry eye, whether the condition results from decreased tear production or increased tear film evaporation, is to lower elevated tear film osmolarity while addressing any concomitant inflammatory lid disease.

Artificial tears

For many years, until it was demonstrated that tear film osmolarity was elevated in dry eye, it was believed s that dry spots—physical drying on the surface of the cornea—caused dry eye. Because of this longstanding belief, most artificial tears are designed to cover only the cornea effectively. Certainly, the dry spots that develop late in the dry eye disease are not therapeutic, but they are a late change resulting from a prolonged and extended elevation of tear film osmolarity.

In 1985, experiments were performed to determine how hypotonic an artificial tear solution needed to be to lower elevated tear film osmolarity effectively [30]. The first artificial tear hypotonic enough to lower elevated tear film osmolarity is TheraTears (Advanced Vision Research, Woburn, MA). Continued treatment with this agent four times a day has been shown to produce a gradual, cumulative decline in elevated tear film osmolarity that is statistically significant at 8 weeks [31,32]. In addition, this agent has been shown to restore corneal glycogen levels and conjunctival goblet cells by decreasing elevated tear film osmolarity and by providing a patented electrolyte balance that precisely matches that found in the human tear film.

LASIK is a refractive procedure that decreases tear production by decreasing corneal sensation [33]. As such it serves as a good model for the group of dry eye cases in which dry eye is caused by conditions that decrease corneal sensation (diabetes, long-term hard contact lens wearing, herpes zoster, LASIK eye surgery, or any surgery that interrupts corneal nerves). In a masked study published in 1999, LASIK patients were divided into two groups, one treated with TheraTears postoperatively and the other treated with a preservative-free control. At 1 week after surgery 87.5% of the TheraTears-treated patients were symptom free, whereas only 12.5% of the control patients were symptom free. At 1 month after surgery 100% of the TheraTears-treated patients were symptom free, but only 20% in the control group were symptom free. In the same study, TheraTears was once again shown to restore conjunctival goblet cells in contrast to the control, which did not [34].

In patients with incomplete lid closure, a thicker artificial tear can be helpful. TheraTears Liquid Gel has been helpful in these patients. For patients with seriously impaired lid closure the additional use of a non-preserved lubricant eye ointment is also frequently helpful.

Omega-3 fatty acids

In 1998 Oxholm and co-workers [35] found that, in a population of patients with Sjögren's syndrome, the higher the level of dietary long-chain omega-3 fatty acids in the serum and cell membranes, the lesser the severity of dry eye. In 2003, Ceramak and co-workers [36] found that patients with Sjögren's syndrome had a significantly lower dietary intake of omega-3 fatty acids than did age-matched controls. Still more recently, Schaumberg's group [37] at the Harvard School of Public Health has studied more than 32,000 female health care professionals and has found that the higher the dietary intake of omega-3 fatty acids, the lower the risk of having clinically diagnosed dry eye from any cause. An open-label clinical trial by Boerner and associates [38] treated 116 patients with omega-3 supplementation and found that 98% of dry eye patients reported an improvement in their symptoms. TheraTears Nutrition for Dry Eyes (omega-3 supplement with fish oil, flaxseed oil, and vitamin E) is a formulation that provides pharmaceutical-grade short-chain and long-chain omega-3 fatty acids based on the summation of what is known today about omega-3 fatty acids and dry eye. Patients typically note an improvement in dry eye symptoms in 6 to 8 weeks.

Punctal occlusion

By lowering elevated tear film osmolarity, punctal occlusion decreases ocular surface staining and improves patient symptoms [39]. Punctal occlusion is not effective in restoring the conjunctival goblet cells that are lost in dry eye [40].

Punctal occlusion used to mean cauterizing the puncta. This procedure was painful, and the puncta frequently reopened and required recautery. For these reasons, punctal cautery has been replaced almost exclusively by the use of punctal plugs. These plugs, which come in a variety of shapes, sizes, and materials, are designed to be inserted either into the puncta with a cap exposed at the lid margin or into the canaliculus. Some canalicular plugs are absorbable, so the effect is temporary.

The advantage of the plugs with caps exposed at the lid margin is that one can tell that the plugs are still in place. It is also relatively easy to remove the plugs should the patient complain of tear overflow. These plugs have an extrusion rate of about 22% [39,40]. Canalicular plugs are generally more comfortable for the patient, but localization of the plug is more difficult, and it is more difficult to confirm that they are still in place.

Warm compresses

Warm compresses have long been recommended to patients with meibomitis to help reduce the inflammation in the eyelids. Recently, warm compresses have emerged as an adjunctive treatment for dry eye. The use of warm compresses on the lids for 5 minutes produces a temporary thickening of the oil layer of the tear film [41,42] and reduces tear film evaporation. The author recommends that dry eye patients use warm compresses once upon awakening in the morning and again in the mid-afternoon.

Lid hygiene

The use of dilute and gentle soaps to wash the eyelid margin has long been recommended for patients with anterior blepharitis—a dandruff-like process at the base of the eyelashes. Recently, research has shown that patients with dry eye have significantly higher bacterial colonization of the eyelids and conjunctiva. In addition, these bacteria decrease the proliferation of conjunctival goblet cells [43]. Lid hygiene is another adjunctive treatment for dry eye.

Humidifiers and moist chambers

The use of humidifiers and moist chambers is another way to reduce tear film evaporation. Humidifiers are practical primarily for patients who spend most of their time in one or two locations. Moist chambers have wider applicability, especially since the introduction of an easy-to-fit product call PanOptx DryEyeWear (PanOptx, Inc., Pleasanton, CA). These frames were developed by a maxillofacial surgeon, and three or four frames provide a virtually custom fit for most whites. Frames for persons of Asian and African-American heritage are reportedly under development.

A scleral lens made of a modern gas-permeable material is now available through the Boston Foundation for Sight and is an effective moist chamber [44]. These lenses are useful in desperate cases where there has been a failure to maintain corneal epithelial integrity using other means. Tarsorraphy is helpful in these desperate cases as well.

Tetracyclines

Many patients with dry eye also have meibomitis. Systemically administered tetracyclines are widely recognized for their ability to suppress the inflammation and improve the symptoms of meibomitis [45,46]. The dose is generally 50 mg doxycycline one time each day. For extremely obese patients, the dose may need to be increased to 100 mg/day. Recent research has shown that the long-term use of systemic tetracyclines is associated with an increasing risk of breast cancer in women based on the amount and

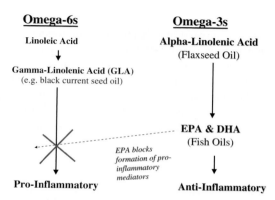

Fig. 3. Omega-3 fatty acids are anti-inflammatory. Omega-6 fatty acids are proinflammatory. Omega-3 fatty acids also block the inflammatory potential of omega-6 fatty acids.

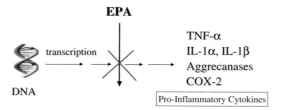

Fig. 4. Eicosapentaenoic acid blocks the gene transcription of the proinflammatory cytokines. COX, cyclo-oxygenase; EPA, eicosapentaenoic acid; IL, interleukin; TNF-α, tumor necrosing factor alpha.

duration of treatment [47]. For this reason, the author begins treatment of patients with mild to moderate meibomitis with TheraTears Nutrition alone, four soft gels in the morning. The omega-3 fatty acids in TheraTears Nutrition suppress inflammation throughout the body by generating anti-inflammatory eicosanoid acids and by blocking the gene expression of proinflammatory cytokines (Figs. 3 and 4). For patients with more severe meibomitis, the author starts treatment with doxycycline and TheraTears Nutrition at the same time. Once the symptoms are under control, the author has had great success stopping the doxycycline and continuing treatment with TheraTears Nutrition.

References

[1] Schaumberg DA, Sullivan DA, Buring JE, et al. Prevalence of dry eye syndrome among US women. Am J Ophthalmol 2003;136(2):318–26.
[2] Schein OD, Munoz B, Tielsch JM, et al. Prevalence of dry eye among the elderly. Am J Ophthalmol 1997;124(6):723–8.
[3] McCarty CA, Bansal AK, Livingston PM, et al. The epidemiology of dry eye in Melbourne, Australia. Ophthalmology 1998;105(6):1114–9.
[4] Dilly PN, Mackie IA. Surface changes in the anaesthetic conjunctiva in man, with special reference to the production of mucus from a non-goblet cell source. Br J Ophthalmol 1981; 65:833–42.
[5] Adams AD. The morphology of human conjunctival mucus. Arch Ophthalmol 1979;97: 730–4.
[6] Diebold Y, Rios JD, Hodges RR, et al. Presence of nerves and their receptors in mouse and human conjunctival goblet cells. Invest Ophthalmol Vis Sci 2001;42(10):2270–82.
[7] Warwick R. Ocular appendages. In: Wolff's anatomy of the eye and orbit. Philadelphia: WB Saunders; 1981. p. 181–237.
[8] Mishima S. Some physiological aspects of the precorneal tear film. Arch Ophthalmol 1965; 73:233–41.
[9] Botelho SY. Tears and the lacrimal gland. Sci Am 1964;211:78.
[10] Jordan A, Baum J. Basic tear flow. Does it exist? Ophthalmology 1980;87:920–30.
[11] Gilbard JP, Dartt DA, Rood RP, et al. Increased tear secretion in pancreatic cholera: a newly recognized symptom in an experiment of nature. Am J Med 1988;85:552–4.
[12] Gilbard JP, Farris RL, Santamaria J II. Osmolarity of tear microvolumes in keratocon-junctivitis sicca. Arch Ophthalmol 1978;96:677–81.

[13] Gilbard JP, Cohen GR, Baum J. Decreased tear osmolarity and absence of the inferior marginal tear strip following sleep. Trans Am Ophthalmol Soc 1991;89:209–14.

[14] Farris RL, Stuchell RN, Mandel ID. Tear osmolarity variation in the dry eye. Trans Am Ophthalmol Soc 1986;84:250–68.

[15] Gilbard JP, Dartt DA. Changes in rabbit lacrimal gland fluid osmolarity with flow rate. Invest Ophthalmol Vis Sci 1982;23:804–6.

[16] Iwata S, Lemp MA, Holly FJ, et al. Evaporation rate of water from the precorneal tear film and cornea in the rabbit. Invest Ophthalmol 1969;8:613–9.

[17] Begley CG, Chalmers RL, Abetz L, et al. The relationship between habitual patient-reported symptoms and clinical signs among patients with dry eye of varying severity. Invest Ophthalmol Vis Sci 2003;44(11):4753–61.

[18] Sjögren H. A new conception of keratoconjunctivitis sicca. Sydney (Australia): Australasian Medical Publishing; 1943. [Hamilton JB, Trans.] 1943.

[19] Abdel Khalek LMR, Williamson J, Lee WR. Morphological changes in the human conjunctival epithelium. II. In: Keratoconjunctivitis sicca. Br J Ophthalmol 1978;62: 800–6.

[20] Gilbard JP, Rossi S, Gray K. A new rabbit model for keratoconjunctivitis sicca. Invest Ophthalmol Vis Sci 1987;28:225–8.

[21] Luo L, Li DQ, Doshi A, et al. Experimental dry eye stimulates production of inflammatory cytokines and MMP-9 and activates MAPK signaling pasthways on the ocular surface. Invest Ophthalmol Vis Sci 2004;45(12):4293–301.

[22] Gilbard JP, Rossi SR, Gray KL, et al. Tear film osmolarity and ocular surface disease in two rabbit models for keratoconjunctivitis sicca. Invest Ophthalmol Vis Sci 1988;29(3):374–8.

[23] Calvillo MP, McLaren JW, Hodge DO, et al. Corneal reinnervation after LASIK: prospective 3-year longitudinal study. Invest Ophthalmol Vis Sci 2004;45(11):3991–6.

[24] Rolando M, Refojo MF. Tear evaporimeter for measuring water evaporation rate from the tear film under controlled conditions in humans. Exp Eye Res 1983;36(1):25–33.

[25] Fox SA. The palpebral fissure. Am J Ophthalmol 1966;62:73–8.

[26] Gilbard JP, Farris RL. Ocular surface drying and tear film osmolarity in thyroid eye disease. Acta Ophthalmol (Copenh) 1983;61:108–16.

[27] Gilbard JP, Rossi SR, Heyda KG. Tear film and ocular surface changes after closure of the meibomian gland orifices in the rabbit. Ophthalmology 1989;96(8):1180–6.

[28] Mathers WD, Shields WJ, Sachdev MS, et al. Meibomian gland dysfunction in chronic blepharitis. Cornea 1991;10(4):277–85.

[29] Mathers WD. Ocular evaporation in meibomian gland dysfunction and dry eye. Ophthalmology 1993;100(3):347–51.

[30] Gilbard JP, Kenyon KR. Tear diluents in the treatment of keratoconjunctivitis sicca. Ophthalmology 1985;92:646–50.

[31] Gilbard JP, Rossi SR, Gray Heyda K. Ophthalmic solutions, the ocular surface, and a unique therapeutic artificial tear formulation. Am J Ophthalmol 1989;107:348–55.

[32] Gilbard JP, Rossi SR. An electrolyte-based solution that increases corneal glycogen and conjunctival goblet cell density in a rabbit model for keratoconjunctivitis sicca. Ophthalmology 1992;99:600–4.

[33] Benitez-del-Castillo JM, del Rio T, Iradier T, et al. Decrease in tear secretion and corneal sensitivity after laser in situ keratomileusis. Cornea 2001;20(1):30–2.

[34] Lenton LM, Albietz JM. Effect of carmellose-based artificial tears on the ocular surface in eyes after laser in situ keratomileusis. J Refract Surg 1999;15(2 Suppl):S227–31.

[35] Oxholm P, Asmussen K, Wiik A, et al. Essential fatty acid status in cell membranes and plasma of patients with primary Sjögren's syndrome. Correlations to clinical and immunologic variables using a new model for classification and assessment of disease manifestations. Prostaglandins Leukot Essent Fatty Acids 1998;59(4):239–45.

[36] Ceramak JM, Papas AS, Sullivan RM, et al. Nutrient intake in women with primary and secondary Sjögren's syndrome. Eur J Clin Nutr 2003;57(2):328–34.

[37] Trivedi KA, Dana MR, Gilbard JP, et al. Dietary omega-3 fatty acid intake and risk of clinically diagnosed dry eye syndrome in women [abstract]. Fort Lauderdale, FL: Association for Research in Vision and Ophthalmology; May 3-8, 2003.

[38] Boerner CF. Dry eye successfully treated with oral flaxseed oil. Ocular Surgery News, October 15, 2000. p. 147–8.

[39] Gilbard JP, Rossi SR, Azar DT, et al. Effect of punctal occlusion by Freeman silicone plug insertion on tear osmolarity in dry eye disorders. CLAO J 1989;15:216–8.

[40] Willis RM, Folberg R, Krachmer JH, et al. The treatment of aqueous-deficient dry eye with removable punctal plugs. A clinical and impression-cytologic study. Ophthalmology 1987; 94(5):514–8.

[41] Olson MC, Korb DR, Greiner JV. Increase in tear film lipid layer thickness following treatment with warm compresses in patients with meibomian gland dysfunction. Eye Contact Lens 2003;29(2):96–9.

[42] Goto E, Monden Y, Takano Y, et al. Treatment of non-inflamed obstructive meibomian gland dysfunction by an infrared warm compression device. Br J Ophthalmol 2002;86(12): 1403–7.

[43] Graham JE, Moore JE, Xu J, et al. Analysis of bacterial flora in dry eye. The Ocular Surface 2005;3(1)S:S68.

[44] Schein OD, Rosenthal P, Ducharme C. A gas permeable scleral contact lens for visual rehabilitation. Am J Ophthalmol 1990;109:318–22.

[45] Browning DJ, Proia AD. Ocular rosacea. Surv Ophthalmol 1986;31:145–58.

[46] Esterly NB, Koransky JS, Furey NL, et al. Neutrophil chemotaxis in patients with acne receiving oral tetracycline therapy. Arch Dermatol 1984;120:1308.

[47] Velicer CM, Heckbert SR, Lampe JW, et al. Antibiotic use in relation to the risk of breast cancer. JAMA 2004;18;291(7):827–35.

ELSEVIER
SAUNDERS

Otolaryngol Clin N Am
38 (2005) 887–902

OTOLARYNGOLOGIC
CLINICS
OF NORTH AMERICA

Botulinum Toxin Management of Upper Facial Rhytidosis and Blepharospasm

Stuart R. Seiff, MD, FACS*, Orin M. Zwick, MD

*Department of Ophthalmic Plastic and Reconstructive Surgery,
University of California San Francisco, 400 Parnassus Avenue, Suite A-750,
San Francisco, CA 94131, USA*

Botulinum toxin is a neuromuscular blocking agent produced by *Clostridium botulinum* that has been proven to be an effective agent in the treatment of facial dystonia and upper facial rhytidosis. Since the original description of the toxin by Alan Scott [1] for strabismus 3 decades ago, the clinical use of this medication has expanded in an exponential fashion. Although the cosmetic benefits of botulinum toxin have become widely known, the full potential of this agent is yet to be realized. Its applications have grown to include treatment of a variety of disorders spanning many subspecialties including gastroenterology, pain management, otolaryngology, ophthalmology, dermatology, and neurology. Botulinum toxin is considered as a potential treatment in any situation involving inappropriate or exaggerated muscle contraction.

The Food and Drug Administration (FDA) approved the use of botulinum toxin (Botox; Allergan Pharmaceuticals, Inc, Irvine, CA) to treat blepharospasm and strabismus in 1989. In December 2000, approval was given to treat cervical dystonia, a neurologic movement disorder causing severe neck and shoulder contractions, in December 1989. In April 2002, the FDA announced the approval of botulinum toxin type A (Botox Cosmetic; Allergan) to improve temporarily the appearance of glabellar lines. The product's manufacturer has marketed botulinum toxin type A for this new indication, and the use of this product has skyrocketed. This article discusses the development of the use of botulinum toxin and then focuses on its benefits in treating facial dystonia and upper facial rhytidosis.

---
* Corresponding author.

E-mail address: seiff@itsa.ucsf.edu (S.R. Seiff).

0030-6665/05/$ - see front matter © 2005 Elsevier Inc. All rights reserved.
doi:10.1016/j.otc.2005.03.005   *oto.theclinics.com*

Botulinum toxin background

Pharmacology

Botulinum toxin paralyzes muscle by inhibiting the release of acetylcholine from the presynaptic nerve terminal of the neuromuscular junction [2]. Muscle weakness may not become evident for 2 to 4 days because of the continued spontaneous release of acetylcholine that is not blocked by the toxin [3]. The toxin occurs in eight immunologically distinct forms—A, B, C_1, C_2, D, E, F, and G—of which type A is the most potent [2]. Therefore, botulinum toxin type A has been used clinically, although types B and F are under study for alternate use. Type F may be a useful alternative for those rare patients who develop blocking antibodies to type A, but its usefulness is limited by its shorter duration of action and greater side effects [4].

Antibody production to botulinum toxin has been detected in humans treated for focal dystonia, blepharospasm, and hemifacial spasm (HFS) [5–7]. Antibody presence may explain the decrease in the effectiveness of botulinum toxin in some patients who have been injected repeatedly. In patients with focal dystonia, Jankovic and Schwartz [7] detected antibodies in 5 of the 14 poor responders (35.7%) and in none of the positive responders. Zuber and colleagues [6] found antibodies in 3 of 96 patients with focal dystonia, with no apparent clinical correlation between the antibodies and decreased botulinum toxin effectiveness. Siatkowski and coworkers [5] did not find a correlation between antibody production and length of treatment, number of injections, or total cumulative dose in patients with blepharospasm and HFS. The clinical effect of the botulinum toxin was not decreased by the presence of antibodies in the serum of 24 of 42 patients [5]. Although botulinum toxin antibodies have been detected, their absolute significance is uncertain.

Botulinum toxin potency, derived from a mouse assay, is measured in units. One unit of botulinum toxin is the quantity that kills 50% (LD_{50}) of a group of Swiss Webster mice [3]. The LD_{50} for monkeys after intramuscular injection of the botulinum toxin is approximately 40 units/kg [6]. The toxic dose for humans is estimated to be similar.

Storage

Commercially available botulinum toxin type A (Botox) comes in vials of 100 units in a lyophilized crystalline preparation. The botulinum toxin is reconstituted to the desired concentration with sterile normal saline just before use. Product labeling for botulinum toxin approved by the FDA recommends that the reconstituted toxin be used within 4 hours and that it not be shaken, because bubbles will cause surface denaturation of the toxin. The manufacturer recommends storing it immediately on receipt at $-5\,^{\circ}C$ or lower. Several studies have investigated the potency and duration of action of botulinum toxin with different lengths of storage [8–10]. Using a rabbit model, Jabor et al [11] evaluated the efficacy of freshly reconstituted and stored botulinum toxin A. They concluded that reconstituted and stored botulinum toxin A retains its initial potency, but the duration of action is affected at some time after 2 weeks of storage in a conventional freezer. Hexsel et al [12] found that botulinum toxin A may be applied up to 6 weeks after reconstitution without losing its effectiveness. The reconstituted vials were stored in a refrigerator at a constant temperature of 4°C. Although there was a concern about the risk of contamination during storage, Hexsel reported no microbiologic contamination in any of the samples analyzed. This information is valuable, because a significant amount of the drug must be discarded if only a small amount is used on a patient.

Anesthesia

Various studies have investigated methods to help reduce the pain of botulinum toxin injection. Topically applied anesthetics such as combined lidocaine 2.5% and prilocane 2.5% (EMLA Cream, Astra UAS, Inc., Westborough, MA) may be used before the injections. EMLA cream has been found to be an effective and safe method to improve comfort in patients who need repeated botulinum toxin for facial dyskinesia [13]. For it to work properly, however, injection should be delayed until approximately 45 minutes after the application of the cream, which limits efficiency in a busy practice. The use of EMLA is advisable for patients with low pain thresholds but is not necessary for all patients. Elamax 4% topical anesthetic (Ferndale Laboratories, Ferndale, MI) has also proven to be a useful nonprescription cream for patients to apply before injection to limit discomfort. Other methods that have been evaluated include using ice before injection and using preserved rather than nonpreserved saline to reconstitute the botulinum toxin. Both these methods have shown efficacy in decreasing the pain of injection [14]. Although the manufacturer recommends reconstitution with nonpreserved saline, the use of preserved saline seemed to have no effect on clinical outcome.

Botulinum toxin and facial spasm

Botulinum toxin has become the treatment of choice for patients with symptomatic facial spasms secondary to benign essential blepharospasm (BEB) and HFS. Although these disorders have different causes, they are grouped together because the treatment and response to the clinical symptoms are similar. The efficacy of treating BEB and HFS with botulinum toxin reached the highest evidence-based medicine degree in a recent critical evaluation [15]. This section describes the clinical features of BEB and HFS, followed by an explanation of the current modalities of treatment. The emphasis is on the use, side effects, duration, and success of botulinum toxin injection.

Benign essential blepharospasm

BEB is an adult-onset, focal dystonia characterized by repeated, involuntary, progressive contractions of the eyelids. This contraction is often so severe that the patient may become functionally blind. The spasms are typically bilateral and absent during sleep. Many patients have discovered "tricks" to get their eyes open, which may include drinking, singing, or pinching the neck [16]. Aside from the typical eyelid squeezing, BEB may be associated with dystonia of the lower face, jaw, and cervical muscles. Some believe that BEB is a forme fruste of the Meige syndrome, an orofacial cervical dystonia with spasms of the eyelids, eyebrows, lower face, mouth, lips, jaw, neck, or soft palate [16]. Approximately 20% of cases remain with isolated eyelid spasm; most present with or progress to more extensive facial dystonias [17]. The diagnosis of BEB is one of exclusion, and it is important to rule out processes of ocular surface irritation that could lead to a reflex blepharospasm. Neurodegenerative disorders, such as Parkinson's disease, Huntington disease, and Wilson's disease, may also cause blepharospasm [2]. The exact pathophysiology of BEB and the Meige syndrome is not clearly defined. Several studies support the hypothesis that BEB is caused by hyperexcitability of brainstem interneurons, as a result of organic dysfunction of the basal ganglia [18]. Blepharospasm is a vicious cycle of eyelid spasms and the facial malpositions caused by the blepharospasm. The eyelid malpositions result from the chronic forceful squeezing and in turn exacerbate the blepharospasm [17]. Patients who present with BEB do not require extensive etiological investigation because it is rarely caused by an identifiable condition.

Because the cause of BEB is unknown, therapy is directed at resolution of the symptoms. The major treatment modalities that have been used to control the symptoms include education and support, medications, surgery, and botulinum toxin injections.

All patients with BEB should be offered conservative treatment options. These include sunglasses to decrease photophobia, lid hygiene to decrease blepharitis, and artificial tears to relieve dry eyes. Patients can be referred to the Benign Essential Blepharospasm Research Foundation (BEBRF, www.blepharospasm.org), which organizes local support groups, distributes a newsletter, and supports research for the disorder. The information provided by the BEBRF, as well as familial and psychologic support, is important to help patients and families understand and manage this progressively debilitating disorder [17].

At present, drugs are used more often as an adjunctive therapy to botulinum toxin or myectomy than as a primary long-term treatment for eyelid spasms [17]. Among the many medications tried for the relief of BEB are clonazepam, tetrabenazine, baclofen, trihexyphenidyl hydrochloride, diphenylhydantoin, levodopa, haloperidol, deanol, amantadine hydrochloride, and meprobamate [16]. The degree and length of improvement with the use of medications has been limited. The medications directed at the central pathophysiology of BEB and facial dystonias are based on unproven pharmacologic hypotheses including cholinergic excess, γ–aminobutyric acid hypofunction, and dopamine excess [17]. Drug therapy directed to the control center of blepharospasm is not available. Pharmacotherapy is most commonly recommended for patients with severe spasm of the middle and lower face, which is difficult to treat with botulinum toxin [19].

Before the development of botulinum toxin, the only modalities for the treatment of blepharospasm were surgical, with the exception of systemic medications. Initially, neurectomy was the primary surgical treatment, but this procedure was technically difficult with a high risk of causing bilateral facial nerve palsies. Anderson [17] described the procedure known as "full myectomy" for BEB, which involves removal of virtually all of the orbicularis muscle, as well as the corrugator superciliaris and procerus muscles. The full myectomy is also a difficult and technically demanding operation, and results are directly related to the meticulous and complete removal of the squeezing muscles. With the successful use of botulinum toxin, the full myectomy is usually reserved for patients who refuse to use botulinum toxin or for whom botulinum treatment fails. A limited myectomy is a useful tool for patients who respond inadequately to botulinum toxin or have cosmetic and functional deformities associated with BEB [17]. A limited myectomy as an adjunct to botulinum toxin improves function and converts many failures to good responses. After limited myectomy, a decreased dosage of botulinum toxin is required, and greater portions of the botulinum toxin can be directed to the residual spasm [17].

Botulinum toxin is now the mainstay of treatment for blepharospasm. The original articles on its use in blepharospasm [16,20–22] proved the effectiveness of botulinum toxin with a duration of 3 months in nonoperated patients and 4 to 6 months in previously operated patients. As described, botulinum toxin temporarily blocks the motor end plate by preventing the release of acetylcholine. Through the motor end plate sprouting of new nerves, and possibly other mechanisms, the effect is overcome in about 3 months [23]. The duration of 4 to 6 months in patients who had a previous myectomy or neurectomy is similar to the duration of effect in patients with HFS. This phenomenon makes intuitive sense, because previously operated patients have an underlying muscle weakness similar to HFS. The serotype A is used. Muscle weakness starts 2 to 7 days after the injection, and relief lasts 3 months in 90% of BEB patients [24].

In injecting botulinum toxin, it is critical to place the toxin in the target muscle. In blepharospasm, the target muscles are the corrugator, procerus, and orbicularis oculi. Because the corrugator and procerus lie deep, the injection is given deep, just anterior to the periosteum. Because the orbicularis oculi is located just beneath the skin, the injection is given as a superficial, intradermal bleb, thereby avoiding the deeper levator palpebrae superioris and Muller's muscle. Injections are given at the medial and lateral portions of the upper eyelid to minimize the effect on the levator muscle and help prevent blepharoptosis. Additionally, an intradermal injection minimizes trauma to the underlying vascular orbicularis oculi muscle and decreases the incidence of hematoma and ecchymosis. Earlier studies showed that 1.25 units/0.1 cm^3 was not an effective dose. Although effective, doses between 2.5 and 5.0 units/0.1 cm^3 showed no difference in therapeutic effect. Injections into the pretarsal muscle have been shown to produce a significantly higher response and longer duration in both BEB and HFS patients [25]. For patients with Meige syndrome, other facial and neck muscles can be directly injected at a level consistent with the muscle targeted. Affected lower facial muscles are injected as necessary with 2.5 to 5 units of botulinum toxin. Injections of the toxin have been shown to be efficacious and safe over a 10-year period in one study [26].

Patients with BEB are treated bilaterally. Injections are given with a tuberculin syringe and a 30-gauge needle. The authors treat each eyelid with 12.5 units botulinum toxin, divided into 5 aliquots of 2.5 units each. Deep injections are given medial to the brow, and superficial blebs are raised at the lateral and medial aspects of the upper and lower eyelids. Nearly all patients develop weakness of the orbicularis muscle after injection. Loss of efficacy is most typically a result of disease progression rather than a true resistance to the toxin. To differentiate a loss of pharmacologic effect from disease progression, affected patients should be evaluated 2 to 3 weeks after initial botulinum toxin treatment and should be tested for weakness of the orbicularis. Patients who do not develop weakness after injection are good candidates for myectomy [19].

Hemifacial spasm

HFS is characterized by periodic, unilateral eyelid and facial spasms that may persist during sleep. There is a generalized facial weakness of the affected side underlying the spasms [27]. The disorder occurs in both men and women, although it more frequently affects middle-aged or elderly women. The initial symptom is usually an intermittent twitching of the eyelid muscle, which can lead to forced closure of the eye. The spasms may slowly progress to involve the muscles of the lower face and cause the mouth to be pulled to one side. Ultimately, the spasms may involve all of the muscles on one side of the face almost continuously. Causes of HFS include facial nerve trauma, tumor compression, or, most commonly, a pulsatile, vascular structure that compresses the seventh cranial nerve in the cerebellopontine angle. The most common blood vessels responsible for this compression are the anterior and posterior inferior cerebellar arteries and vertebral artery [19]. A surgical cure can often be attained through intracranial vascular decompression of the seventh nerve (Janetta procedure) [28].

Although neuroimaging is not a necessary step in the evaluation of BEB, it is an important tool in HFS. The imaging study of choice is MRI to evaluate the cerebellopontine angle and posterior fossa to rule out intracranial pathology causing compression of the seventh nerve. Although mass lesions are uncommon (incidence of approximately 1%), any patient with HFS whose general clinical course could justify intervention should be considered for imaging studies [29]. Imaging is definitely indicated in patients who present with other cranial neuropathies, progression of the spasms, or recurrence or increasing severity of disease.

The Hemifacial Spasm Association (www.hfs-assn.org) is an online support community that provides information, understanding, and support to individuals and families dealing with HFS. There is no role for pharmacologic management of HFS, because no medications have proven effective. Surgical modalities have been described previously and include vascular decompression if this cause is found on imaging. In addition, surgery can be performed for excision of a tumor compressing the seventh nerve and for traumatic decompression, if necessary.

Injection of botulinum toxin has become the procedure of choice for managing the symptoms of HFS. Patients with HFS are treated with botulinum toxin only on the affected side. The standard dosage of botulinum toxin for HFS is 2.5 to 5.0 units/0.1 cm^3, using an injection technique similar to that described for blepharospasm (Fig. 1). Because there is underlying weakness of the affected side of the face, overtreatment with botulinum toxin can precipitate a facial paralysis. Therefore, careful attention to dose and effect are necessary initially in these patients. Injections can also be given targeting the lower face and mimetic muscles, but results are variable. Overtreatment of the lower facial muscles may unmask a facial palsy, leading to difficulty with speech, drooling, and asymmetric facial animation. Patients with HFS experience a more prolonged symptom-free period, 4 to 6 months [16]. This duration of effect is similar to that seen in the original studies of blepharospasm patients who had undergone facial-weakening procedures [16].

Botulinum toxin injections have been accepted as a safe and effective treatment of both BEB and HFS. Complications of botulinum toxin treatment include ptosis, blurred vision, diplopia, and other minor side effects that usually improve in days to weeks. Effectiveness and side effects may be influenced by the location of the injection sites around the orbicularis [18]. The most common side effect of the injections is bruising. Toxin spreading to the levator muscle can cause ptosis. This effect can be avoided by injecting anteriorly in an intradermal fashion and sparing the central portion of the eyelid. Other side effects are corneal exposure, lagophthalmos, ectropion, entropion, epiphora, photophobia, diplopia, and lower facial weakness. Allergies to the drug, infection in the injection site, uncooperative patients, coagulopathies, myasthenia gravis, and pregnancy and breastfeeding are relative contraindications to botulinum toxin.

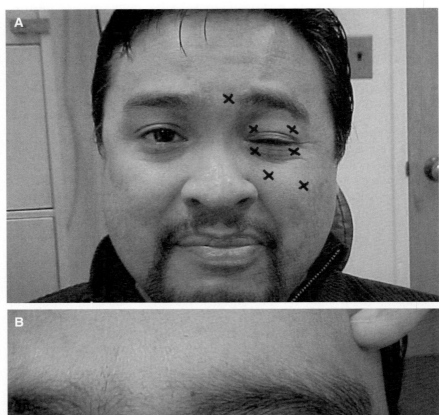

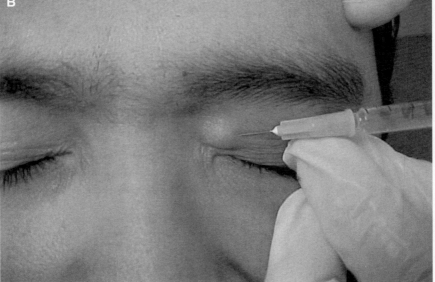

Fig. 1. (*A*) Botulinum toxin injection sites (*x*) in a patient with hemifacial spasm. (*B*) The superficial, intradermal bleb ideal for the orbicularis oculi muscle injections.

Botulinum toxin and facial rhytidosis

In the early 1990s, Alistair and Jean Carruthers began using botulinum toxin to treat facial rhytids after their blepharospasm patients joked that they were "back to get the wrinkles out" when they returned for re-treatment [30]. The use of botulinum toxin, as a primary procedure or as an adjunct to other procedures, has revolutionized cosmetic treatment of facial hyoids. The FDA approved the use of botulinum toxin for managing glabellar wrinkles in 2002, but its cosmetic use has expanded to manage forehead wrinkles, crow's feet, and perioral wrinkles successfully.

Cosmetic background

Skin changes associated with the aging face may be classified broadly into two types: wrinkles and lines [31]. Wrinkles consist of many multidirectional superficial indentations of the skin. Lines are single distinct depressions of the skin and may be classified further as creases and furrows. Creases are shallow lines that extend into the dermis, whereas furrows are deeper, more pronounced lines that extend into the subcutaneous tissues. Many factors are responsible for these skin changes, including aging and actinic damage that result in break down of dermal collagen. Facial movement, gravity, and sleep positions are additional factors that contribute to involutional skin changes. Lines induced by facial expression arise perpendicular to the direction of action of contracting facial muscles. Crow's feet, creases in the lateral periorbital region, are produced by the repeated contraction of the orbicularis oculi muscle. Forehead creases or furrows are created by contraction of the frontalis muscle, and glabellar frown lines by contraction of the corrugator superciliaris and procerus muscles.

Aesthetic techniques used to decrease the appearance of wrinkles and lines include chemical peels, carbon dioxide laser resurfacing, fillers, hyaluronic acid gel, and surgical procedures such as rhytidectomy, eyebrow lift, and blepharoplasty. Chemical peels and laser resurfacing are more beneficial for the treatment of wrinkles than of lines. Fillers may be used to smooth creases and furrows. Botulinum toxin injections, unlike other methods used to treat the deep lines of facial expression, address the cause of the creases and furrows: the contraction of the underlying muscles. With this minimally invasive and rapid procedure, the injected muscles are weakened, thus smoothing the overlying skin and minimizing the appearance of the deep lines of the upper face [32].

Treatment of facial rhytidosis

Glabellar lines, also called frown lines, occur because of contraction of the corrugator superciliaris and procerus muscles [33]. The paired corrugator muscles arise from the superomedial orbital rim and insert laterally and superiorly into skin and muscle of the medial eyebrow. The corrugator muscles contract when a person frowns, and this contraction pulls the medial eyebrow inward and downward, producing vertical lines in the skin of the glabellar region. The procerus muscle is a continuation of the frontalis muscle into the midline glabellar region. Its vertically oriented fibers originate from the nasal bone and interdigitate with the frontalis muscle. Contraction of the procerus muscle moves the medial brow downward and generates horizontal lines in the overlying skin. Injection of botulinum toxin into the corrugator muscle smoothes the vertical frown lines, whereas injection into the procerus improves the horizontal creases [32]. The location of the injections should be modified for each patient. Foster and colleages [34] studied botulinum toxin injection of the glabellar region and found objective improvement of the glabellar lines at rest in 6 of 11 patients and similar improvement with attempted muscle contraction in all 11 patients. A multicenter, double-blind, randomized, placebo-controlled study demonstrated that botulinum toxin A is effective in reducing the severity of glabellar lines [33]. The orbicularis oculi muscle, organized in an elliptical pattern, has pretarsal, preseptal, and orbital portions. Contraction of the pretarsal and preseptal orbicularis muscle, which overlies the upper- and lower-eyelid tarsi and orbital septum, results in eyelid closure and blinking. The orbital section of the muscle is involved in facial expression and forced eyelid closure. Squinting or smiling, associated with contraction of the orbital orbicularis, produces deep lines or crow's feet in the lateral periorbital region. Minimal subcutaneous tissue exists between the skin and underlying orbicularis muscle. Keen and associates [35] reported 11 patients injected with botulinum toxin or saline in a double-blind, placebo-controlled study for forehead lines and crow's feet. Of the 11 subjects, 9 experienced significant improvement, and 2 had moderate improvement in severity of facial lines. In a bilateral, double-blind, randomized study, Lowe and associates [36] demonstrated that botulinum toxin A is a safe and effective treatment for crow's feet with high patient satisfaction and occasional mild side effects.

The frontalis muscle arises from within the galea aponeurotica, interdigitates with the orbital orbicularis muscle, and inserts into the skin of the eyebrow. With contraction of the frontalis muscle, the eyebrows are raised, and horizontal forehead lines are created. Weakening the frontalis muscle with botulinum toxin, especially close to the eyebrow, may cause eyebrow ptosis. In contrast, the medial brow may lift slightly after the corrugator and procerus muscles are injected, because of the relatively unopposed action of the frontalis muscle. Particular attention must be paid to the position and nature of the eyebrows and eyelids in patients with forehead lines. If a patient has underlying blepharoptosis or excessive dermatochalasis, the consistently contracted frontalis muscle may be elevating the eyelid margin or redundant upper-eyelid tissue to clear the visual axis. If deep forehead lines are treated with botulinum toxin, the frontalis muscle will relax, which could exacerbate the ptosis or the apparent amount of excess upper-eyelid tissue.

Injection

Immediately before the procedure, the lyophilized botulinum toxin can be reconstituted in a variety of concentrations. Concentrations typically used for blepharospasm (2.5–5 units/0.1 cm^3) are quite effective for aesthetic purposes. The patient is asked to frown, squint, or smile so that the overacting muscle can be visualized beneath the deep lines. Use of a 30-gauge needle minimizes patient discomfort and bruising. The location and depth of the injections depend on the facial region to be treated. The corrugator and procerus muscles can be identified when the patient frowns. With contraction, the muscles shorten and become more prominent. Two intramuscular injections for each corrugator muscle and one midline procerus injection are suggested to relax these muscles (Fig. 2). The first corrugator injection should be at the superomedial aspect of the eyebrow, and the second should be just lateral to it, along the superior aspect of the brow. Because these muscles are deep in the scalp flap, the injection is given just anterior to the periosteum to achieve maximum effect. The dose may need to be adjusted for the specific patient and the degree of overaction [32].

For crow's feet, the lateral orbicularis oculi muscle is weakened with a superficial, intradermal bleb of botulinum toxin. The injections are placed adjacent to the deep lines, after the patient has squinted to allow better localization of the portion of the muscle to be treated (Fig. 3). The authors administer two or three injections to each side, so that 5.0 to 7.5 units of botulinum toxin are evenly spaced over the lateral orbital rims.

Forehead furrows require careful injection of the frontalis muscle to avoid significant brow ptosis. The injections should be spaced evenly and symmetrically over the upper forehead. The region of the insertion of the frontalis muscle near the brows should be avoided. Titration of the dose may be necessary to achieve the desired affect.

Patients must understand that botulinum toxin is not a line filler. Its effect depends on a lack of muscle movement so the overlying skin does not have to fold, allowing the line to relax and become less evident. Therefore, some improvement in dynamic facial lines will be noted relatively quickly after muscle paralysis occurs. Deep, static lines take several months to improve. The authors suggest a dose of 2.5 units/0.1 mL at each site, making injections as close as possible to the target muscle. This dose, the same as used to treat blepharospasm and HFS, gives excellent cosmetic efficacy and duration. Patients must understand that the onset of muscle weakening occurs 2 to 7 days after injection. After the first injection, the patient is instructed to return for follow-up re-injection in 3 months, whether movement has returned or not. The patient returns again 3 months later, to allow 6 total months for the creases to soften. If there is still a crease after 6

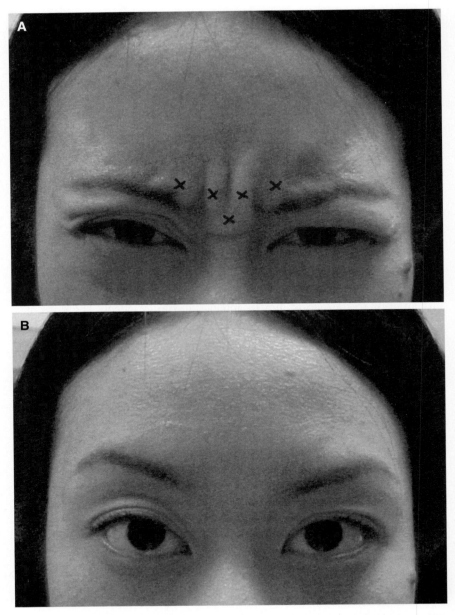

Fig. 2. (A) Glabellar lines demonstrated by frowning, with identification of the overactive corrugator and procerus muscles. Note the botulinum injection sites (x) target the muscles, not the lines. (B) Marked limitation of corrugator and procerus muscles on attempted frowning 5 days after botulinum toxin injection.

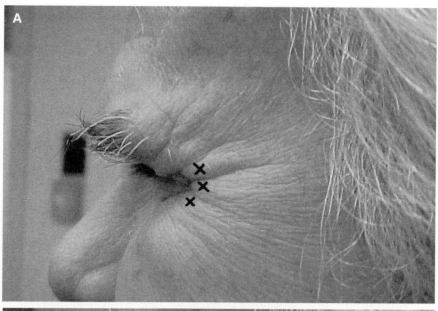

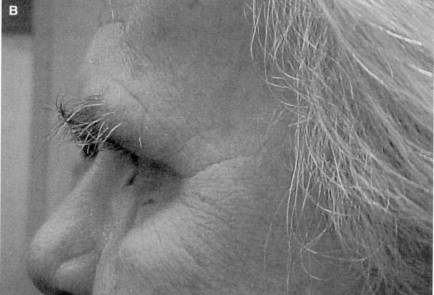

Fig. 3. (*A*) Crow's feet demonstated by squinting, with botulinum injection sites marked with an *x*. (*B*) Limited movement on attempted squinting with decrease in lines 5 days after injection. For the crow's feet to disappear completely, the affected area should be completely paralyzed for at least 6 months.

months, a filler can be injected into the affected areas. After 6 months, the patient is instructed to return for repeat injections before the complete return of muscle function, to enhance the smoothing effect of the botulinum toxin on the overlying skin. Part of the art of botulinum injection is to weaken the muscles of facial expression enough to smooth the overlying skin while still preserving facial animation. Titration of the dose for the individual patient is essential. The effect of botulinum toxin injections lasts from 3 to 6 months, depending on the degree of muscle weakening. It is emphasized to patients that botulinum toxin is most useful for dynamic lines and works by paralyzing the muscle that causes the repetitive folding of skin. The deeper, static lines are better treated with fillers.

Adverse effects

Adverse effects of botulinum toxin injections are few. Most commonly, local bruising or hematoma formation may occur at the injection site. Blepharoptosis has been observed after injection of the glabellar region [36,37]. Injections performed at the proper location and depth should minimize this occurrence. If the crow's feet are overtreated with botulinum toxin, paralysis of the orbicularis oculi muscle may result in an inability to close the eye completely. As with the corrugator region, if the injections are not placed properly or if diffusion of the botulinum toxin occurs, ptosis or even diplopia could occur [8]. Frontalis muscle weakness may cause eyebrow ptosis of varying degrees. If a patient has preexisting blepharoptosis or visually significant dermatochalasis of the upper eyelids, even subtle brow ptosis may create a problem.

In addition, a full medical history, including allergies and current medications, should be obtained. Patients with known allergies to botulinum toxin or albumin should not be injected, because the solution before lyophilization contains human serum albumin. Additional contraindications to botulinum toxin injections include pregnancy or neuromuscular disorders such as myasthenia gravis.

Summary

The injection of botulinum toxin is a nonsurgical technique that interferes minimally with a patient's daily life. The botulinum toxins have revolutionized the treatment of patients with BEB, HFS, and other facial dystonias. The success rate has been reported to be greater than 90% [26]. Patient acceptance of the injections is high. Patients with BEB are typically injected every 3 to 4 months, whereas those with HFS have injections every 4 to 6 months.

Botulinum toxin treatment of deep lines of facial expression is an effective, rapid, relatively painless office procedure. Many investigators have demonstrated positive results in decreasing glabellar lines, crow's feet, and forehead lines. The procedure itself has an excellent safety profile and takes minutes. The patient may resume daily activity immediately after the treatment. Other than the possibility of a small hematoma at the injection site, the patient's appearance is practically unchanged immediately after the injections. These benefits are significant advantages in today's society.

References

[1] Scott AB. Botulinum toxin injection into extraocular muscles as an alternative to strabismus surgery. Ophthalmology 1980;87:1044–9.

[2] Simpson LL. The origin, structure, and pharmacological activity of botulinum toxin. Pharmacol Rev 1981;33:155–88.

[3] Greene P, Kang U, Fahn S, et al. Double-blind placebo-controlled trial of botulinum injections in the treatment of spasmodic torticollis. Neurology 1990;40:1213–8.

[4] Mezaki T, Kaji R, Nohora N, et al. Comparison of therapeutic efficacies of type A and F botulinum toxins for blepharospasm: a double-blind, controlled study. Neurology 1995;45: 506–8.

[5] Siatkowski RM, Tyutyunikov A, Biglan AW, et al. Serum antibody production to botulinum A toxin. Ophthalmology 1993;100:1861–6.

[6] Zuber M, Sebald M, Bathien N, et al. Botulinum antibodies in dystonic patients treated with type A botulinum toxin: frequency and significance. Neurology 1993;43:1715–8.

[7] Jankovic J, Schwartz K, Donovan DT. Botulinum toxin treatment of cranial-cervical dystonia, spasmodic dysphonia, other focal dystonias and hemifacial spasm. J Neurol Neurosurg Psychiatry 1990;53:633–9.

[8] Gartlan MG, Hoffman HT. Crystalline preparation of botulinum toxin type A (Botox): degradation in potency with storage. Otolarygol Head Neck Surg 1993;108:135.

[9] Garcia A, Fulton JE. Cosmetic denervation of the muscles of facial expression with botulinum toxin. Dermatol Surg 1996;22:39.

[10] Sloop RR, Cole BA, Escutin RO. Reconstituted botulinum toxin type A does not lose potency in humans if it is refrozen or refrigerated for 2 weeks before use. Neurology 1997;48:149.

[11] Jabor MA, Kaushik R, Shayani P, et al. Efficacy of reconstituted and stored botulinum toxin type A: an electrophysiologic and visual study in the auricular muscle of the rabbit. Plast Reconst Surg 2003;111:2419–26.

[12] Hexsel DM, Almeida AT, Rutowitsch M, et al. Multicenter, double-blind study of the efficacy of injections with botulinum toxin type a reconstituted up to six consecutive weeks before application. Dermatol Surg 2003;29:523–9.

[13] Soylev MF, Kocak N, Kuvaki B, et al. Anesthesia with EMLA cream for botulinum A toxin injection into eyelids. Ophthalmologica 2002;216:355–8.

[14] Kwiat DM, Bersani TA, Bersani A. Increased patient comfort utilizing botulinum toxin type a reconstituted with preserved versus nonpreserved saline. Ophthal Plast Reconstr Surg 2004;20:186–9.

[15] Jost WH, Kohl A. Botulinum toxin: evidence based medicine criteria in blepharospasm and hemifacial spasm. J Neurol 2001;248(Suppl 1):21–4.

[16] Shorr N, Seiff SR, Kopelman J. The use of botulinum toxin in blepharospasm. Am J Ophthalmol 1985;99:542–6.

[17] Anderson RL, Patel BC, Holds JB, et al. Blepharospasm: past, present and future. Ophthal Plast Reconstr Surg 1998;14:305–17.

[18] Frueh BR, Musch DC. Treatment of facial spasm with botulinum toxin: an interim report. Ophthalmology 1986;93:917–23.

[19] McCann JD, Ugurbas SH, Goldberg RA. Benign essential blepharospasm. Int Ophthalmol Clin 2002;42:113–21.

[20] Freuh BR, Felt DP, Wojno TH, et al. Treatment of blepharospasm with botulinum toxin: a preliminary report. Arch Ophthalmol 1984;102:1464–8.

[21] Scott AB, Kennedy EG, Stubbs HA. Botulinum A toxin injection as a treatment for blepharospasm. Arch Ophthalmol 1985;103:347–50.

[22] Tsoy EA, Buckley EG, Dutton JJ. Treatment of blepharospasm with botulinum toxin. Am J Ophthalmol 1985;99:176–9.

[23] Holds JD, Alderson K, Fogg SG, et al. Motor nerve sprouting in human orbicularis muscle after botulinum A injection. Invest Ophthalmol Vis Sci 1990;31:964–7.

[24] Dutton JJ, Buckley EG. Long-term results and complications of botulinum A toxin in the treatment of blepharospasm. Ophthalmology 1988;95:1529–34.

[25] Cakmur R, Ozturk V, Uzunel F, et al. Comparison of preseptal and pretarsal injections of botulinum toxin in the treatment of blepharospasm and hemifacial spasm. J Neurol 2002; 249:64–8.

[26] Defazio G, Abbruzzese G, Girlanda P, et al. Botulinum toxin A treatment for primary hemifacial spasm: a ten year multicenter study. Arch Neurol 2002;59:418–20.

[27] Auger RG. Hemifacial spasm. Clinical and electrophysiologic observations. Neurology 1979;29:1261.

[28] Janetta PJ, Abbasy M, Maroon JC, et al. Etiology and definitive microsurgical treatment of hemifacial spasm. J Neurosurg 1977;47:321.

[29] Sprik C, Wirtschafter JD. Hemifacial spasm due to intracranial tumor. An international survey of botulinum toxin investigators. Ophthalmology 1988;95:1042–5.

[30] Scott AB. Development of botulinum toxin therapy. Dermatol Clin 2004;22:131–3.

[31] Stegman SJ, Tromovitch TA, Glogau RG. Cosmetic dermatologic surgery. Chicago: Year Book Medical Publishers; 1990. p. 5–15.

[32] Carter SR, Seiff SR. Cosmetic botulinum toxin injections. Int Ophthalmol Clin 1997;37: 69–79.

[33] Carruthers JA, Lowe NJ, Menter MA, et al. A multicenter, double-blind, randomized, placebo-controlled study of the efficacy and safety of botulinum toxin type A in the treatment of glabellar lines. J Am Acad Dermatol 2002;46:840–9.

[34] Foster JA, Barnhorst D, Papay F, et al. The use of botulinum A toxin to ameliorate facial kinetic frown lines. Ophthalmology 1996;103:618–22.

[35] Keen M, Blitzer A, Aviv J, et al. Botulinum toxin A for hyperkinetic facial lines: results of a double-blind, placebo controlled study. Plast Reconst Surg 1994;94:94–9.

[36] Lowe NJ, Lask G, Yamauchi P, et al. Bilateral, double-blind, randomized comparison of 3 doses of botulinum toxin type A and placebo in patients with crow's feet. J Am Acad Dermatol 2002;47:834–40.

[37] Guyuron B, Huddleston SW. Aesthetic indications for botulinum toxin injection. Plast Reconstr Surg 1994;93:913–8.

ELSEVIER
SAUNDERS

Otolaryngol Clin N Am
38 (2005) 903–919

OTOLARYNGOLOGIC
CLINICS
OF NORTH AMERICA

Current Techniques of Entropion and Ectropion Correction

Ira Eliasoph, MD, FACS[a,b,c,d,e,f,*]

[a]Department of Ophthalmology, Mount Sinai School of Medicine,
New York, NY, USA
[b]Veterans Hospital, Bronx, NY, USA
[c]Beth Israel Hospital, New York, NY, USA
[d]Jewish Home and Hospital, Bronx, NY, USA
[e]Manhattan Eye, Ear, and Throat Hospital, Manhattan, NY, USA
[f]Mount Sinai Hospital, New York, NY, USA

Writing about entropion and ectropion gives one the opportunity to discuss the "ins and outs" of eyelid surgery. These two conditions are tied together insofar as the same anatomic structures are involved and certain pathophysiology is shared. Constant awareness of the eye itself guides our plans and their execution. Although cosmetic benefits result from most eyelid operations, correction of these specific defects is for restoration of the function of the lids as protectors of the eye. Some of the anatomy and physiology is reviewed as pertains to these conditions and their origin and repair. The major coverage is for the adult and aged patient and for situations that facial plastic surgeons encounter rather than rare cases handled by experienced oculoplastic specialists. The history of operations for these conditions includes time-honored names in the field, including the ancient writers Hippocrates, Susruta, and Celsus as well as Adams [1], Arlt, Arruga, Blaskovics, Elschnig, Fox, Gaillard, von Graefe [2], Hotz, Hughes, Jones, Kirby, Kuhnt, Meek, Snellen, Spaeth, Stallard, Streatfeild, Weeks, Wheeler, and Ziegler. This list reveals a fraction of the interest and efforts that have been put into solutions for these common disorders.

Some pertinent points follow. The relation between the skin and orbicularis layer and the layer of tarsus and conjunctiva shifts with aging. There is less tight adherence, along with general laxity of connective tissue elements. It has been clearly demonstrated that the lateral canthal tendon elongates as we grow older. This is readily understood if one places

* 133 East 73rd Street, New York, NY 10021.
  E-mail address: eyedoctor21@mac.com

0030-6665/05/$ - see front matter © 2005 Elsevier Inc. All rights reserved.
doi:10.1016/j.otc.2005.05.003   *oto.theclinics.com*

a fingertip lightly on the skin at the lateral canthus and then forcefully closes the eye. There is a discernible pull toward the nose, which, repeated over decades, stretches the attachments. The canthus drifts forward and down [3,4], and the lid margin is no longer snug against the globe (Fig. 1). This allows the hammock of the lower lid to turn in or out, depending on the laxity of the lower lid retractors and the downward pull of the lower lid-cheek complex (Fig. 2). With older individuals, loss of orbital fat results in some enophthalmos, which may favor the development of entropion. The possible role of diminished corneal sensation is not clear. The loss of facial animation in Parkinson's disease aggravates surface dryness problems. In contrast, with marked rapid weight loss and thinning of the cheek fat pad, ectropion has been reported as a consequence.

Anyone operating on the lower eyelid should be aware of how slight a bit of traction draws the lid margin down and of the serious consequences of this deformity. An average palpebral fissure is approximately 25 mm wide and presents an area of approximately 125 mm^2 to the air. Dropping the lower lid margin by 1 mm increases the area by 25 mm^2 (or approximately 20%). This not only increases evaporation but shifts the tear meniscus so that the upper lid may not dip into it and thus not spread the tear film, particularly the lipid secretion from the Meibomian glands, over the eye surface. It is evident that a patient undergoing lower lid blepharoplasty, who does not have dry eye symptoms before surgery, should not be symptomatic after surgery, regardless of the Schirmer test results. If the level of the outer canthus relative to the medial is lower and any hint of scleral show is

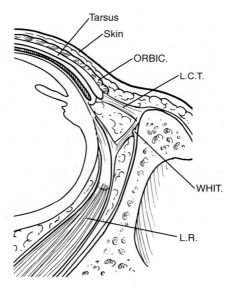

Fig. 1. Lateral orbit, canthal tendon emphasized.

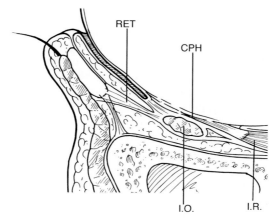

Fig. 2. Lower lid cross section, retractors emphasized.

present, these are danger signals. By gently pulling on the lower lid and observing the return to its initial position, laxity is easily revealed and steps are planned to keep this from becoming a complication.

Examination of the face starts with a general view in regard to the overall appearance, symmetry, and blemishes. The eyelids, brows, cheeks, and their condition are examined. The eyelids are evaluated, and pathologic findings like entropion and ectropion are carefully noted. The patient's complaints and history are essential to determine what steps are appropriate for therapy. Proper medical evaluation, cessation of use of aspirin and similar agents that may promote bleeding, photographs, and chart notations of the pathologic findings are all seen to before surgery.

Entropion

There are several subdivisions of entropion, which is an abnormal inward rotation of the eyelid. Congenital entropion is rare and may really be epiblepharon or excess of the skin and orbicularis overlying and inverting the margin. Entropion may occur after trauma and scar contraction or after surgery, particularly on the inner lamina of the lid, with shortage of tissue. Long-term use of medications, such as some for glaucoma, may produce tissue shrinkage and entropion (and punctal stenosis). This may happen with enucleation and shortage of conjunctiva.

In many parts of the world, trachoma is still endemic; the upper lid is usually involved and curls in, with fibrosis and contraction. This is a problem of serious interest to the World Health Organization and charity groups of international scope. More than 5 million people are blind, or near blind, from trachoma. On the Internet, there are more than 30,000 items that appear in response to a "trachoma/surgery" inquiry. Thousands of operations are performed each year, for example, in Vietnam and Tanzania [5,6]. In my own experience as a Navy medical officer, the donation of a bottle of tetracycline to the port doctor, to be used for trachoma treatment, ensured our swift passage through the Egyptian control station of the Suez Canal. For many decades, the United States Immigration Service officers were the experts on trachoma. Crowded conditions and poor hygiene in parts of Europe made for transmission of trachoma to many people. It was a reason for exclusion from the United States.

In this part of the world, we see lower lid entropion frequently. The condition is usually symptomatic, with eye discomfort to the point of pain, tearing, photophobia, discharge, secondary infection, and varying degrees of corneal surface breakdown (with visual loss). Occasionally, the lid is inverted so much that the lashes are tucked down into the fornix, but the eye is not particularly uncomfortable. Frequent use of lubricating eye ointment as well as taping the lid into a relatively normal position may serve as effective temporary palliation.

The pathophysiology has been commented on for centuries, and so have surgical procedures. There are three changes that must be assessed in each case. The first is thinning out and weakening of the pull of the lower lid retractors (see Fig. 2). The second is the elongation and stretching of the lateral canthal tendon. The third component is the shift and contraction of the pretarsal orbicularis muscle toward the margin of the lid.

Examination of the lid and manipulating it with a cotton-tipped applicator or fingertip demonstrates the changes as well as what may be needed surgically. When the condition is intermittent, asking the patient to close the eyes forcefully brings out the problem and the need for correction. Pressing at the level of the inferior orbital rim may evert the margin easily and leave the margin in proper apposition to the globe at the lower limbus. This may indicate that only rotation is needed. If the lid margin and the lateral canthus are displaced down and medially, laxity of the tendon needs to be addressed. The lateral canthus should be slightly above the medial to provide a low slope toward the nose and the lacrimal drainage system. A rounded and thickened margin may require resection and realignment of a band of orbicularis muscle, and possibly of skin. There are features in common with what has been termed *reverse ptosis* of the lower lid [7]. This failure of the lower lid to retract on downgaze causes obstruction of vision and needs restoration of the function of the retractors. With entropion, the patient should be instructed to look down, and movement of the lid should be observed to assess retractor function.

For an unimaginable time, entropion was treated by many reputable surgeons with a double line of hot cautery burns into the lid. This "Ziegler" cautery procedure was done by my chief when I started my residency [8]. I can remember vividly the hissing sound, the steam and smoke, and the smell of burning flesh. I was dismayed that what I envisioned as a field of precise and exacting surgery involved this crude and barbaric assault. The fact that the procedure often worked was based on the fibrous adhesions achieved between the skin and the lower lid retractors.

Trichiasis, or misdirected eyelashes, is treated by simple epilation, microelectrolysis, laser ablation, cryosurgery, and, sometimes, surgical excision. Microelectrolysis is generally the best alternative and is easily done, with minimal local anesthesia and a small electrosurgical unit, at the slitlamp microscope. Epilation is prone to regrowth. Cryosurgery produces a lot of tissue reaction. Laser ablation poses extra risk to the eye and the lid margin. Surgical excision is usually performed in posttrauma cases with some distortion of the lid margin, which requires repair.

Upper lid entropion

Upper lid entropion with cicatricial changes can be helped by a marginal rotation procedure. The Wies procedure involves making an incision through the full thickness of the lid, approximately 3 mm from the lash line and extending from just lateral to the punctum to the end of the tarsus [9]. After careful hemostasis is accomplished, sutures are placed to bring the skin edge on the marginal side of the incision to the conjunctival edge on the main lid side of the cut. This turns the margin and lashes away from the globe and eliminates the source of the irritation. The bare area on the inner side of the lid epithelializes after a short time. Several variations of this operation are used in different parts of the world.

A marginal rotation of the tarsus can be done with lesser rotation by making a skin incision 2 mm from the lashes. A wedge of tarsus can be cut out through this incision along the length of the tarsus, and the gap so formed can be sutured closed, with outward turning of the margin. The skin can then be closed, often with excision of a long thin band of skin to enhance the effect.

In cases in which the skin and some orbicularis muscle have migrated over the lashes and turned them in, skin and orbicularis removal, with sutures to the tarsus further from the lid margin, can correct the defect. This procedure and the prior technique can be combined with an upper lid blepharoplasty or ptosis correction.

Lower lid entropion

This extremely common deformity has been the source of an endless parade of operative procedures. There is hardly a name known in the fields of ophthalmology and plastic surgery without an article and procedure attached. Fine strips of bamboo or other materials have been stitched to the surface to turn the lid outward. Cautery, as referred to previously, was used for centuries. In a more humane and rational time, some suture methods have been proposed. The method developed by Feldstein [10,11] is based on the pathophysiology and was designed to do what that percentage of successful cauteries did, namely, to bring the lower lid retractors back into play. Other procedures place sutures obliquely through the lid and may provide some improvement; however, the improvement is not adequate in most cases, with less probability of lasting effect.

Correction of congenital entropion, or epiblepharon, is treated with sutures as in the Feldstein procedure [10,11] or supplemented by excision of a spindle-shaped segment of skin and orbicularis muscle as determined by the pinch technique.

Entropion surgery

Feldstein suture procedure

After appropriate local and topical anesthesia is given, sutures of 4-0 chromic are placed; as they are absorbed by the body, they leave a track of fibroblasts that contract and produce an adhesion. The needle is introduced downward into the inferior conjunctival fornix and inserted to catch the retractor tissue. The needle is then rotated so that the point passes up through the lid to exit the skin just below the level of the lower tarsal border. The second arm is passed a couple of millimeters to the side of the first and exits the skin similarly spaced from the first. The suture is tied firmly on the skin, dimpling the surface, and the ends are cut off. Three such sutures are usually required, but, on occasion, two may suffice. The lid should be slightly everted at the end of the procedure. No dressing or ointment is required. The suture knots fall away in a few days, and in a month, no external sign of the operation usually remains.

The Feldstein suture method is used widely even in veterinary surgery [12] but is usually attributed to Quickert and Rathbun [13]. Feldstein's method was published much earlier. Quickert subsequently stated that the procedure as described by Feldstein was better than the technique he had reported. In seeking simplicity, this is certainly achieved. No dissection is needed, and no tissue is excised. The result can last for many years, but other more elaborate operations also have recurrences. This operation may be done at the bedside in debilitated patients and can easily be repeated if necessary. The elaborate operations make repeat correction much more difficult. In myasthenia gravis, there may be total failure of the retractor fibers comparable to loss of levator function. Surgical correction thus cannot rely on the retractors.

Horizontal suture repair

The observation that with entropion, the lid margin is tucked in and the middle part of the lid bulges forward gave Schimek [14] the idea of tightening the orbicularis along this meridian. With two short horizontal incisions carefully placed medially and laterally, a band of orbicularis is tightened. At each incision, orbicularis muscle is dissected and sutured with a suture passed across the lid under the skin and muscle. This shortens the bowed-out arc of the muscle and snugs the lid toward the globe. This tightening is akin, in a sense, to tightening with a base-down triangle excision (see section on tarsal excision).

External imbrication of the retractors

This method advocated by Schaeffer [15] is performed through an incision across the length of the lid approximately 6 mm below the lash line. Dissection exposes the lower tarsal border and the thinned or dehisced aponeurosis of the retractor. Five silk sutures are spaced along the lid, going through the upper skin edge, the tarsus, the aponeurosis, and finally out through the lower skin edge. When the sutures are tied, they bring together the aponeurosis and the skin edges. The proper pull may then be restored, and the lid is kept from its abnormal rotation. Schaeffer [15] states that the sutures may need supplementation by tightening the lateral canthal tendon and, at times, the medial canthal tendon. He stated, rather dogmatically, that "this is the only procedure that directly attacks the retractor pathophysiology" [15]. The procedure was reported by Jones and colleagues [16] in 1972.

Lower eyelid reverse ptosis shares in the tissue changes of entropion [7] and requires re-establishing the function of the attenuated or dehisced lower lid retractors, much as is done in the Jones operation.

Orbicularis redirection procedures

Several different patterns of preparing a tongue or tongues of muscle and suturing to the orbital rim have been used [17]. A lower lid incision across the lid is made, and the skin is dissected free of the underlying muscle. A 4-mm wide band or tongue of the muscle is dissected and cut free at one end, which then is drawn across to the orbital rim and stitched to the periosteum. The placement is planned to pull the external layers of the lid down and to the side, causing outward rotation of the lid margin. Some horizontal tightening may be achieved as well. The muscle strips are variable in the resulting tension, and there is a marked tendency for the lid margin to be pulled down, causing scleral show and added exposure.

Tarsal excision

Removal of a segment of tarsus has been used for many years [1]. The removal of a base-down triangle of conjunctiva and tarsus was performed, and with a modification by Fox [18,19], a triangle of skin at the lateral end of the lid was added. A procedure designed to shorten the lid and rotate the margin devised by Quickert [20] could deal with severe lid laxity and entropion. An incision is made through the full thickness of the lid lateral to the limbus, and from the lower end of this incision, cuts are made nasally and temporally. The tongue of tissue on the nasal side is drawn temporally to overlap, indicating what segment is to be removed. The overlap is cut off, and closure is then achieved. Along the horizontal incision line, sutures as in the Wies procedure are used to provide further eversion, and the vertical incision is then closed in the usual manner. The lid is turned from its abnormal rotation, but the lateral canthus is pulled medially and the punctum is pulled laterally. The horizontal length of the palpebral fissure is shortened, and the punctum may be out of position, impairing its function.

Cicatricial entropion

When there is scarring, the initial surgical step is to open the scar and excise scar tissue as is done elsewhere in the body. Some intervening material must then be placed to fill the gap and allow restoration of contour. Materials used have been banked sclera, mucous membrane, dermis-fat grafts, and synthetic implant materials. Ear cartilage in the substance of the lid has also been used but is often unsightly, because the thickness required is not accommodated within the usual thin eyelid structure.

The occurrence of entropion associated with aging often needs correction of the stretched lateral canthal tendon. If this is not recognized and taken care of, along with something like the Feldstein sutures, the operation is doomed to failure. In the subsequent section on ectropion, I have included my method of lateral canthal suspension.

Ectropion

Ectropion is defined as a turning out of the eyelid. This can be of varying degree and may involve only a portion of the eyelid margin. There may be only punctual eversion, a degree of scleral show, or a frank rotation with the conjunctival surface facing out.

There are many causes of this condition and many recommended corrective procedures. The aging process is at the root of many cases, which occur spontaneously. A great number of cases of serious concern are those that result from surgical interventions of different sorts. The most frequent disappointment or complication of lower lid blepharoplasty is scleral show, ocular discomfort, and tearing, basically an ectropion. The deformity of the eyelids in mandibulofacial dysostosis (Treacher-Collins syndrome) is severe lower lid ectropion. Ectropion has been reported with acute weight loss, as stated previously [21]. In cases of orbital fat presenting under the temporal conjunctiva on the globe, there is obviously a defect in the connective tissue. This fat is easily removed with a small conjunctival incision; however, ectropion may be present and need repair when the bulge has been taken away. There are recurrent reports of ectropion caused by the lower rim of the patient's spectacles touching the upper cheek or the lid skin and pushing the lid down [22]. This is the reverse of the intentional (but questionable) use of a ptosis crutch for the upper lid. Conditions affecting the facial skin, such as burns or ichthyosis, result in contractions that evert the lid. The recent use of laser energy to resurface facial and eyelid skin is also the culprit in shrinking the lid and pulling the margin down. Direct trauma, such as lacerations, dog bites, and blunt trauma, may end up with lid shortening and eversion. The use of malar implants is a recent cosmetic procedure of great popularity. The malar implant lifts the overlying tissues to achieve a new contour. The surgeon must precisely determine whether or not the lid margin is going to be shifted from its normal position. Damage to the eyelid innervation has occurred, and scleral show and ectropion have also resulted [23]. The lid retraction of thyroid disease is in a special category but similarly needs correction. With seventh nerve palsy, there is often brow ptosis, lagophthalmos, and ectropion. Associated conjunctival chemosis or conjunctivochalasis needs care. In almost all cases, the anophthalmic socket develops a sagging lower lid over time attributable to the weight of the prosthetic shell.

Ectropion of the upper eyelid is infrequent and often attributable to an abnormal pull on the skin. Trauma to the upper lid is often followed by contracted scars, which need skin grafting and other reconstructive techniques. There are rare congenital upper lid eversions and colobomas. Correction of upper lid ptosis can turn the lid margin out and pull the lid away from the globe. In most current texts, the frontalis suspension operation shown is not physiologic. The three incisions just above the lash line for placement of the suspensory ribbon are unsightly and, worse, produce a pull at the lid margin. This can be compared with the can-can dancer grasping the hem of her skirt to flip it up. Above the brow, the temporal incision is inappropriately placed lateral to the frontalis muscle. Upper lid retraction is comparable to scleral show below and is the hallmark of thyroid ophthalmopathy. In myasthenia gravis, uncommonly, there is weakness of the orbicularis muscle and retained good function of the levator, producing lid lag.

Temporary palliation with teardrops and ointment is critical for corneal protection, even if the patient's complaint is tearing. Taping the lid into position, a frost suture, or a temporary tarsorrhaphy with sutures or glue may be useful. Eye shields, which seal in the moisture, particularly for nighttime, are often a big help. In some cases of postoperative ectropion, placing a scleral ring that lies in the fornices and repeatedly massaging over this stretches out the skin and the subjacent scar and corrects the problem.

The pathophysiology is based on stretched canthal tendons, loss of retractor pull, and downward pull on the outer layers of the eyelid. A short septum, often the result of surgery, can be a significant causative factor.

Ectropion surgery

A time-honored method of correction of ectropion is the Snellen suture technique. This is simply passing sutures through the lower fornix and out on the skin inferiorly. This is like inverting a trouser pocket that was pulled out. Using chromic suture material gives some fibrosis and a longer lasting result. Snellen sutures alone fail in many cases because the other anatomic changes have not been addressed. After a drop or two of anesthetic to the eye, a moistened cotton-tipped applicator or a muscle hook inserted inside the lid can show what Snellen sutures can be expected to accomplish. This suture technique, possibly with some excision of conjunctiva, is used to correct conjunctival chemosis or conjunctivochalasis, a cause of "moist eye" and tearing.

The concept of eyelid shortening is often incorrect in re-establishing normal anatomy. When the lateral canthal tendon has elongated, that is the anatomic structure needing correction. A century ago, a wedge of full-thickness eyelid was removed to treat this deformity. This created a new, and sometimes worse, situation with a central lid scar contracted and pulling the margin down. Taking out a triangle of skin at the lateral end of the lid and a triangle of tarsus and conjunctiva in the center of the lid followed. Many variants and names accompanied this operation.

An elaborate procedure sometimes used in severe cases is a modified Tripier flap [24]. This is also called a "bucket handle flap" because it remains attached at both ends. It is done by making two parallel incisions across the full extent of the upper lid and swinging the tissue in between into a prepared bed in the short lower eyelid.

Less complex but also infrequently performed is placement of a ribbon of fascia from the medial canthal tendon through the space under the orbicularis to the lateral canthal tendon. This strip can be adjusted and can be enhanced by Snellen sutures and other procedures.

Skin grafts are often used with donor sites from another eyelid as well as retroauricular, supraclavicular, and other areas of fine hairless skin. Tissue expansion is not often used but is helpful in certain cases and can be accomplished by repeat injections that stretch out the skin. Vertical shortage of tissue in the lid is often really downward migration of the cheek with the aging process. Through a classic blepharoplasty incision, or otherwise, a cheek lift can be done, sometimes just with one or two stitches anchored to the lower orbital rim periosteum.

Horizontal shortening

The hammock of the lower lid can be better approximated to the globe by shortening the lid. This is not always desirable, however, because the procedures often leave their own new blemish where a vertical full-thickness incision has been made and the horizontal length of the palpebral fissure is significantly shortened. There is widespread use of the tarsal strip or modified Bick procedure to shorten the lower lid [25]. The surgeon prepares a narrow piece of the lateral tarsus by removing the skin and other tissues at the margin. This shortens the palpebral fissure by at least 5 mm. The cut end of the tarsus is then supposed to be stitched inside the lateral orbital rim. Often, the stitches are not well placed, and the lateral-most part of the lid is not in apposition to the globe. The horizontal dimension of the palpebral fissure is shortened instead of restored to the state before stretching out of the lateral canthal tendon. The outer portion of the upper lid can be seen to override the lower, a kind of pseudoptosis.

The most popular procedure for the nasal third of the lid has come to be known as the "lazy-T" operation. In 1975, English and Keats published *Reconstructive and Plastic Surgery of the Eyelids* [26]. They present a clear description of what they called the double-wedge technique for everted punctum. A vertical full-thickness incision is made just lateral to the punctum. "The temporal fragment is drawn nasalwards and the redundant tissue highlighted by the resultant overlap. This full thickness wedge of eyelid is removed, restoring the horizontal dimension to normal. Now, with a probe placed in the lower canaliculus to ensure there is no injury to the drainage mechanism, a horizontally oriented wedge of tarsus is outlined on the nasal fragment from a conjunctival approach and dissected out. Closure of this defect rolls the punctum in a backward direction. After the required amount has been removed, interrupted 6-0 silk sutures close the wound, and the other defect is then bridged by primary anastomosis. When completed, the combined maneuver restores the inferior punctum to its anatomical location" [26]. The following year, 1976, witnessed the publication of a report on the double-wedge resection under a new name, "the lazy-T procedure," by Smith [27], who had written the foreword to English and Keat's book.

Meltzer reported a method of medial ectropion repair with a special rotating flap that eliminates the need for a free graft (which does not match the lid skin as well) [28].

Lid shortening procedures are necessary at times. Certain principles must be followed to avoid a bad result. In Wiener's book [29], a method is shown for closure of a through and through laceration of the lid. On each side of the cut, the tissue is freshly cut out along an arc from the margin to the nether end of the defect. This alters the geometry by providing a closure line along the arc longer than the chord length. At closure, this produces a small protrusion of the margin. This counteracts the anticipated scar shrinkage, which would cause a notch. Hecht [30] called this a "bowlegs" procedure, and others called it a "corncrib" operation [31]. Later, the pentagonal procedure for tumor excision was proposed. The pentagonal technique relies on the divergence of the cuts from the lid margin into the lid. Diagrams showing parallel sides (the configuration of a baseball home plate) are not correct. A true geometric pentagon (one edge being the lid margin) has obtuse angles. A five-pointed star (a true pentagon rather than a square with parallel sides) can be inscribed neatly into the pentagon.

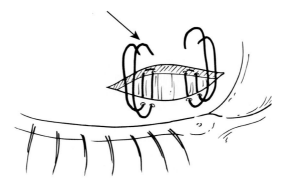

Fig. 3. Suture closure of medial spindle, arrow indicates needle pass through, to be tied on the skin.

Medial spindle excision

When the punctum is everted, it is possible to correct this with removal of a diamond or ellipse of conjunctiva and deeper tissue from inferior to the canaliculus. This can be done with an initial incision and then overlap to determine how much needs to be removed, followed by suture closure. The closure is accomplished with one or two fine double-armed sutures (eg, 6-0 Vicryl). The suture is first passed at the inferior edge of the excision through the deep tissue and then out through the upper conjunctival edge. The needles are next passed through the full thickness of the lid just below the lower incisional edge and then down and out to be tied on the skin (Fig. 3). This adds an element of suture rotation to the method.

Lateral canthal correction

Several currently popular operations are based on the Bick procedure [25]. Webster and colleagues [32] used a suture at the outer canthal area as part of a lower lid blepharoplasty. Shorr and Fallor [33] have advocated what they have called the "Madame Butterfly" lateral canthal lift. Small [34] has proposed the "extended" blepharoplasty with the lower lid incision longer temporally, with a deep suspending suture.

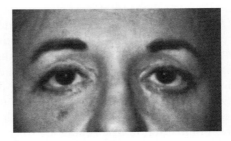

Fig. 4. Bilateral scleral show, low lateral canthi, post blepharoplasty.

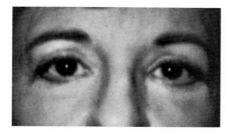

Fig. 5. Bilateral 3D canthal correction done.

Lateral canthal suspension

A lateral canthal suspension procedure has been my operation for more than 30 years and 200 cases [35]. A postblepharoplasty patient presented with a severe lower lid ectropion. The lid was not shortened, as easily shown with an applicator gently rotating it into normal position. It was evident that the lateral canthal tendon support was lost. The operation can give lateral, upward, and posterior pull inside the orbital rim—the third dimension (Figs. 4–9).

Eliasoph three-dimensional canthal correction

The lateral end of the tarsus is inspected. Local anesthesia is given (into the lateral one third of each lid and a small amount into the orbit). A 5-mm incision is made approximately 3 mm below and parallel to the lash line (near the lateral end of the tarsus). Each arm of a doubly armed suture of 5-0 white braided polyester is passed through the lateral end of the tarsus from the conjunctival side to exit through the skin incision. Adequate tarsal tissue must lie in the loop. (The conjunctiva is sealed over the suture by the next day). The needles are removed, and the suture ends are threaded on a half-curved cutting needle approximately 25 mm long. This needle is introduced into the incision pointing laterally and deep to the orbicularis.

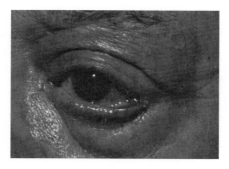

Fig. 6. Male patient, ectropion post blepharoplasty.

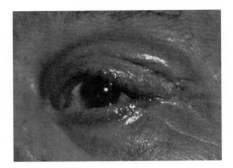

Fig. 7. Male patient, after 3D canthal correction.

The plane of the needle is shifted to point into the orbit just inside the rim and deep to the anterior portion of the lateral canthal tendon. The needle is advanced along its curve, hugging the inside of the orbit, and is brought around to tent up the upper lid skin. Here, an incision approximately 15 mm long is made (or previously made) along a natural skin line, and the suture is drawn through.

The bony orbital rim is exposed. One arm of the suture is threaded on a small needle, and a firm bite of periosteum is taken inside the orbit. Both ends of the suture are drawn up to tighten as needed and tied securely, and the tag ends are cut away. Skin sutures are placed as needed, and cold compresses are applied.

Graefe forceps are effective to hold the lid margin and evert it as needed. A heavy surgeon's needle holder is needed for the big needle to control it properly. When the big needle has been passed most of the way, lifting meets great weight, almost lifting the patient's head. If the needle wiggles and comes up easily, it was not passed deeply enough. There is, however, no significant resistance to passing the needle around its curve and out the upper incision. The anchoring bite in the periosteum is not critical in its placement, but care must be taken in doing this, because improper rotation

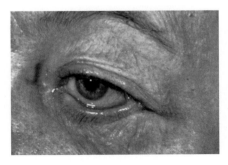

Fig. 8. Ectropion post blepharoplasty.

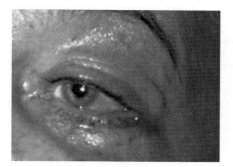

Fig. 9. After 3D canthal correction.

can break the needle or tear the tissue. The pass should be inside the rim (so that the knot is deep and better periosteum is found) and taken pointing away from the globe. If traction on the suture, before anchoring it, shows an unsuitable direction, it can be pulled and replaced or cut and redone. Often, there is a bit of folding of the skin at the canthus, but this always smoothes out. Some transient edema of the conjunctiva may occur. If performed in conjunction with a lower lid blepharoplasty, any excision of skin must be done after this. The superior incision can be the lateral extent of an upper lid blepharoplasty incision. A cheek lift with this gives good results.

Summary

The entities of entropion and ectropion have some important common factors in their genesis. Preoperative examination requires similar careful assessment and planning. The need for surgery must first be established, and the changes in the anatomy must be evaluated. Prior local trauma or surgery, conjunctival or skin changes, septal shortening, weakness of muscles, retractor thinning or dehiscence, orbicularis muscle shift, and, most importantly, the status of the lateral canthal tendon must all be considered. In performing any eyelid surgery, entropion or ectropion should not be produced, and preventive techniques must be incorporated into such undertakings. Anesthetic injections should be subcutaneous and only as deep as needed. The amount injected should not be excessive, because distortion or stretching can occur. Dealing with orbital fat should never involve any pulling, which can shear off a deep orbital vessel with serious consequences. Immediate and adequate measures for intraorbital bleeding should be familiar to the surgeon and instituted without delay. Restoration of lid anatomy with precise surgical methods yields improved lid function, comfort, and cosmesis.

References

[1] Adams W. Entropion correction by excision of a triangle of tarsus and conjunctiva. Practical Obs on Ectrop 1812, p. 4. Cited by Beard CH. Ophthalmic surgery. 2nd edition. Philadelphia: P. Blakiston's Son & Co.; 1914. p. 286.

[2] von Graefe A. Bemerkungen zur Operation des Entropium und Ectropium. Archiv fur Ophthalmologie 1864;10:221–32.

[3] Gioia VM, Linberg JV, McCormick SA. The anatomy of the lateral canthal tendon. Arch Ophthalmol 1987;105:529–32.

[4] Ousterhout DK, Weil RB. The role of the lateral canthal tendon in lower eyelid laxity. Plast Reconstr Surg 1982;69:620–3.

[5] Ngerwamungu E, Kilima P, Munoz B. Gender equity and trichiasis surgery in the Vietnam and Tanzania national control programmes. Br J Ophthalmol 2004;88:1368–71.

[6] Win WN. Surgery for trachoma in Burma. Br J Ophthalmol 1963;63:113–6.

[7] Bartley GB, Frueh BR, Holds JB, et al. Lower eyelid reverse ptosis repair. Ophthal Plast Reconstr Surg 2002;18:79–83.

[8] Ziegler SL. Galvanocautery puncture in ectropion and entropion. JAMA 1909;53:183–6.

[9] Wies FA. Spastic entropion. Trans Am Acad Ophthalmol Otolaryngol 1955;59:503–6.

[10] Feldstein M. A method for correction of entropion in aged persons. Eye Ear Nose Throat Mon 1960;39:730–1.

[11] Feldstein M. Correction of senile entropion. Ophthalmic Surg 1970;1(3):20–3.

[12] Williams DL. Entropion correction by fornix-based suture placement: use of the Quickert-Rathbun technique in ten dogs. Vet Ophthalmol 2004;7:343–7.

[13] Quickert MH, Rathbun E. Suture repair of entropion. Arch Ophthalmol 1971;85:304–5.

[14] Schimek RA. A simplified entropion operation. Presented at the Meeting of the Wilmer Residents Association, The Johns Hopkins Hospital. Baltimore, April 2, 1955.

[15] Schaeffer AJ. Variation in the pathophysiology of involutional entropion and its treatment. Ophthalmic Surg 1983;14:653–5.

[16] Jones LT, Reeh MJ, Wobig JL. Senile entropion: a new concept for correction. Am J Ophthalmol 1972;74:327–9.

[17] Wheeler JM. Spastic entropion corrected by orbicularis transplantation. Trans Am Ophthamol Soc 1938;5:157–62.

[18] Fox SA. A Modified Kuhnt-Szymanowski procedure. Am J Ophthalmol 1966;62:533.

[19] Fox SA. Idiopathic blepharoptosis of lower eyelid. Am J Ophthalmol 1972;74:330–1.

[20] Quickert MH. Malpositions of the eyelid. In: Sorsby A, editor. Modern ophthalmology, vol. 4. 2nd edition. London: Butterworth & Co.; 1972. p. 941–3.

[21] Amalong RJ. Tarsal conjunctival exposure following weight loss. Am J Ophthalmol 1968;65: 930–1.

[22] Chalfin J, Putterman AM. Ectropion produced by eyeglass frames. Arch Ophthalmol 1979; 97:306.

[23] Logani SC, Conn H, Logani S, et al. Paralytic ectropion; a complication of malar implant surgery. Ophthal Plast Reconstr Surg 1998;14:89–93.

[24] Siegel RJ. Severe ectropion: repair with a modified Tripier flap. Plast Reconstr Surg 1987;80: 21–8.

[25] Bick MW. Surgical management of orbital tarsal disparity. Arch Ophthalmol 1966;75:386–9.

[26] English FP, Keats WF. Reconstructive and plastic surgery of the eyelids. Springfield, MO: Charles C Thomas; 1975. p. 49–51.

[27] Smith B. The "lazy-T" correction of ectropion of the lower punctum. Arch Ophthalmol 1976;94:1149–51.

[28] Meltzer MA. Medial ectropion repair. Ophthal Plast Reconstr Surg 1989;5:182–5.

[29] Wiener M. Surgery of the eye. 2nd edition. New York: Grune and Stratton; 1949. p. 292–4.

[30] Hecht SD. Bowlegs procedure for recurrent and primary senile entropion. Ann Ophthalmol 1981;13:119–21.

[31] Mauriello JA, Abdelsalam A. Modified corncrib (inverted T) procedure with Quickert suture for repair of involutional entropion. Ophthalmology 1997;104:504–7.

[32] Webster RC, Davidson TM, Reardon EJ, et al. Suspending sutures in blepharoplasty. Arch Otolaryngol 1979;105:601.

[33] Shorr N, Fallor MK. "Madame Butterfly" procedure: combined cheek and lateral canthal suspension procedure for postblepharoplasty, "round eye," and lower eyelid retraction. Ophthal Plast Reconstr Surg 1985;1:229–35.

[34] Small RG. The extended lower lid blepharoplasty. Arch Ophthalmol 1981;99:1402–5.

[35] Eliasoph I. Put the lateral canthus back—3D correction [poster]. Presented at the American Society of Ophthalmic Plastic and Reconstructive Surgery Annual Meeting. New Orleans, LA; November 7, 1998.

ELSEVIER
SAUNDERS

Otolaryngol Clin N Am
38 (2005) 921–946

OTOLARYNGOLOGIC
CLINICS
OF NORTH AMERICA

Ptosis Evaluation and Management

Brenda C. Edmonson, MD*, Allan E. Wulc, MD

847 Easton Road, Suite 1500, Warrington, PA 18976

Drooping of the upper eyelids is one of the most common complaints in oculoplastic practice. Other related complaints include difficulty seeing due to the attendant visual field obstruction and prefrontal headaches due to chronic use of the frontalis muscle in an attempt to lift the eyelids [1]. This anatomic and morphologic state is termed *ptosis*, from the Greek "to fall."

Ptosis causes a simultaneous cosmetic deformity that is apparent both to the patient and to others. A recent study suggested that photographs of patients with droopy lids are subjectively perceived by others as less intelligent and more negatively than their counterparts when compared with photographs after having undergone ptosis correction [2].

Ptosis surgery can be challenging for even the most experienced eye and facial plastic surgeon. The rate of reoperation in most series of acquired ptosis varies from 5% to 35% [3–5]. The correction of ptosis of more complex etiology, and congenital ptosis may even be more elusive. To minimize reoperations and maximize postoperative symmetry, detailed preoperative assessment and intraoperative anatomic dissection with respect to tissue planes and hemostasis are necessary. This article discusses some of the more common types of ptosis and provides an introduction to the evaluation and management of the ptosis patient. Complications of ptosis surgery and recent innovations in ptosis surgery are discussed.

Terminology

The eyelid fissure is a measurement of the opening of the eyelid when the eye is in primary position (looking straight ahead). It is measured in millimeters at the center of the eyelid from the bottom of the upper lid to the top of the lower lid. The normal measurement is 9 to 10 mm. Ptotic eyes are defined as those with eyelid fissures less than 9 mm.

---

* Corresponding author.
E-mail address: bcmiller72@pol.net (B.C. Edmonson).

Marginal reflex distances (MRDs) are measurements that are often useful as well. MRD_1 is the distance from the upper eyelid to the corneal light reflex. Measurements less than 4 mm are considered abnormal; an MRD_1 of 2.5 or less is usually considered vision-impairing. MRD_2 the distance from the corneal light reflex to the lower eyelid. A normal measurement is 4 to 5 mm; a measurement of more than 5 mm represents a lower eyelid that is too low and can be caused by eyelid retraction or ectropion. A patient can have a ptotic upper eyelid and a normal eyelid fissure if the lower eyelid position is abnormally low. All three measurements are therefore important.

Levator function is a measurement of how well the levator muscle works. Normal function is greater than 11 mm. A measurement greater than 11 mm is considered very good, 8 to 10 mm is considered good, 5 to 7 mm is considered fair, and 4 mm or less is considered poor.

Classification of ptosis

Ptosis can occur for a variety of reasons. *Congenital ptosis* may be diagnosed shortly after birth. *Mechanical ptosis* due to dermatochalasis and brow ptosis is often seen in the aging population and can accompany many of the other types of ptosis. Myogenic ptosis, aponeurotic ptosis, neurogenic ptosis, and neuromyogenic ptosis (eg, ocular myasthenia) can all present in adults and present rarely in children as well [1]. The most common type of ptosis in adults is involutional ptosis secondary to acquired dehiscence or detachment of the levator aponeurosis from the tarsus [1,6]. Ptosis in children is most often myogenic in origin and due to levator muscle maldevelopment [1,6,7].

Myogenic ptosis

Myogenic ptosis occurs when levator strength has diminished [1]. The most common myogenic ptosis is simple congenital ptosis, which can occur as an autosomal dominant or, more often, sporadically [7]. Simple congenital ptosis is usually secondary to levator muscle maldevelopment. Approximately 30% of patients who have congenital ptosis will also have ocular motility disturbances, the most common being weakness of the ipsilateral superior rectus muscle [6–8]. Congenital myogenic ptosis is usually unilateral with no other associated facial abnormality (Fig. 1A) [7].

In acquired myogenic ptosis, levator function is usually moderate but may be normal early on in the course [1,6]. In congenital myopathic ptosis, lag on downgaze can be seen due to fibrosis of the levator, and lesser degrees of levator function are commonly seen.

Congenital ptosis can also accompany craniofacial syndromes. Most common among these are blepharophimosis syndrome and Marcus Gunn jaw wink syndrome [1,6,7]. Blepharophimosis can be inherited as an autosomal dominant trait. The signs of blepharophimosis are bilateral ptosis,

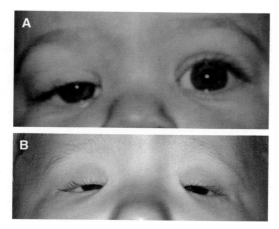

Fig. 1. (*A*) A 6-month-old patient showing congenital ptosis of the right upper eyelid. (*B*) A child with blepharophimosis. Note the ptosis, epicanthal folds, and telecanthus.

decreased horizontal fissure size, epicanthal folds (epicanthus inversus), telecanthus, and ectropion of the lower lateral eyelids (Fig. 1B) [7].

Marcus Gunn Jaw winking is caused by a miscommunication between the third cranial nerve that innervates the levator and the fifth cranial nerve that innervates the muscles of mastication. The result is a unilateral ptosis that resolves or improves when the patient opens the mouth or moves the lower jaw in a contralateral direction (Fig. 2A, B) [7].

Other less common craniofacial syndromes associated with a congenital ptosis are Turner's syndrome, Noonan's syndrome, Smith-Lemli-Opitz syndrome, Rubenstein-Taybi syndrome, Saethre-Chotzen syndrome, and

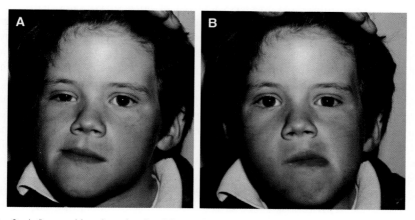

Fig. 2. A 5-year-old patient showing Marcus Gunn syndrome. Patient with ptosis of the right upper eyelid (*A*) that resolves with contraction of the ipsilateral masseter muscle (*B*).

fetal trimetadione [9,10]. Because of their rarity, these syndromes are beyond the scope of this article.

In adults, trauma can give rise to myopathic ptosis when the muscle itself is injured. More often, traumatic ptosis involves injury to the aponeurosis, the third cranial nerve supplying the levator muscle, or the bones adjacent to the levator (mechanical ptosis) impinging on the excursion of the muscle itself, or due to orbital injury with consequent enophthalmos [1,6]. Orbital roof fractures, in particular, often give rise to ptosis. If bony injury is suspected, the patient should be evaluated accordingly with appropriate neuroimaging studies. Edema of the eyelid after trauma can mimic ptosis; therefore, the diagnosis of a true ptosis may be delayed. Any lacerations of the eyelid involving the levator should be repaired as soon as possible unless the original injury is not found until weeks after the injury. At this time it is best to wait 3 to 6 months to see if there is any improvement in the ptosis before embarking upon surgical correction [6].

Patients may also present with myopathic ptosis following blepharoplasty surgery. This type of traumatic ptosis may be due to lid edema, hematoma, levator aponeurosis injury from cautery, or careless removal of the post septal fat from septal suturing, septal levator adhesions, or a blepharoplasty technique that involves supratarsal fixation [11,12]. Ptosis repair may be difficult, because the anatomy of the eyelid has been disrupted from the previous surgery. Mild ptosis may improve with time. Ptosis existing after 3 months should be repaired with the correct surgical procedure based on levator function [11].

Other types of myogenic ptosis seen in adults include oculopharyngeal dystrophy, chronic progressive external ophthalmoplegia (CPEO), myotonic dystrophy, and infiltrative ptosis [6]. Oculopharyngeal dystrophy is more commonly found in patients of French Canadian ancestry [7]. These patients have ptosis and also difficulty swallowing secondary to weakness of the oropharyngeal muscles. CPEO is inherited in 50% of patients, with signs and symptoms beginning in childhood [7]. CPEO results in ptosis and ophthalmolplegia and can be associated with retinal pigmentary problems and heart block. The classic presentation is a patient with ptosis and ophthalmoplegia without diplopia [6]. Most patient present with a bilateral, symmetric ptosis with decreased levator function [8]. The extraocular muscle become involved later in the course of the disease. Patients with ptosis and ophthalmoplegia of unknown etiology should have a cardiac workup including an electrocardiogram to rule out Kearn Sayre syndrome. Myotonic dystrophy has an autosomal dominant inheritance and is usually associated with ptosis, orbicularis weakness, and extraocular muscle weakness and may also be associated with cardiac conduction defects [13].

Myogenic ptosis can also be caused by infiltrative processes such as amyloidosis. Amyloidosis may affect other muscles, including the extra-ocular muscles, where it can be confused with orbital myositis [8]. Biopsies of the levator muscle or extraocular muscle can help establish the diagnosis.

The diagnosis can be made through the demonstration of birefringence and dichroism with Congo red stain [8]. Other stains including crystal violet and thioflavin-T may help with the diagnosis [8]. Treatment should include a systemic workup and referral to the appropriate specialist.

Biopsies of the levator muscle in congenital ptosis usually show an inversely proportional relationship between the amount of ptosis and the density of striated muscle [8,9].

The surgical correction of myopathic ptosis involves levator advancement surgery in patients with moderate to good to function, or frontalis sling where levator function is more compromised. In general, the authors prefer autogenous slings in children above the age of 4, and favor giving adults the choice between adjustable silicone slings or autogenous slings based on the overall clinical situation.

Aponeurotic ptosis

The most common type of aponeurotic ptosis is involutional ptosis secondary to stretching, attenuation, or detachment of the levator aponeurosis from its tarsal attachments (Fig. 3) [1,6,7]. Examination of these patients usually reveal a normal levator function and a high eyelid crease [6,7]. The ptosis is normally bilateral and symmetric but may be unilateral and asymmetric. Patients with involutional aponeurotic ptosis should not have motility or pupillary abnormalities [1,6]. Stretching of the levator aponeurosis occurs commonly in patients who wear contact lenses and in patients who are constantly rubbing their eyes such as those with Down syndrome and in patients with ocular allergy [8].

Up to 6% of patients who have undergone cataract surgery can develop aponeurotic ptosis [8]. The mechanism of postcataract ptosis is thought to be trauma to the levator aponeurosis or the superior rectus muscle complex, which shares strong intermuscular fascial connections to the levator muscle and can be disrupted either by postcataract eyelid swelling or by the eyelid speculum used to separate the eyelids at the time of surgery [12].

The preferred surgical procedure in these patients is levator aponeurotic advancement.

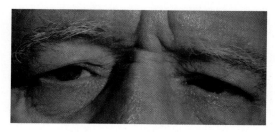

Fig. 3. A 62-year-old patient showing bilateral dermatochalasis and aponeurotic ptosis.

Neurogenic ptosis

Neurogenic etiologies of ptosis include myasthenia gravis, III cranial nerve palsy, and Horner's syndrome [7].

Myasthenic ptosis is due to a problem at the neuromuscular junction and therefore can be classified as neurogenic or myogenic (Fig. 4) [6,7]. Myasthenic ptosis is an autoimmune disease due to diminished acetylcholine receptors at the neuromuscular junction. It may be unilateral or bilateral and often involves the extraocular muscles. Ocular myasthenia is a form of myasthenia that only affects the extraocular muscles, the levator muscle or the orbicularis oculi muscle without systemic involvement [14]. The hallmark of myasthenia is the variability of the ptosis [6,7]. The ptosis usually worsens with fatigue and usually improves with the ice test or edrophonium test [1,7]. Other signs include ptosis that worsens in the evening, paradoxical eyelid retraction, and Cogan's lid twitch, which is eyelid retraction that occurs after sustained downgaze.

Third-nerve palsies can be caused by tumors, vascular lesions, or inflammatory or neurotoxic diseases [7]. Palsies of the third cranial nerve present with ptosis, hypotropia, and extraocular motility disturbance that spare the lateral rectus and superior oblique muscle (Fig. 5A) [1,6]. Pupillary involvement resulting in a mydriatic pupil is seen with aneurysms of the posterior communicating artery. Aberrant regeneration may occur in patients with third-nerve palsy and is a sign of etiologies other than those that are ischemic, such as hypertension or diabetes. Patients with aberrant regeneration should be suspected to have intracranial tumors until proved otherwise and require neuroimaging. Work-up for patients with third-nerve palsies depends on the patient's age and whether or not the pupil is involved. If the pupil is involved, an aneurysm of the posterior communicating artery should be presumed until ruled out by neuroimaging [14]. An MRI/MRA should be performed. If the MRI/MRA is negative and aneurysm is

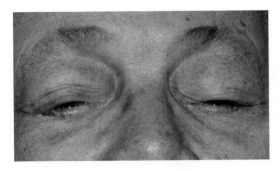

Fig. 4. A 54-year-old patient showing bilateral ptosis secondary to myasthenia gravis. The ptosis worsens with fatigue.

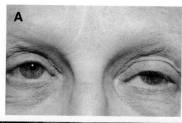

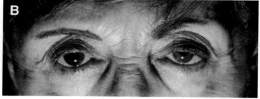

Fig. 5. (*A*) This 52-year-old patient has a left-sided third-nerve palsy. Note the ptosis and mydriatic pupil on the left side. (*B*) This 50-year-old female has left-sided congenital Horner's syndrome. Note the left ptosis, miosis, and lighter-colored iris.

considered, emergent angiography should be performed (MRA is not always sensitive enough to exclude an aneurysm) [15].

In children under 10 years of age, the most common cause of third-nerve palsy is congenital third-nerve palsy, which is usually incomplete and associated with aberrant regeneration. Third-nerve palsy in children can also be caused by ophthalmoplegic migraine.

In adults under 50 years of age, all third-nerve palsies are evaluated with an MRI, erythrocyte sedimentation rate, serologic syphilis testing, Lyme titer, glucose, and antinuclear antibody to rule out vasculitis and infection [8]. A spinal tap to rule out infection, meningiomatosis, and metastatic disease may also be required. After the etiology has been discovered, the patient should be given 6 to 12 months for spontaneous recovery of the palsy.

Levator function in third cranial nerve palsies may be absent or almost normal [6]. The most common surgical procedure in third cranial nerve palsies is the frontalis sling, particularly when levator function is absent or severely reduced. Any strabismus problem should be repaired before eyelid surgery, because alteration of globe position may result in a change in eyelid position [8].

Horner's syndrome is due to damage to the sympathetic supply to the orbit from tumors, aneurysms, or inflammations. It results in ptosis, anhidrosis, and miosis (Fig. 5B) [6]. Horner's syndrome can be present at birth and can present with concomitant third-nerve palsy [1,7]. The ptosis is often of a minor nature, up to 2.5 mm, and levator function is normal. In addition to ptosis, anhidrosis, and miosis, patients who have congenital Horner's syndrome may have heterochromia, in which the affected eye has a lighter-colored iris [8].

The workup for acquired Horner's syndrome includes pharmacologic testing with cocaine and hydroxyamphetamine. Cocaine prevents reuptake of norepinephrine and can aid in the diagnosis of Horner's syndrome. In a patient with ptosis and anisocoria due to Horner's syndrome, the instillation of 5% or 10% cocaine hydrochloride into the eyes will cause a dilation of the mydriatic pupil and only mild dilation of the miotic pupil, therefore increasing the amount of pupil inequality. Hydroxyamphetamine 1% eye drops help determine the location of the lesion along the sympathetic pathway; these drops should be used at least 48 hours after the cocaine test. Miotic pupils from preganglionic lesions or central lesions will dilate normally or more than the normal pupil after instillation of hydroxyamphetamine. Miotic pupils from postganglionic lesions do not dilate at all. Hydroxyamphetamine drops do not help the localization of the lesion in infants [8]. Postganglionic lesions are usually caused by benign vascular headaches (such as cluster headaches) or carotid dissection, and thus it is important to determine the cause of postganglionic lesions. Preganglionic lesions can be from malignant metastases or lung apex tumors. A Horner's syndrome acquired in infancy can be caused by neuroblastoma [8]. Because of the magnitude of the ptosis, the preferred surgical correction for patients with ptosis from Horner's syndrome is either a mullerectomy or an external levator aponeurotic advancement [8].

Mechanical ptosis

Mechanical ptosis is most commonly due to excess skin that hangs over the eyelid margin and decreases the visual field [6,7]. It can also be secondary to masses or scars that physically weigh down the lid or obstruct free movement (Fig. 6) [1,6,7].

Surgery for these patients involves the removal of the underlying abnormality such as excess skin, mass, or scar. Residual ptosis can be corrected by levator aponeurosis advancement in patients with normal levator function [8].

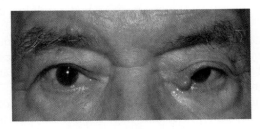

Fig. 6. A 60-year-old patient with a mass of the medial left upper eyelid resulting in left-sided ptosis.

Pseudoptosis

Pseudoptosis is an eyelid that seems ptotic but is not [7]. Causes of pseudoptosis include hemifacial spasm, facial nerve palsy with aberrant regeneration, contralateral lid retraction contralateral proptosis, enophthalmos, anophthalmos with superior sulcus deformity, and lower eyelid ptosis (Fig. 7) [1,7]. Floppy eyelid syndrome usually occurs in obese men, and its etiology is unknown. The tarsus of the eyelid becomes lax, resulting in redundant and "floppy" eyelids. The flaccid eyelids are easily everted and may present as dermatochalasis or pseudoptosis [8].

Examination of the patient with ptosis

History

A patient who has ptosis usually complains of heaviness of the lids, headache from constant use of the frontalis muscle, difficulty reading, difficulty seeing the superior visual field, and looking tired [1,6,7]. The duration of ptosis is significant to the history. Congenital ptosis, of course, will present early in life, but it may not be perceived by the patient's parents; thus in all patients with a long history of ptosis, old photographs may be useful in the determination of the duration of the ptosis. Acquired types of ptosis are predominantly chronic and slowly progressive. Acute onset ptosis, in contrast, can be associated with eye or eyelid infection, allergy, angioneurotic edema, and, when associated with hypotropia, can signal aneurysm of the posterior communicating artery [15].

Ptosis may occur following surgery or other types of trauma, and a thorough past surgical history is mandatory. As discussed, both previous eyelid surgery and intraocular surgery can cause aponeurotic ptosis. Surgical sympathectomy or endarterectomy can also give rise to Horner's syndrome.

Patients should be asked if the amount of lid droopiness varies throughout the day. Ptosis that worsens toward the end of the day or with fatigue can represent myasthenia gravis [7]. Patients should be asked about double vision; diplopia can be seen in myopathic ptoses such as diplopia in myasthenia gravis, CPEO, and third-nerve palsy [6,7].

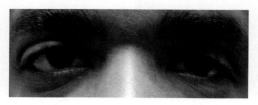

Fig. 7. A 28-year-old patient with left-sided pseudoptosis. He sustained an orbital floor and medial wall fracture resulting in enophthalmos of the left globe and pseudoptosis.

Patients should also be queried about other eye problems, especially dry eyes and contact lens use. History should include any history of smoking, allergies, anticoagulant use, herbal medicine use, vitamins, and prescription medicines. Past medical history should query for sleep apnea and floppy eyelid syndrome. Family history may be relevant if oculopharyngeal dystrophy is entertained as a diagnostic possibility.

Examination

When examining a patient who has ptosis, several important measurements must be made that are critical to management and have a direct impact on surgical planning. The examination of the ptotic patient should also involve the normal side, if there is one, because symmetry is the desired goal if surgery is indeed performed.

Lid height or palpebral fissure is the distance from the bottom of the upper eyelid margin to the top of the bottom eyelid margin taken at the center of the eyelid. A normal measurement ranges from 8 to 10 mm.

Levator function is obtained by measuring the movement of the upper eyelid from down-gaze to up-gaze while stabilizing the eyebrow/frontalis muscle (Fig. 8A, B). Normal levator function is considered to be greater than 11 mm [7].

The eyelid crease is the measurement of the distance from the eyelid margin to the eyelid crease when the patient is looking down at a 45° angle. The normal crease measurement is 7 to 8 mm in males and 9 to 10 mm in females [1,6].

MRD_1 should be measured and is particularly helpful if lower eyelid position is assymetric (Fig. 9) [1,6].

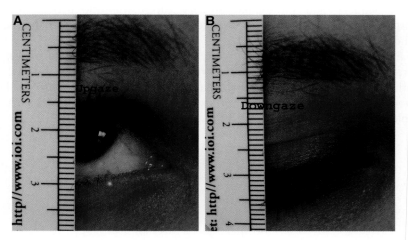

Fig. 8. Levator function is a measurement of the upper eyelid from up-gaze (*A*) to down-gaze (*B*).

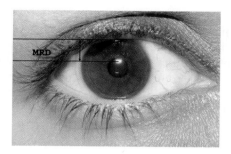

Fig. 9. MRD$_1$ is a measurement from the central upper eyelid to the pupillary light reflex.

Determination of the patient's dominant eye is valuable because levator muscle tone is influenced by ocular dominance in ptotic patients [16].

In the authors' practice, most adult patients who have acquired ptosis are tested with neosynephrine to determine whether the ptosis diminishes following its instillation. After instilling a drop of 2.5% neosynephrine in the abnormal eye, the upper eyelid position is rechecked after 5 minutes. If the ptotic lid elevates by 2 to 3 mm, the patient may benefit from a tarsal-conjunctival resection or a conjunctival-Muller's muscle resection surgery [13]. If external levator aponeurosis surgery is planned, determination of neosynephrine sensitivity allows one to plan for a greater intraoperative overcorrection, as the effects of neosynephrine in general mimic the effect of intraoperative epinephrine administered with the amide anesthetic.

In patients who are suspected of having a ptosis secondary to myasthenia, the ptosis should improve with the ice test and tensilon or the edrophonium test [1,7]. Applying an ice pack to the ptotic eyelid for 5 minutes should improve the ptosis in a patient who has myasthenic ptosis [13]. The tensilon test is performed by injecting 2 mg of tensilon IV to rule out an adverse reaction. This is followed by a second injection of 8 mg 30 seconds later. The ptotic eyelid should elevate within 1 to 5 minutes in a patient with myasthenic ptosis. In case of adverse reaction, it is recommended that injectable atropine be on hand to be administered intravenously [13]. A large percentage of patients who have myasthenia will also have acetylcholine receptor antibodies in their blood, which can be easily checked with a routine blood test [13]. Between 70% and 80% of patients with systemic myasthenia gravis will have autoantibodies to acetylcholine receptors. An electromyogram can also be performed in patients with suspected myasthenic ptosis and is the most specific study. Patients who have myasthenia will demonstrate a decreased amplitude of muscle action potentials [17].

Bell's phenomenon must also be evaluated; this is the ability of the eyeball to move upward with eyelid closure. Orbicularis strength is tested by having the patient tightly close their eyes and resist the examiner's efforts to open them.

The position of the lower eyelid is also important and should be noted. The lower eyelid may be higher then normal in patients who have Horner's syndrome or may be lower than normal in patients with facial nerve palsy.

The amount of excess eyelid skin and fat and brow position are important preoperative parameters and should be recorded. Patients who have ptosis and excessive eyelid skin and fat may be better served with an anterior approach that enables the surgeon to address these problems simultaneously. Patients who have brow ptosis may benefit from a concurrent brow lift.

Ancillary examination

The patient should be examined for pupil abnormalities and motility problems. It is exceedingly important to assess the status of the cornea, as patients with drying of the cornea or instability of the precorneal tear film may have exacerbation of their symptoms following any type of ptosis procedure. Tests to rule out dry eye include Schirmer testing, as well as a slit lamp examination looking at the cornea and the precorneal tear film. Assessing corneal and conjunctival staining patterns with fluorescein, rose bengal, or lissamine green are also valuable adjuncts [8]. All patients with ptosis should be examined by an ophthalmologist before eyelid surgery.

Documentation of ptosis before surgery

In patients with ptosis, insurance companies usually require specific documentation before the surgery. Photographic documentation of the patient looking in primary gaze, down-gaze, up-gaze, and side views of the patient while looking in primary gaze all may be required and often are useful postoperatively to document the preoperative condition, because patients quickly forget the severity of their condition.

Visual fields of the patient illustrating defects in the superior visual field are usually also required. The visual field is performed on each ptotic eyelid with the eyelids in their natural position and again with the eyelids taped up to simulate the postsurgical response. Insurers usually require a difference of at least 12° between the two fields, but different states and different insurances vary in their requirements. Recent studies have demonstrated that manual kinetic visual field testing (Goldmann) and automated static visual fields (Humphrey) are equally effective at demonstrating ptosis. However, the automated static testing may be less sensitive and also has a longer examination time [18].

Interestingly, there is a rationale to the requirements of visual field to document field loss and severity of ptosis. A recent study has shown that the degree of ptosis is proportional to the superior field depression with both static and automated perimetry [19].

Surgical management

The most common procedure performed for all types of ptosis in our practice with few exceptions is levator advancement. This versatile procedure can be used on patients with all but the most severe impairment in levator function. At the time of ptosis surgery, we explore the levator muscle and aponeurosis to determine anatomic relationships and try to use existing anatomy to obtain more favorable eyelid position. The effectiveness of this approach can be verified at the time of surgery, and the adequacy of eyelid curve and contour can be ascertained simultaneously. External surgery also allows the surgeon to remove excess skin and fat which often improve the aesthetic outcome.

Levator advancement

This procedure is the most common technique of ptosis surgery in our practice [20]. For adults, monitored anesthesia is recommended to be able to adjust lid height with the patient's cooperation. Patients with dry eyes are usually better served with a modest correction instead of a maximum correction.

Anesthetic eye drops are instilled in each eye. The patient's natural eyelid crease is marked using a sterile marking pen and symmetry to the fellow eyelid crease is verified (Fig. 10A), after which 0.5 to 1.0 mL of local anesthetic is injected subcutaneously and allowed to diffuse using gentle massage. The patient is prepped and draped in the usual sterile manner. A skin incision is made in the marked eyelid crease site. The edges of the orbicularis are tented upward with two 0.5 tissue forceps (Fig. 10B). A skin muscle flap is dissected superiorly, exposing the point of fusion of the levator with the septum, and continued till preaponeurotic fat is visualized beneath the septum. This natural anatomic plane can be dissected either with a cautery, a scissors, or bluntly with a cotton tip. The septum over the pre-aponeurotic fat pad is incised with sharp Wescott and opened completely. The pre-aponeurotic fat is then swept off the aponeurosis gently. The superior tarsal border is exposed and the levator aponeurosis is then dissected off the superior aspect of the tarsus using Wescott scissors (Figs. 10C and 10D). The inferior edge of the aponeurosis is grasped and dissected off Muller's muscle by moving the aponeurosis edge superiorly and inferiorly. A nonabsorbable suture such as 6-0 silk on a tapered or spatulated cutting needle is used to attach the levator aponeurosis to the superior tarsal border, creating an edge-to-edge reapproximation of the levator aponeurosis to the tarsal leading edge (Figs. 10E and 10F). The knot is secured with a slip knot initially. The eyelid is everted to assure the surgeon that no penetration of the needle through conjunctiva occurs; if it does, the needle should be removed and repassed. The patient is then asked to open and close the eyes. Contour is best assessed with the patient sitting

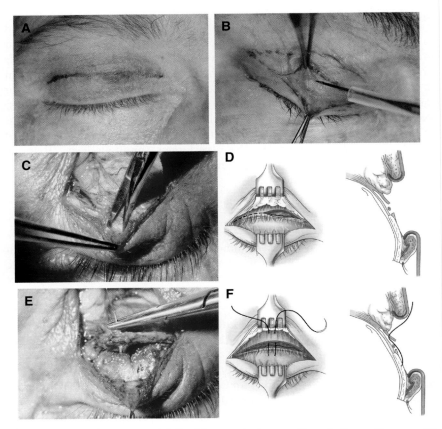

Fig. 10. Levator advancement. (*A*) Eyelid crease is drawn with a sterile marking pen. (*B*) Tenting of the orbicularis to facilitate dissection of the muscle from the orbital septum. (*C,D*) Identification of the superior tarsal border. (*E,F*) Passage of a nonabsorbable suture through the levator aponeurosis.

up, though it is often difficult to do this in the partially sedated patient unless it is planned for in the intraoperative period, the surgical table allows it, and sterility is assured. A slight overcorrection of 1 to 1.5 mm is desired.

If the eyelid is still ptotic, an advancement of the levator aponeurosis on the front surface of the tarsus is performed. A larger bite of aponeurosis is now taken, and this leading edge is advanced and attached to the front surface of the tarsus in horizontal mattress fashion, performing an edge-to-edge imbrication of advanced levator onto the tarsus. Again, the edges are tied in a single slip knot. The leading edge of the levator is trimmed once eyelid height and contour have been verified in the upright position.

The contralateral side is operated simultaneously so that both sides can be assessed, because the laws of reciprocal innervation apply both postoperatively and in the operating room [7]. The authors prefer to attach the levator using a single suture technique; many surgeons may prefer to secure the levator using two to three sutures.

Once eyelid height and contour have been verified and symmetry is created, the sutures are trimmed when the desired height is achieved. A blepharoplasty can also be performed at this time if needed. The skin is closed with several 6-0 absorbable interrupted sutures, incorporating a small bite of aponeurosis to reform the eyelid crease. A 6-0 running suture is then used to close the skin and antibiotic ointment is applied both into the eyes and onto the surfaces of the wounds (Figs. 11 and 12).

Levator advancement surgery in children is performed in much the same manner, though intraoperative assessment is more difficult without the patient's cooperation while under general anesthesia. As a consequence, the results can be more unpredictable because the level of the eyelid cannot be checked intraoperatively. There are two popular methods used to estimate the amount of levator advancement necessary. Levator function can be used to assess the amount of surgery function technique, which bases the height on the levator function [6]. If the levator function is 5 to 6 mm, the height of the lid is adjusted to the desired level and fissure height; in situations in which levator function is less, the lid must be adjusted higher. An alternative to this approach involves using MRD_1 to calculate the amount of levator advancement. With this technique, the levator is advanced a specific amount based on the patient's preoperative MRD [6].

Levator resection

Levator resection is a procedure that can be used in children who have congenital ptosis or in adults who have acquired ptosis. The amount of

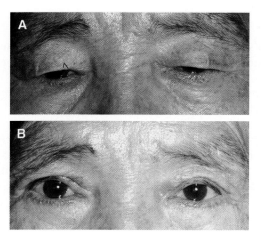

Fig. 11. A 61-year-old patient showing bilateral aponeurotic ptosis preoperatively (*A*) and after levator advancement surgery (*B*).

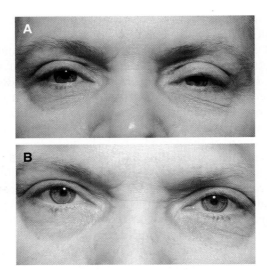

Fig. 12. A 63-year-old patient showing bilateral but asymmetric aponeurotic ptosis pre-operatively (*A*) and after levator advancement surgery (*B*).

levator resected is determined preoperatively by levator function and the level of ptosis. Dissection is often extensive and involves dissecting the levator from the underlying Muller's muscle and the conjunctiva, as well as disruption of the medial and lateral horns of the levator. Because the authors are often are able to achieve our aesthetic and reconstructive aims with advancement surgery or Whitnall's slings, both less invasive procedures, levator function is not performed in our practice.

Whitnall's sling

A Whitnall's sling is performed in a similar manner to levator advancement surgery. It is used in patients with ptosis with poor levator function and as an alternative to brow suspension.

The eyelid crease is marked, local anesthesia is administered, the eyelid is incised, the orbital septum is incised, and the levator aponeurosis is identified. Whitnall's ligament is identified and the aponeurosis is separated from Muller's muscle as in levator advancement. A permanent silk or nylon suture is then passed through Whitnall's ligament and is attached directly to the superior border of the tarsus. Closure is the same as in the levator advancement procedure.

Conjunctivo-mullerectomy

If a patient has a positive response to 2.5% or 10% Neosynephrine, a mullerectomy can be performed to correct a mild to moderate amount of ptosis. After administering local anesthesia, the eyelid is everted over a desmarres retractor. Two 4-0 silk sutures are placed at the lateral and medial aspect of the conjunctiva and Muller's muscle and held at a 45° angle to tent the conjunctiva and Muller's muscle. A Putterman mullerectomy clamp (Karl Ilg, Chicago, IL) is placed to incorporate Muller's muscle and conjunctiva only. Local anesthesia is injected to balloon up and separate Muller's muscle from the levator aponeurosis. A double-armed suture is passed from lateral to medial through conjunctiva and Muller's muscle. A 15 blade is used to remove the conjunctiva and Muller's just inferior to the suture. The sutures are then weaved back through the conjunctival edges in running fashion, being careful to avoid exposure of the suture to prevent corneal irritation. The ends of the suture are brought anterior through the skin and loosely tied over the eyelid crease. Often a collagen shield is placed to protect the cornea.

New algorithms are created as techniques are created or improved. A fairly easy algorithm to use for ptotic patients with a positive Neo-synephrine test has been developed. The formula estimates the amount of conjunctiva and Muller's muscle to be resected. The formula is 9 mm of conjunctiva and Muller's plus x mm of tarsus, where x is equal to the distance of ptosis undercorrection after phenylephrine testing. The study presenting the rew formula had a 0% overcorrection rate and a 3% reoperative rate [21].

Tarsoconjunctival/superior tarsal resection

Tarsoconjunctival/superior tarsal resection or the modified Fasanella-Servat procedure is a surgical option for patients who have mild ptosis and good levator function such as in Horner's syndrome. This procedure is not recommended for patients who have moderate dry eye, because a portion of the conjunctiva and basic tear secretors will be resected [1,6].

Because of this objection, we have not performed this procedure in practice over the past 20 years, though it is employed by many surgeons and will be described below for completeness.

The procedure is performed after the upper eyelid is injected with local anesthetic. The eyelid is everted over a Desmarres retractor. Two small curved hemostats are used to grasp conjunctiva, Muller's muscle, tarsus, and occasionally a small amount of levator fibers (Fig. 13A). The hemostats are placed on the tarsus about 3 mm from the superior edge with the blades of the hemostats running parallel to the tarsus border. A 5-0 suture with a reverse cutting needle is passed from medial to lateral through the eyelid approximately 1 to 1.5 mm above the hemostats (Fig. 13B). The hemostats are removed and the tissue is removed above the suture in the midportion of the clamped area (Fig. 13C). One must be careful to avoid cutting the running suture. The suture is then passed lateral to medial within the crushed remaining tissue. Both needles are passed through the anterior

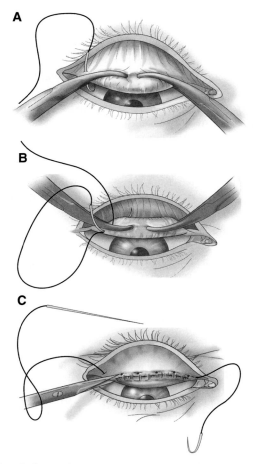

Fig. 13. Tarsoconjunctival resection. (*A*) Two clamps are placed to grasp the conjunctiva, Muller's muscle, and superior tarsus. (*B*) The running suture is passed through all three tissues. (*C*) The clamped tissue is excised while making sure the suture is not cut.

surface of the eyelid skin and tied loosely across the upper eyelid. The final results can be seen in 2 weeks to 2 months.

Frontalis sling

The frontalis sling is commonly used to treat a ptotic child or adult with poor levator and good frontalis function [6,7]. The purpose of the procedure is to use a sling material such as silicon or autogenous or allograft fascia lata to connect the upper eyelid tarsus to the frontalis muscle [6,7]. The patient then employs the frontalis muscle to open the eyelid. The choice of sling material depends on the age of the patient and the duration of the need for the sling. Fascia lata can be harvested from the patient's thigh or obtained from a fascia bank.

Two sling strips are usually needed for each eyelid. Fascia lata harvested from the patient is normally long enough to be used after a child has grown past the age of 4. Silicone or suture slings can be used in small children until their growth allows fascia to be harvested [7].

The surgery is usually performed under general anesthesia for children and monitored anesthesia in cooperative adults.

To obtain fascia, a 3-cm skin incision is made on the lower lateral thigh with the leg and foot internally rotated after infiltration with local anesthetic. The incision is made 1 cm above the knee in a line between the anterior iliac crest and the head of the fibula in adults and adolescents and 2 cm above the knee along the same line in children [21]. The incision is made above the knee joint in an imaginary line between the head of the fibula and the anterior superior iliac spine (Fig. 14A). The skin and subcutaneous tissue is dissected to reveal the fascia lata, which is white. A scalpel is used to make parallel incisions on the fascia about 5 to 8 mm apart. A long scissors is passed between the plane of the fascia and subcutaneous tissue superiorly and beneath the fascia. A fascia stripper can then be inserted and the fascia is thread into the stripper (Fig. 14B). The fascia is severed with the sharp edge of the stripper or a blade, then removed. The usual length is about 10 cm. The fascia is then cleaned of connective tissue and can be divided into 2- to 3-mm strips to be used for ptosis repair (Fig. 14C). The fascia layer does not have to be closed. The site is closed with deep subcutaneous sutures and skin closure with staples or sutures. Steri-strips followed by a pressure dressing are then applied. Ambulation can resume 12 to 24 hours after surgery.

The strip can be positioned in the shape of a pentagon using only one strip (Fox technique) or using two strips shaping each one in the shape of the triangle (Crawford technique) [22]. The Crawford technique, the authors' preferred technique, will be described herein.

The placement of the strips begins with marking of the incision site (Figs. 14D and 14E). Using a sterile marking pen, the eyelid crease is marked. Three additional marks are made: one approximately at the level of the superior brow hairs nasal to the pupil 1 to 2 cm, one approximately above the lateral canthus immediately above the brow hairs, and one just lateral to the medial canthus above the brow hairs. Local anesthesia with adrenaline is then injected and the patient is prepped and draped in the usual fashion. A #15 blade is used to incise skin down through the dermis to the subcutaneous plane at the three premarked brow incisions, beveling the blade so as to avoid injury to the brow hair follicles. The incision is then dissected to the level of the frontalis using a blunt scissors.

An eyelid crease incision is made through skin and is deepened through the orbicularis and septum to identify the levator muscle/aponeurosis, which can be rudimentary in the case of patients who have severe ptosis. The

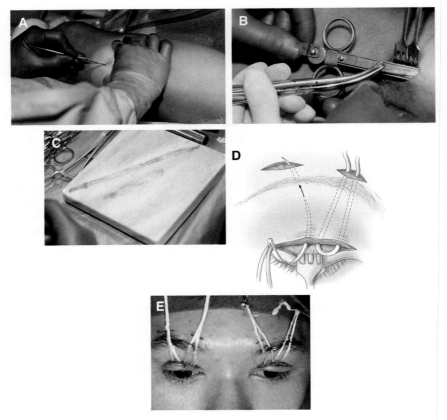

Fig. 14. Fascial sling procedure. (*A*) Incision of the leg. (*B*) Harvesting of the fascia with the stripper. (*C*) Cutting the strips into the correct size. (*D,E*) Correct placement of the fascial slings in the Crawford technique.

superior half of the tarsus is exposed by sharp dissection. The central aspect of the sling is sutured to the upper third of the tarsus in the point of greatest curvature in the eyelid, slightly nasal to the pupil. It is then sutured medially to the tarsus, slightly medial to the limbus. The second strip is attached to the tarsus at the peak, the two strips are overlapped, and the second strip is sutured approximately at the level of the lateral limbus. The strips are then passed with a large cutting free needle or a fascia passer under the septum, out the corresponding brow incisions laterally, and sutured to the frontalis after checking eyelid contour. The location of the fascia with respect to the frontalis may be altered with suture to achieve symmetry and contour. The skin crease incision is then closed with interrupted 6-0 absorbable sutures, attaching the skin directly to the fascia to create an eyelid crease. The interrupted sutures can be used to form an eyelid crease by passing the suture through the skin edge, incorporating a small bite of tarsus and then passing it out the other skin edge. A running 6-0 absorbable suture is then placed. The strips are then pulled superiorly to adjust the lid height at the level of the superior limbus. Each strip is tied with a square knot over a piece of 5-0 nonabsorbable suture and fixated to frontalis to assure that the knot will not slip. One end of the strip is then cut 1 cm from the knot and each long end is then passed out the central brow incision with the passer or the free needle. The two long sides are then tied and the ends are trimmed. The ends under the frontalis muscle with forceps and the brow incisions are closed with 6-0 nonabsorbable nylon or prolene sutures. A frost suture can be placed to prevent exposure in the early postoperative period (Fig. 15A, B).

Silicone slings

A silicone rod can also be used instead of fascia with a few differences in the procedure. A single rod is used so it is attached to the tarsus and passed through the same marked incisions and/or overlapped over a silicone sleeve that is sutured to the central brow incision. Silicone is a good choice in patients that require adjustment, such as patients who have myopathic ptosis or severe ptosis accompanying dry eye. Silicone can easily be adjusted with a small incision in the central forehead incision,

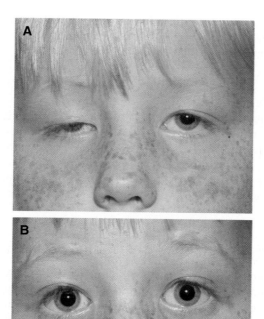

Fig. 15. A 5-year-old patient showing right-sided congenital ptosis preoperatively (*A*) and after ptosis surgery with a fascial sling (*B*).

and either tightened or loosened. The silicone does not scar into the tissues as much as fascia, making it easier to adjust or remove, but it can become infected. It also may cheese wire through tissue, making it less effective over time.

Special cases

Unilateral ptosis in Marcus Gunn syndrome

Patients who have Marcus Gunn syndrome have a unilateral ptosis and other problems to address other than the ptosis. When the ipsilateral pterygoid muscle is stimulated, the ptotic eyelid retracts and makes the ptosis improve [17]. The treatment of the ptosis can be addressed with the Fasanella-Servat procedure (in patients with good levator function), but this often worsens the eyelid retraction associated with jaw movement. More commonly, some type of sling procedure is required. The surgeon has multiple options that often must be discussed with the parents. A unilateral sling may be performed, or bilateral surgery can also be performed, which improves the overall asymmetry. In this situation, either disinsertion of the abnormally innervated levator either alone or accompanied by the contralateral disinsertion of the normal levator can be performed [17]. According to one study, the best procedure is performing a bilateral fascial sling procedure with a disinsertion of the contralateral (the nonptotic side) levator muscle [17]. Most parents in our practice, however, prefer not to have the contralateral normal levator disturbed, at least at the time of the primary procedure.

Third-nerve palsy

Most patients with a third-nerve palsy are more concerned about the motility abnormality than the ptosis. The ptosis surgery may not be performed if the motility abnormality cannot be corrected, because the patient may experience diplopia. The ptosis is usually best corrected with a frontalis sling or levator advancement [7]. All patients must be evaluated for aberrant regeneration before ptosis surgery to select the correct surgical procedure.

Unilateral ptosis

Unilateral ptosis should be managed based on its etiology and the levator function. Preoperative evaluation is especially important in these patients so that the surgeon can ascertain that the ptosis is truly unilateral. Often correction of a unilateral acquired ptosis will reveal a contralateral ptosis, especially if the dominant eye is ptotic, as the drive to elevate the fellow eye will disappear once the dominant eye ptosis is corrected. In patients who have severe unilateral ptosis, it is often difficult to make both eyes "match," because even when the eyes are symmetric in the primary position, lid closure may be compromised and ptosis will remain in upgaze.

Any of these ptosis procedures can be combined with blepharoplasty if redundant skin or fat is present. Blepharoplasty techniques are discussed elsewhere in this issue.

New advances

Small incision surgery

Small incision surgery consists of a levator advancement or resection with an incision only 8 mm in length instead of across the entire length of the upper eyelid [23]. The surgery is performed as the regular levator advancement surgery, except that extra skin and fat are not excised. Patients needing a blepharoplasty or who have had prior eyelid surgery are not ideal candidates for this procedure [23]. The goal of the minimal incision surgery is to speed recovery time [23].

Adjustable suture surgery

Given the inherent inaccuracy of adjustable techniques, the possibility of performing this surgery on adjustable sutures is an intriguing one and has been explored by several investigators [3]. The theory behind the adjustable suture is to decrease the amount of reoperations. One recent technique uses a "hang-back" suture similar to the adjustable suture that is used in adult strabismus surgery [3]. A double-armed 5-0 silk suture is passed horizontally, incorporating a bite of midline aponeurosis 5 to 6 mm in length. The suture ends are passed through the tarsus 6 to 10 mm apart, straddling the midline of the tarsus. The suture is tied loosely in a bow and is brought to the skin surface, where it is secured with a prolene suture. The patient uses ice compresses at home and undergoes adjustment by postoperative day 4. The results from these initial studies are encouraging, with somewhat lower reoperation rates [3].

Postoperative care

The authors usually recommend applying ice compresses to the eyelids for 48 to 72 hours after surgery and applying an ophthalmic antibiotic ointment to the incisions twice a day for 3 days. The patient can shower the day after surgery, taking care not to let the water from the shower head hit directly on the eyelids. The authors also recommend that the patient avoid exercise or heavy lifting for 2 weeks. Patients can resume their preoperative prescriptions medicines the day after surgery—with the exception of blood thinners, which can be resumed at 2 weeks, unless they are deemed essential by the patient's internist.

Complications of ptosis surgery

The most common "complications" of ptosis surgery are not true complications but instead are part of the inherent inaccuracy of the procedure; that is, undercorrections and overcorrections [1]. The rate of occurrence of overcorrections or undercorrections varies from 5% to 35% depending on the series. In the authors' experience, undercorrections are much more frequent than overcorrections. Overcorrections are more worrisome because in addition to the inherent cosmetic defect, patients can suffer from exposure keratopathy and are frequently uncomfortable. Overcorrection is usually more common in bilateral, aponeurotic ptosis; undercorrection is more common in congenital ptosis [4]. Massaging the eyelid downward may resolve or reduce an overcorrection [18]. Reoperating on patients with overcorrections should be done within 2 weeks of the original surgery after edema has resolved but before scarring has taken place [1,4,24].

True complications in ptosis surgery can also be seen accompanying overcorrections, making this postoperative state undesirable. These include lagophthalmos, lid lag, exposure keratitis, corneal ulceration, and visual loss [1].

Lagophthalmos can occur in the absence of overcorrection if sutures incorporate the septum and the levator aponeurosis, resulting in a "hangup" with eyelid closure [1]. Exposure keratitis can cause permanent vision loss and should be treated aggressively. Lubrication with artificial tears and ointments, bandage contact lenses, moisture shields, and temporary tarsorraphy can help treat the problem. If these more conservative approaches do not work, overcorrection surgery with levator recession is indicated [1]. The decision to reoperate is usually made within 2 to 6 months after the original surgery [1,6]. Studies by Dortzbach and colleagues [25], however, have shown that lid height 1 week postoperatively is comparable to that at 3 months postoperatively; thus there is a rationale to early revision within the first week of surgery, when tissue planes are freshly created. This principle is often used in the authors' practice in the willing patient with overcorrection.

Hemorrhage in the postoperative period can negate the improvement following ptosis surgery and also cause vision loss. All patients should be warned about increasing swelling, bleeding, postoperative pain, and vision changes signaling hemorrhage [1,7]. Any of these occurrences should be reported to the physician immediately. Meticulous hemostasis should be maintained throughout the surgery to avoid this problem. Patients should also discontinue all blood thinners for 2 weeks before and 2 weeks after surgery with their doctor's permission. If a patient has a tense or tight orbit and eyelids, proptosis, vision changes, or pupillary defect after surgery, the original surgical incision should be opened and all bleeding stopped with cautery before reclosure. An emergent canthotomy and cantholysis of the lateral canthal tendon can be performed but usually is not necessary once bleeding is controlled.

Infection can occur but is unlikely, because the eyelids have an excellent blood supply. To avoid problems, many surgeons recommend application of an antibiotic ointment to the incision site during the immediate postoperative period [1,6,7]. Moist healing has been shown to be the quickest means of healing, and we recommend the use of occlusive ointments in the first 48 hours postoperatively. Blepharitis should be resolved or minimized before surgery to lessen the risk of infection.

Another important complication is the temporary change in vision after ptosis surgery [25]. Rarely, this change can be permanent [26]. The etiology of visual change relates to astigmatism from changes in the cornea related to the change in eyelid position. Most patients will have some degree of persistent astigmatism 3 months after surgery, but most have resolved by 12 months [26].

Other important but uncommon complications include entropion, ectropion, eyelid crease abnormality, lid margin notching, eyelash loss, symblepharon, conjunctival prolapse, and diplopia from damage to the superior rectus or oblique muscle [1,7].

Notching or tarsal kinks usually occur due to poor release of adjacent levator tissue, or advancement too far down on the front surface of the tarsus, and are a consequence of overly ambitious levator advancement. Ectropion and conjunctival prolapse can also be seen when aponeurotic advancement is overly robust. Management often involves takedown of the original procedure, excision of a small portion of tarsus, or excision of conjunctival prolapse.

All potential complications should be discussed with the patient before surgery. The risk of reoperation should be emphasized, because patients who submit themselves to a surgical procedure with the expectation of taking care of the problem with a single surgery are often discouraged to be informed that further intervention is required.

References

[1] Schaefer AJ, Schaefer DP. Classification and correction of ptosis. In: Stewart WB, editor. Surgery of the eyelid, orbit, and lacrimal system. American Academy of Ophthalmology; 1994. p. 84–133.
[2] Bullock JD, et al. Psychosocial implications of blepharoptosis and dermatochalasis. Trans Am Ophthalm Soc 2001;99:65–71.
[3] Meltzer MA, Elahi E, Taupeka P, et al. A simplified technique of ptosis repair using a single adjustable suture. Ophthalmology 2001;108:1889–92.
[4] McCulley TJ, Kersten RC, Kulwin DR, et al. Outcome and influencing factors of external levator palpebrae superioris advancement for blepharoptosis. Ophthal Plast Reconstr Surg 2003;19:388–93.
[5] Whitehous GM, Grigg JR, Martin FS. Congenital ptosis; results of surgical management. Aust N Z J Ophthalmol 1995;23:309–14.

[6] Nerad JA. Evaluation and treatment of the patient with ptosis. In: Krachner JH, editor. Oculoplastic surgery the requisites in ophthalmology. St. Louis (MO): Mosby Inc.; 2001. p. 157–92.

[7] Putman JR, Nunery WR, Tanenbaum M, et al. Blepharoptosis. In: McCord CD Jr, Tanenbaum M, Nunery WR, editors. Oculoplastic surgery. New York: Raven Press; 1985. p. 175–220.

[8] Yanoff M, Duker JS. Ophthalmology. London: Mosby; 1999.

[9] Larned DC, Flanagan JC, et al. The association of congenital ptosis and congenital heart disease. Ophthalmology 1986;93:492–4.

[10] Bartlett SP, Mackay GJ. Craniosynostosis syndromes. In: Aston SJ, Beasley RW, Thorne CHN, editors. Grabb and Smith's plastic surgery. Philadelphia: Lippencott-Raven; 1997. p. 295–304.

[11] Wolfort FG, Poblete JV. Ptosis after blepharoplasty. Ann Plas Surg 1995;34:64–6.

[12] Lemke BN, Stasior OG, Rosenberg PN. The surgical relations of the levator palpebral superioris muscle. Ophthal Plast Reconstr Surg 1988;4:25–30.

[13] Tomsak RL, Levine MR. Handbook of neuro-ophthalmology and orbital disease. Philadelphia: Butterworth Heinemann; 2004.

[14] Weinberg DA, Lesser RL, Vollmer TL. Ocular myasthenia: a protean disorder. Surv Ophthalmol 1994;39:169–210.

[15] Renowden SA, Harris KM, Hourihan MD. Isolated atraumatic third nerve palsy. Br J Radiol 1993;66:1111–7.

[16] Lyon DB, Gonnering RS, Dortzbach RK, et al. Unilateral ptosis and eye dominance. Ophthal Plast Reconstr Surg 1993;9:237–40.

[17] Doucet TW, Crawford JS. The quantification, natural course, and surgical treatment; results in 57 patients with myasthenia gravis syndrome. Am J Ophthalmol 1981;92:702–5.

[18] Riemann CD, Hanson S, Foster JA. A comparison of manual kinetic and automated static perimetry in obtaining ptosis visual fields. Arch Ophthalmol 2000;118:65–9.

[19] Meyer DR, Stern JH, Jarvis JM, et al. Evaluating the visual field effects of blepharoptosis using automated static perimetry. Ophthalm 1993;100:651–8.

[20] Wulc AE. Oculoplastic surgery, an overview. J Derm Surg Oncol 1992;18:1033–8.

[21] Perry JD, Kadakia A, Foster JA. A new algorithm for ptosis repair using conjunctival Mullerectomy with or without tarsectomy. Ophthal Plast Reconstr Surg 2002;18:426–9.

[22] Jordan DR, Anderson RL. Obtaining fascia lata. Arch Ophthal 1987;105:1139–40.

[23] Lucarelli MJ, Lemke BN. Small incision external levator repair: technique and early results. Am J Ophthalm 1999;127:637–44.

[24] Mauriello JA Jr, Abdelsalam A. Modified levator advancement with delayed postoperative office revision. Ophthal Plast Reconstr Surg 1998;14:266–70.

[25] Dortzbach RK, Kronish JW. Early revision in the office for adults after unsatisfactory blepharoptosis correction. Am J Ophthalm 1993;115:68–75.

[26] Shao W, Byrne P, Harrison A, et al. Persistent blurred vision after blepharoplasty and ptosis repair. Arch Facial Plast Surg 2004;6:155–7.

ELSEVIER
SAUNDERS

Otolaryngol Clin N Am
38 (2005) 947–984

OTOLARYNGOLOGIC
CLINICS
OF NORTH AMERICA

Comprehensive Management of Eyebrow and Forehead Ptosis

Jonathan A. Hoenig, MD[a,b]

[a]Private Practice, 5400 Balboa Boulevard, #127, Encino, CA 91316, USA
[b]Jules Stein Eye Institute, University of California-Los Angeles Medical Center,
Los Angeles, CA, USA

The forehead and eyebrows are under the constant influence of downward forces of gravity and the periorbital protractor muscles (orbicularis oculi, procerus, corrugator, and depressor supercilii). These downward forces are opposed by the elevating action of the frontalis muscle. In time, this constant "tug of war" between the downward and upward forces leads to a series of wrinkles in the forehead and downward displacement of the eyebrows and eyelids (Fig. 1).

The inferior displacement of the eyebrows results in apparent redundancy of the upper eyelid skin and hooding in the multicontoured areas of the medial and lateral canthal regions. Patients often present to the aesthetic surgeon complaining of dermatochalasis and request blepharoplasty. When the eyebrows are raised to their normal position, however, there is often less redundant upper eyelid skin than anticipated and blepharoplasty may not be necessary or appropriate [1,2].

Correction of the redundancy in the periorbital multicontoured regions represents a great challenge to the aesthetic surgeon. It is imperative that the surgeon and patient understand that excision of the upper eyelid and lateral canthal skin without elevating or fixating the eyebrow pulls the eyebrow down. This results in further ptosis of the eyebrows and canthal webbing [3,4]. This can give the eyebrows an appearance of being sutured to the eyelids (Fig. 2). The re-establishment of the structural integrity of the eyebrow is fundamental to achieving an aesthetically acceptable surgical result for cosmetic and functional periocular surgery [5]. For these reasons, an increasing percentage of blepharoplasties are performed in conjunction with eyebrow lifts [6].

E-mail address: hoeing@msn.com

0030-6665/05/$ - see front matter © 2005 Elsevier Inc. All rights reserved.
doi:10.1016/j.otc.2005.05.006
oto.theclinics.com

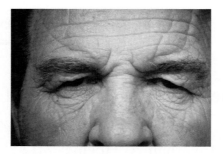

Fig. 1. Classic "squinter and squeezer." This patient demonstrates periorbital and forehead rhytids and eyebrow ptosis.

Eyebrow structure and position

Facial expression is determined by the contour and position of the eyebrows and mouth. Although we may not consciously be aware of a person's eyebrow position, we subconsciously assess eyebrow shape and thereby determine a person's mood. Changing eyebrow position changes the entire facial expression. For example, low and flat eyebrows that hang over the eyes denote fatigue. Eyebrows that are low laterally give a sad appearance. Eyebrows that are low medially denote anger, and properly positioned and slightly arched eyebrows denote happiness (Fig. 3).

It is difficult to describe a "normal" or "abnormal" eyebrow position and contour. As one looks through our popular fashion magazines, we can easily see that eyebrows come in all shapes and sizes. In fact, the aesthetically pleasing eyebrow varies with the times, styles, and cultures. Even within one racial group and one sex, there are totally different combinations of normal structural arrangements that society recognizes as beautiful [6,7].

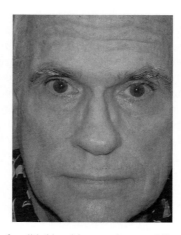

Fig. 2. Excessive resection of eyelid skin without eyebrow stabilization leads to the appearance of the eyebrows being sutured to the eyelids.

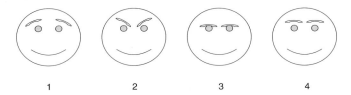

Fig. 3. This drawing illustrates the role of brow position in facial expression: 1 denotes a sad mood, 2 denotes an angry mood, 3 denotes a tired look, and 4 denotes a happy look.

Despite the variety of eyebrow shapes and sizes, there are still some general principles that are common to all aesthetically pleasing eyebrows. In men and women, the youthful eyebrow tends to be full and projects anteriorly from the bone. This fullness is secondary to the suborbicularis fat pad known as the retro-orbicularis oculi fat (ROOF). In general, the female eyebrow has a high arch, whereas the male eyebrow is flatter with a lesser arch. The high point of the female brow lies along a vertical line that intersects the lateral limbus when the eye is in the primary position.

Patient evaluation

All patients who are considering eyebrow and forehead surgery require a thorough history and physical examination. It is important to ask patients if they are taking aspirin, nonsteroidal anti-inflammatory medications, vitamin E, or herbal supplements. Many of these medications and supplements have an effect on platelet function, which can lead to increased bleeding and prolonged clotting time. Patients are questioned for a history of tearing, chronic ocular irritation, or a "sandy" sensation of their eyes. This could represent dry eyes and may be a contraindication for surgery.

A physical examination, including measurement of visual acuity, tear film evaluation, corneal status, and a 5-minute basal tear secretion test, is performed. Frontalis and orbicularis muscle strength is assessed as well as the position and contour of the eyebrows and eyelids. The eyebrows are manually elevated to their proper anatomic position, allowing the surgeon and patient to see if and how much excess eyelid skin is present. The distance between the superior cilia of the eyebrow and the hairline is measured. In general, distances greater than 6 cm indicate that the patient has a "long" forehead. Because some eyebrow elevation techniques displace the hairline superiorly, it is imperative that forehead length be determined before surgery. In patients with long foreheads, a technique that shortens the forehead length while raising the eyebrows should be considered. It is also imperative to examine the scalp and determine if there is any evidence of alopecia. Men with a history of male-pattern baldness and women with thinning hair may not be candidates for certain eyebrow lifting procedures.

Malposition of the eyebrows can often be overlooked. Many patients reflexively raise the eyebrows with their frontalis muscles to lift the eyebrow and eyelid tissue out of the visual axis. These patients develop furrows in the forehead region because of the constant contraction of the frontalis muscles. It is the surgeon's task to ensure that the patient's frontalis muscles are completely relaxed before assessing the eyebrow position [8]. The position of the upper eyelid must also be carefully assessed, because eyelid ptosis invariably results in recruitment of the frontalis muscle to raise the eyebrow and the eyelid (Fig. 4). Patients with eyelid ptosis almost always have eyebrow malposition. Unfortunately, if the patient is not examined properly before surgery, this eyebrow malposition is not discovered until after the eyelids have been raised.

Eyebrow malposition can be easily assessed by asking the patient to bring in photographs from each decade of his or her life. The patient and doctor can then determine how the eyebrow position has changed. Some patients realize that their eyebrows have been low their entire life. These congenital low-eyebrow patients may wish to augment their normal look by having their eyebrows raised to a higher and more pleasing position. The patient's skin type is assessed, and the different skin types are reviewed with the patient. Patients with thick oily skin can expect less improvement than patients with thinner and smoother skin. Fair-complexioned patients are informed that their incision scars are likely to be more erythematous and raised than in other patients.

As part of the physical examination digital and Polaroid photographs are taken from front, side, and oblique views. The Polaroid pictures are reviewed with the patient. Polaroid snapshots also have an added benefit in that their use avoids the difficulties of explaining surgical goals while looking in the mirror. Polaroid pictures are also hung in the operating room at the time of surgery, adding perspective to the repositioning of the eyelids and eyebrows at the time of surgery.

Once the surgeon and patient have decided on surgery, the anticipated postoperative course is discussed. Patients should expect to be swollen and bruised for several weeks. Stitches, staples, and screws are usually removed

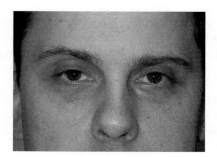

Fig. 4. This patient has right upper eyelid ptosis. He elevates his right eyebrow to compensate for the ptosis. When the ptosis is corrected, the stimulus to open the eye is decreased and the eyebrow falls.

within 7 to 14 days. Patients are advised to refrain from wearing contact lenses during the initial healing process. A written consent form is signed after reviewing the realities, risks, complications, and expectations. An extensive list of medications and supplements that increase bleeding is given to the patient. The patients are informed that these medications must not be taken for 2 weeks before and 1 week after surgery.

Forehead and eyebrow anatomy

From a surgical anatomic standpoint, it is probably best to divide the forehead and scalp into central and lateral portions. The temporal line, the insertion of the temporalis muscle onto the skull, is the boundary between the central and lateral portions. Centrally, the scalp consists of five layers. The first layer is the skin, which tends to be quite thick and well vascularized. The next layer is a subcutaneous layer of fibrofatty tissue that is densely adherent to the skin and underlying muscle. The middle layer consists of the galea aponeurotica, which is a tendinous aponeurosis that forms a sheath around the frontalis muscles. The fourth layer consists of loose areolar tissue that connects the galea aponeurosis to the periosteum of the skull. This relatively avascular layer provides an excellent dissection plane in cosmetic surgery. The deepest layer is the periosteum of the skull and is known as the pericranium. The layers of the scalp can be remembered by the mnemonic SCALP: S for skin, C for connective tissue, A for aponeurosis, L for loose areolar tissue, and P for pericranium.

Laterally, the anatomy is slightly more complex and variable (Fig. 5). The lateral scalp consists of skin, subcutaneous tissue, and the temporalis muscle with its fascial coverings. The temporalis muscle is a fan-shaped muscle that originates from the temporal line on the side of the skull. Inferiorly, it becomes tendinous and inserts onto the mandible. The temporalis is a muscle of mastication and is innervated by cranial nerve V. The muscle is covered by several layers of fascia—the superficial and deep temporal fascias. The terminology of the fascial layers is quite confusing and variable throughout the literature (Table 1) [9–12]. The superficial temporal fascia is continuous with the galea aponeurosis and contains the superficial temporal artery, the frontal branch of the facial nerve, and the auriculotemporal nerve. The superficial temporal fascia is separated from the deep temporal fascia by loose areolar tissue, which is sometimes known as the subgaleal fascia. The deep temporal fascia is thick and has a white glistening surface. Several centimeters above the zygomatic arch, the deep temporal fascia (temporal fascia proper) splits into two layers. These layers are called the intermediate temporal fascia and the deep temporal fascia. The intermediate fascia inserts onto the anterosuperior aspect of the zygomatic arch, whereas the deep temporalis fascia inserts onto the posterosuperior aspect of the arch. Located between these two layers is a fat pad known as the intermediate temporal fat pad or Yasergill's fat pad [13]. Dissection in the

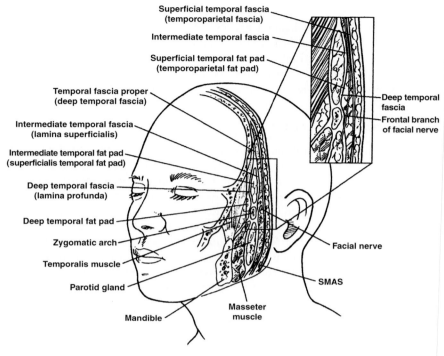

Fig. 5. Anatomy of the temporal region.

temporal region is along the intermediate deep temporal fascia so as to avoid injury to the temporal branch of the facial nerve.

A detailed understanding of the anatomy of the facial nerve [10,11,13–18] is essential to any surgeon who is performing facial surgery. Careful

Table 1
Nomenclature of fascial coverings of the temporalis muscle

Current nomenclature	Old nomenclature	Other nomenclature	Other nomenclature
Superficial temporal fascia	Temporoparietal fascia	Epicranial aponeurosis	Galeal extension
Subgaleal fascia	Areolar fascia	Innominate fascia	Subaponeurotic plane
Superficial temporal fat pad			
Temporal fascia proper	Deep temporal fascia	Temporal fascia	Investing fascia of temporalis
Intermediate temporal fascia	Superficial deep temporal fascia		Innominate fascia
Intermediate temporal fat pad	Superficial temporal fat pad		Yasergill's fat pad
Deep temporal fascia	Deep temporal fascia		

attention to anatomic landmarks and selection of safe dissection planes should greatly reduce the likelihood of damaging branches of this nerve. The branch of the facial nerve most vulnerable during brow lifting is the frontal branch. The frontal and zygomatic branches exit the parotid region and course over the zygomatic arch 1 to 2 cm anterior to the ear. The most posterior ramus lies anterior to the superficial temporal vessels, whereas the most anterior ramus is approximately 2 cm from the anterior end of the zygomatic arch [14,19]. At the temple, the nerve runs in the superficial temporal fascia approximately one fingerbreath above the eyebrow (Fig. 6). The zygomatic branches innervate the inferior portion of the orbicularis oculi muscle. The temporal branch supplies the anterior and superior auricular muscles, the frontal belly of the occipitofrontalis, the superior portion of the orbicularis oculi, and the corrugator muscles.

Sensory innervation to the scalp and eyebrow is derived from the supratrochlear and supraorbital nerves. Both nerves cross the orbital rim anterior to the periosteum and move into more superficial layers as they course superiorly. The supraorbital neurovascular bundle exits the orbit through a foramen in approximately one in four cases and through a notch in approximately three in four cases. There are up to four branches of the supratrochlear nerve, with considerable variability.

Forehead and eyebrow movement is governed by five sets of muscles: the occipitofrontalis, procerus, corrugator supercilii, orbicularis oculi, and depressor supercilii [9]. The occipitofrontalis muscle is the elevator of the eyebrow. The other four muscles are the depressors of the eyebrow.

The ROOF (Fig. 7) is a fat pad that lies posterior to the muscles of the eyebrow [17]. It is densely attached to the underlying periosteum of the

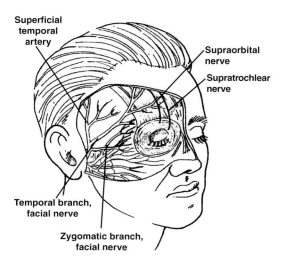

Fig. 6. Course of the temporal and zygomatic branches of the facial nerve.

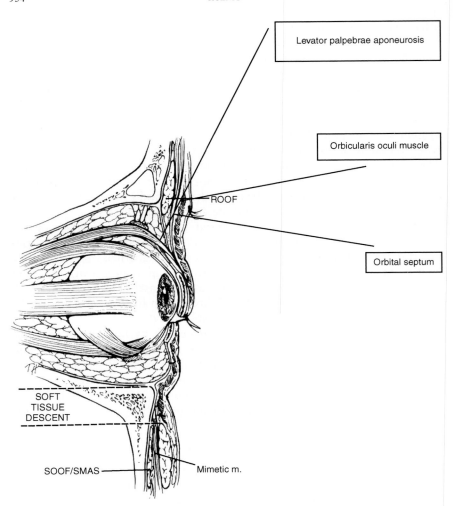

Fig 7. The subbrow fat pad, known as the ROOF, sits posterior to the orbital portion of the orbicularis oculi muscle. This fat pad atrophies and descends as we age, which results in aging in the periorbital region.

medial two thirds of the supraorbital ridge. The fat pad enhances motility by permitting vertical sliding of the overlying skin and muscle. It is most prominent laterally and may extend inferiorly into the suborbicularis preseptal plane of the upper eyelid.

Selection of surgical procedures

There are eight general types of eyebrow elevation procedures (Table 2): (1) standard direct eyebrow elevation, (2) paralytic eyebrow lift (variation of

Table 2
Forehead and eyebrow lifting procedures

Procedure	Advantages	Disadvantages
Direct eyebrow lift	Accurate and excellent elevation Corrects eyebrow asymmetry Vertically shortens forehead Low incidence of forehead hypesthesia	Possible visible scar Does not treat glabella region
Gull-wing direct	Same as above Treats medical eyebrow ptosis Treats glabellar region	Visible scar in glabellar region
Midforehead	Corrects eyebrow asymmetry Incision hidden in forehead furrows	Possible visible forehead scar May lower frontal hairline

Temporal lift	Improves the lateral eyebrow
	
	Lifts temporal region
	Scar hidden in hairline
		Does not address mideyebrow,
		  midforehead, or glabellar
		  regions

Coronal lift	Corrects eyebrow, forehead, and glabella Scar hidden in hairline	Large incision Possible alopecia Possible hypesthesia of scalp Moves hairline posteriorly Limited use in balding patients

Endoscopic
  coronal
	Corrects eyebrow, forehead,
	  and glabella
	Small incisions
	Can be used in balding patients
	Less hypesthesia and alopecia
		Special instrumentation required
		
		Moves hairline posteriorly

Eyebrowpexy	Performed through
	  blepharoplasty incision
	
	Prevents post blepharoplasty
	  eyebrow descent
		Limited eyebrow elevation
		
		Does not address medial eyebrow,
		  glabella, or forehead
		Pain around suture site

Orbicularis
  plication
	Performed through small
	  forehead incision
	Prevents post blepharoplasty
	  eyebrow descent
		Mild eyebrow elevation
		
		Does not address medial
		  eyebrow, glabella, or forehead

direct eyebrow lift), (3) orbicularis plication, (4) midforehead eyebrow lift, (5) temporal eyebrow lift, (6) coronal forehead and eyebrow lift, (7) endoscopic forehead and eyebrow lift, and (8) internal eyebrowpexy and transeyelid eyebrow lift.

Direct eyebrow lift

The direct eyebrow lift affords the greatest elevation per millimeter of tissue excised. It is useful in those men who do not select endoscopic eyebrow and forehead lifts and in whom coronal or temporal lifts are not advised because of the tendency toward, and progression of, male-pattern baldness. The standard direct eyebrow lift is an excellent procedure for lifting the lateral eyebrow in men and women. It removes skin superior to the eyebrow and therefore elevates the eyebrows and vertically shortens the forehead. It does not, however, address medial eyebrow ptosis, nor does it reduce vertical glabellar folds or significantly reduce horizontal folds. Its main drawback is that potential visible scarring can occur. It is usually reserved for men with full and dark eyebrow cilia (Fig. 8).

Direct eyebrow lift: paralytic eyebrow

Eyebrow ptosis may also be seen in patients with seventh nerve palsies. Surgical intervention is indicated when the eyebrow ptosis is long standing and reinnervation of the nerve has not occurred (Fig. 9). Because lagophthalmus is often present with seventh nerve palsies, it is imperative that eyelid closure be considered and that the eyebrow not be overly elevated. Furthermore, it is imperative that little or no eyelid skin be removed in conjunction with the brow lift. This would worsen the lagophthalmus. The essential part of paralytic eyebrow surgery is permanent suture suspension of the eyebrow to the periosteum. Traditionally, this has been accomplished through a direct eyebrow lift approach. Recently, the endoscopic forehead lift procedure has been used to correct paralytic eyebrow ptosis as well.

Orbicularis plication eyebrow lift

The orbicularis plication lift achieves mild elevation of the central and lateral eyebrow. It is generally reserved for patients who need brow stabilization while undergoing concurrent blepharoplasty (Fig. 10). Through a small 1.5-cm incision above the brow, the orbital portion of the orbicularis is plicated superior to the periosteum. The incision in the forehead is hidden

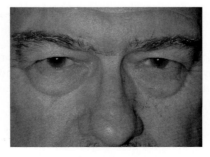

Fig. 8. Ideal candidate for the direct brow lift. This patient has thick eyebrow cilia that can hide the scar.

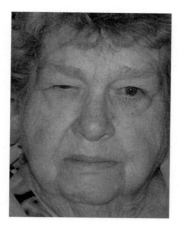

Fig. 9. Right facial nerve palsy patient with paralytic right eyebrow ptosis.

by a horizontal fold lateral to the central portion of the brow. The scarring is usually minimal, although it can take 2 to 3 months to settle.

Midforehead eyebrow lift

The midforehead lift is effective in correcting eyebrow ptosis and glabellar folds. The incision can be hidden in a prominent forehead furrow. Because the procedure may lower the frontal hairline, it is generally reserved for men with prominent forehead furrows and a high and sparse frontal hairline (Fig. 11). Patients with no forehead furrows are poor candidates for

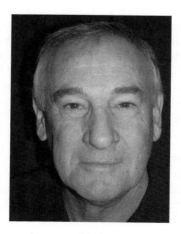

Fig. 10. This patient has requested an upper blepharoplasty. He has moderate eyebrow ptosis. Excision of the upper eyelid skin only will pull his brows down. Stabilizing the brows is paramount to achieving an acceptable result.

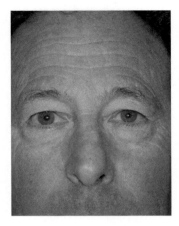

Fig. 11. Patient with significant eyebrow ptosis and severe laxity of the forehead tissues. Extensive rhytids in the forehead are used to hide a midforehead lift incision.

this procedure, because a prominent scar may be seen. A midforehead scar is always going to be visible, to at least some degree; thus, the procedure should be undertaken with the most thorough and detailed patient explanation and consent. I often combine a lateral direct brow lift and a central midforehead lift. This combination avoids an incision in the medial suprabrow region, which has a tendency to scar. The central midforehead incision is usually 3 to 4 cm long and heals quite well.

Temporal eyebrow lift

The temporal eyebrow lift is especially useful in patients with lateral eyebrow ptosis and lateral canthal ptosis. Because the temporal eyebrow is poorly supported anatomically and is the first part of the eyebrow to become ptotic, this procedure is often used in relatively young women (Fig. 12). The incision is hidden in the temporal hairline, minimizing visible scarring. There is no elevation of the medial eyebrow, and a slight elevation of the temporal hairline occurs with this procedure.

Open coronal eyebrow and forehead lift

The coronal eyebrow and forehead lift effectively raises the medial and lateral eyebrow, reduces glabellar folds, and smoothes the forehead. With the standard procedure, the incision is placed entirely within the hair-bearing scalp, camouflaging the scar. The procedure is most appropriately used in women or in men older than 55 years of age who have no familial tendency toward male-pattern baldness (Fig. 13). In men, the coronal incision is modified to a coronal gull-wing configuration to keep the incision line more posterior in the area of typical temporal thinning. The hairline is

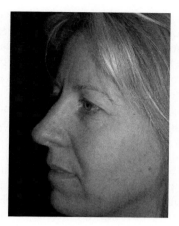

Fig. 12. Young patients with temporal brow ptosis are good candidates for isolated temporal lifts.

commonly elevated by this procedure. In a woman with a low hairline and vertically short forehead, the standard coronal eyebrow lift often improves the aesthetic balance and appearance of the face. In men or women who are concerned with elevation of the hairline, the anterior portion of the incision may be placed along the hairline, effectively lowering it. This variation of the coronal lift is called the pretrichial coronal eyebrow and forehead lift.

Endoscopic or small incision forehead and eyebrow lift

The endoscopic forehead and eyebrow lift has now become the most popular method of raising the eyebrows and forehead. This procedure achieves the aesthetic success of an open coronal lift without the need for

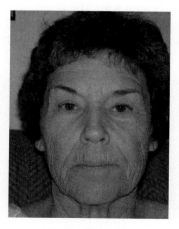

Fig. 13. Ideal candidate for a coronal forehead lift. This patient has thick hair and a vertically short forehead.

a large incision. The indications for endoscopic eyebrow and forehead lifting are essentially the same as for the standard open coronal technique, although younger patients with brow ptosis often elect to have the endoscopic approach (Fig. 14). The endoscopic eyebrow and forehead lift can achieve elevation of the eyebrows and glabella and reduction of forehead furrows and glabellar folds.

The main advantages of the endoscopic technique versus the open coronal technique include minimal incisions with decreased bleeding and scarring, reduction or elimination of postoperative alopecia (ie, a procedure good for thin-haired male or female patients), decreased postoperative sensory neuropathy, less postoperative discomfort, and more rapid recovery. The endoscopic procedure also elevates the hairline less than the open coronal technique because it works by releasing the protractor muscles rather than myotomizing the frontalis muscle. The main disadvantage is that specialized training in the use of endoscopic equipment is required.

There are several variations of the endoscopic forehead and eyebrow lift technique. The procedure can be combined with excision of pretrichial skin to shorten the forehead vertically. The surgery can also be performed through a transeyelid approach without the use of the endoscope. The entire periosteum can be undermined through an eyelid approach and the forehead flap anchored with incisions placed similar to those of a standard endoscopic eyebrow lift. This procedure has an advantage in that it does not rely on expensive endoscopic equipment. It is more difficult to perform, however, and some dissection is not done under direct visualization.

Transblepharoplasty eyebrowpexy

Internal eyebrowpexy plicates the eyebrow to the periosteum at or above the level of the superior orbital rim. The plication is combined with upper blepharoplasty and is accomplished through the upper blepharoplasty incision. Significant elevation of the eyebrow cannot be achieved with the

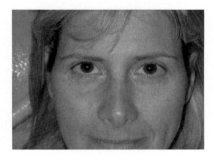

Fig. 14. Middle-aged woman with fine hair and significant eyebrow ptosis. Many younger patients do not want to have a large coronal incision and are worried about postoperative hair loss.

procedure without creating a pleating or corrugation of the skin above the eyebrow. Therefore, the main advantage of the eyebrowpexy is that it limits postblepharoplasty eyebrow descent. The main disadvantage is that tenderness and dimpling of the eyebrow can occur in the region of the plication.

A modification of the internal eyebrowpexy involves suturing the superior cut edge of the orbicularis muscle to the superior lateral arcus marginalis. This technique prevents the descent of the ROOF fat pad and adds some fullness to the lateral brow. This technique does not elevate the eyebrow but prevents the brow tissues from extending into the eyelid space.

Current practice trends

Currently, I find the endoscopic forehead lift to be the most versatile of all procedures. It is an excellent procedure for most women, and the results are long lasting. In men or women with significant laxity of the forehead tissues, a coronal forehead lift is still an excellent choice. It cannot be used in patients with thinning hair. Men with bushy eyebrows who do not want extensive surgery are still good candidates for the direct brow lift. As mentioned previously, I often limit the direct lift to the lateral portion of the brow and raise the central portion with a small midforehead lift. I rarely perform the full midforehead lift, except on patients with severe wrinkling of their foreheads. I find the orbicularis plication lift to be quite useful, especially in men who are undergoing functional blepharoplasty and who choose not to have a brow lift.

Operative procedures

Direct eyebrow lift

The direct eyebrow lift is the simplest and most direct approach to raising the eyebrow. Technical variations have been described by Pierce [19], Bames [20], and Castanares [21]. The procedure is most commonly performed with local anesthesia and intravenous sedation. The surgeon must take into account that the position of the eyebrow at the termination of surgery is usually higher than the final result. Postoperative edema is usually quite minimal. A faint scar at the top of the eyebrow is usually present for several months after surgery. A thin application of eyebrow pencil makeup can usually camouflage the scar if it persists. Standard scar management, including dermabrasion or laser resurfacing, can also be used if the scar is objectionable to the patient.

Surgical technique

Step 1: With the patient in the sitting position, the proposed incision site is marked just above the most superior eyebrow hairs. An ellipse measuring, on average, 15 mm is demarcated with the marking pen (Fig. 15).

Step 2: The eyebrow region is infiltrated with 2% lidocaine with 1:100,000 epinephrine and hyaluronidase. Fifteen minutes are allowed to pass for adequate vasoconstriction. The incision is performed using a no. 15 Bard-Parker blade along the previously demarcated lines. The blade should be held perpendicular to the skin surface. It is not necessary to bevel the incision, as some have suggested in the past [22,23]. (The theoretic advantage of beveling is to avoid damage to the eyebrow hairs. The advantage of not beveling the incision is that it is easier to achieve accurate wound closure, and thus a minimized scar, when the wound edges are perpendicular.) The depth of the incision is carried to a plane just superficial to the frontalis muscle in the region of the supraorbital nerve to avoid damage to the nerve. In patients with extreme lateral eyebrow ptosis, the excised ellipse of tissue can extend more laterally than the lateral eyebrow. The depth of the incision in the lateral portion is just through the skin to avoid damage to the temporal branch of the seventh nerve, however. Scissors, a Colorado needle-cutting cautery, or laser dissection is used to remove the ellipse of tissue. Hemostasis is achieved with the unipolar cautery.

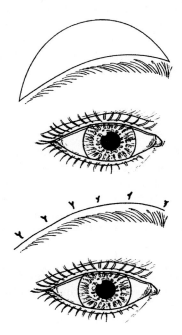

Fig. 15. The inferior portion of the ellipse for the direct brow lift is placed just above the eyebrow cilia. The superior portion of the ellipse is determined by the degree of eyebrow ptosis. After closure of the defect, the incision should form a line parallel to the eyebrow cilia.

Step 3: The wound is closed with a deep layer of buried, subcuticular, interrupted 4-0 Vicryl suture on a P-3 needle. This should perfectly approximate the skin edges. The width of the margin separation at this point determines the final postoperative width of the scar.

Step 4: Multiple, interrupted, vertical mattress sutures of 4-0 nylon or Prolene (polypropylene) are then used to approximate the wound edges. Eversion of the wound edge is important to avoid a depressed scar. Finally, a running 6-0 nylon or Prolene suture on a P-1 needle may be used to close and evert the skin edges. The wound is dressed with antibiotic ointment, and ice compresses are applied four times a day for 2 to 3 days. The running 6-0 suture is removed in 5 to 7 days, and the vertical mattress sutures are removed in 7 to 10 days.

If only lateral eyebrow ptosis is evident, a segmental direct eyebrow lift can be performed (Fig. 16). The eyebrow elevation is marked, incised, and closed in a similar manner. The lateral eyebrow is less well supported than the medial eyebrow; therefore, it falls first. This procedure finds particular application in middle-aged men with lateral eyebrow ptosis (Fig. 17). The direct eyebrow lift in a properly chosen patient provides an excellent structural, functional, and cosmetic result (Fig. 18).

Paralytic eyebrow lift

Reconstruction of the ptotic eyebrow is an integral part of the rehabilitation of the seventh nerve palsy patient. Because of the palsy of the frontalis muscle, the only forces on this eyebrow are in a downward direction. Thus, these eyebrows need to be overcorrected because they are going to fall with time. This surgery can be performed in conjunction with gold weight insertion into the upper eyelid and reconstruction of the lower eyelid.

Surgical technique

Step 1: The patient is examined in the sitting position to determine the preoperative level of the eyebrow. A crescent-shaped area above the eyebrow is demarcated with the marking pen, as described for the

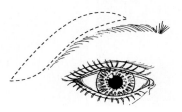

Fig. 16. A modification of the direct brow lift can be performed by excising an ellipse of tissue in the lateral portion over the eyebrow.

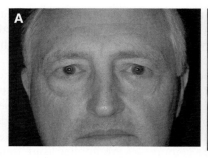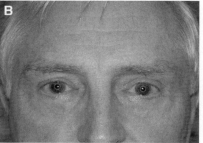

Fig. 17. Preoperative (*A*) and postoperative (*B*) photographs demonstrating a lateral direct brow lift and upper blepharoplasty. The patient also underwent a lower blepharoplasty at the same time.

direct eyebrow lift. The paralytic eyebrow should be overcorrected because it is going to fall with time.

Step 2: After infiltration of 2% lidocaine with 1:100,000 epinephrine and hyaluronidase to the eyebrow area, the previously demarcated crescent of skin is excised, as described for the direct eyebrow lift.

Step 3: Permanently buried 4-0 Prolene sutures are then placed between the elevated eyebrow tissue (at the leading edge of the advancement flap) and the periosteum of the frontal bone. 5-0 Vicryl sutures are used in an interrupted and buried subcuticular fashion to approximate the subcutaneous and muscular layers. The skin is closed in the same fashion as described for the direct eyebrow lift.

Orbicularis plication eyebrow lift

The orbicularis plication lift is a simple method to raise the central and lateral portions of the brow moderately. The main indication of this particular technique is to stabilize the brow and prevent postblepharoplasty

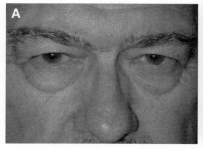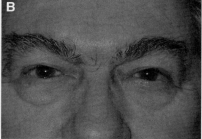

Fig. 18. *A, B,* Standard direct brow lift can significantly elevate the brow centrally and laterally. It does not, however, address the glabella region.

brow descent. The procedure is most commonly performed with local anesthesia and intravenous sedation. The incision is placed in a rhytid 1 to 1.5 cm above the brow. A faint scar is usually present for several months after surgery. Standard scar management, including dermabrasion or laser resurfacing, can also be used if the scar is objectionable to the patient.

Surgical technique

Step 1: With the patient in a sitting position, the proposed incision site is marked in a rhytid 1 to 1.5 cm above the lateral one half of the brow (Fig. 19). The region is infiltrated with 2% lidocaine with 1:100,000 epinephrine and hyaluronidase. Fifteen minutes are allowed to pass for adequate vasoconstriction. The incision is performed using a no. 15 Bard-Parker blade along the previously demarcated lines. The depth of the incision is just posterior under the subcutaneous fat. The dissection is carried inferiorly to the superior portion of the brow. The orbicularis muscle becomes evident at this point, and vertical spreading with tenotomy scissors avoids injury to the muscle as well as excessive bleeding. Hemostasis is achieved with the unipolar cautery.

Step 2: The orbicularis muscle is grasped and pulled superiorly. The vector of pull is determined. Often, the orbicularis is pulled superior and medial, which helps to elevate the tail of the brow. A 5-0 polydioxanone (PDS) mattress suture (Ethicon, Somerville, NJ) is used to secure the orbicularis to the periosteum. One or two sutures are placed.

Step 3: A small amount of skin in the central portion of the wound is then removed. The skin is closed with a deep layer of buried, subcuticular, interrupted 5-0 Vicryl suture on a P-3 needle. This should perfectly approximate the skin edges. A running 6-0 nylon or Prolene suture on a P-1 needle is used to close and evert the skin edges. The wound is dressed with antibiotic ointment, and ice compresses are applied four times a day for 2 to 3 days. The running 6-0 suture is removed in 5 to 7 days (Fig. 20).

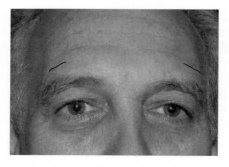

Fig. 19. A 1-cm incision is placed in a rhytid 1 to 1.5 cm above the eyebrow. These incisions heal well and are barely perceptible in several months.

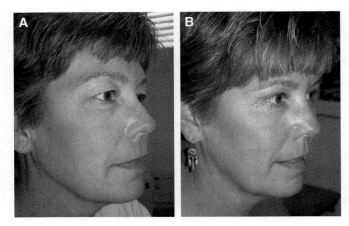

Fig. 20. *A, B*, Photographs of a patient who underwent an orbicularis plication brow stabilizing procedure. This procedure does not raise the brow but reduces postblepharoplasty eyebrow descent.

Midforehead lift

Variations of the midforehead eyebrow lift have been described by Brennan and Rafarty [24], Rafaty and colleagues [25], Ellenbogen [26], and Johnson and Waldman [27]. The midforehead lift may be useful in cases of isolated eyebrow ptosis, glabellar ptosis, and midforehead frown lines. Midforehead scarring is a concern; thus, this procedure is reserved for patients with thin nonsebaceous skin and prominent forehead furrows.

Surgical technique

Step 1: A prominent eyebrow furrow is selected for the superior incision line and is marked with a surgical marker (Fig. 21). One can also break up the incision line by placing the incision in two separate eyebrow furrows (Fig. 22). Alternatively, a running "W" plasty rather than a straight incision line breaks up the scar line. It adds length to the incision and time to the procedure but is beneficial in selected cases. If a large resection is anticipated in severe eyebrow ptosis, the incision line should be carried across most of the forehead to permit adequate closure. If significant lateral eyebrow ptosis exists, the incision can be carried temporally following the inferiorly curved eyebrow furrow.

Step 2: It is often difficult to determine before surgery the amount of tissue to be resected; however, this is often the distance between two prominent eyebrow furrows.

Step 3: Lidocaine 2% with 1:100,000 epinephrine and hyaluronidase is injected as a bilateral supraorbital nerve block. Lidocaine 1% with 1:100,000 epinephrine and hyaluronidase is injected along the incision site, superior eyebrow, and glabellar region. Fifteen minutes are allowed to elapse for adequate vasoconstriction.

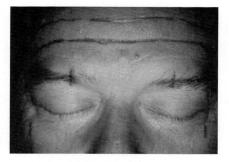

Fig. 21. Prominent rhytids in the forehead are demarcated for the proposed incision for a midforehead lift.

Step 4: A no. 15 Bard-Parker blade is used to make a full-thickness incision in the previously demarcated lines. The incision is carried down through the galea aponeurosis to the loose areolar space. In the temporal region, beyond the lateral extent of the frontalis muscle, the depth of the incision includes skin only. Blunt and sharp dissection is performed in the loose aponeurotic layer inferior to the superior orbital rims. Dissection of the corrugator and procerus muscles may be performed as indicated to eliminate glabellar furrows.

Step 5: The flap is then elevated to the desired height. When appropriate, horizontal relaxing incisions may be made in the posterior muscular lamella using cutting cautery. The redundant forehead tissue is then excised full thickness as appropriate to eliminate eyebrow ptosis. The tissue can be excised in an asymmetric fashion to correct asymmetric eyebrow ptosis or medial or lateral eyebrow ptosis.

Step 6: The wound is closed in two layers, as described for the direct eyebrow lift. Antibiotic ointment is applied, and a Telfa dressing is

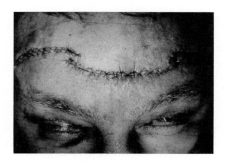

Fig. 22. The midforehead lift incision can be broken up by placing the incision in two separate rhytids.

placed over the wound for 48 hours. Ice compresses are used four times a day for 4 days to reduce swelling and ecchymosis. Sutures should be removed within 7 to 10 days.

Temporal lift

The temporal lift procedure has been described by Gleason [28]. Patients with early eyebrow ptosis and lateral canthal ptosis and rhytids are candidates for this approach. The incisions are hidden in the temporal hairline. Patients are asked to wash their hair with antibacterial shampoo the evening before surgery. In the preoperative holding area, the hair is parted along the coronal line.

Surgical technique

Step 1: With intravenous sedation, several milliliters of 2% lidocaine with 1:200,000 epinephrine and hyaluronidase are given as a supraorbital nerve block. Ten milliliters of 0.5% lidocaine with 1:200,000 epinephrine and hyaluronidase is infiltrated along the proposed incision line. Fifteen minutes are allowed to elapse for maximal vasoconstriction.

Step 2: A no. 15 Bard-Parker blade is used to make an incision approximately 6 cm long. The incision is along the standard coronal line, beginning 1 to 2 cm superior to the interface of the ear and extending to the scalp (Fig. 23). The incision is made to the level of the deep temporalis fascia.

Step 3: Dissection with a large flat periosteal elevator or large blunt scissors is carried along the plane of the temporalis fascia toward the eyebrow. The temporal branch of the facial nerve is located in the flap. Damage to the nerve is avoided if the dissection is carried deep to the nerve along the intermediate temporalis fascia. The temporal flap is

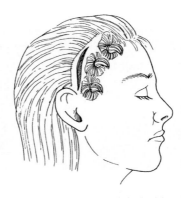

Fig. 23. Drawing illustrates the position of the incision for a temporal lift.

undermined to the level of the eyebrow and lateral canthus. To prevent damage to the facial nerve, the use of cautery is avoided.

Step 4: After the flap is developed, it is advanced and rotated slightly until satisfactory elevation of the eyebrow is noted. Redundant tissue is then excised

Step 5: The wound is closed in a single layer with wide skin staples. No drains are used. Antibiotic ointment is placed on the wound, and fluffs are placed over the flap. Gauze dressings are placed as a head wrap. Ice compresses are placed over the eyes and forehead four times a day for four days. The staples are removed in 10 to 14 days.

Coronal eyebrow and forehead lift

Patients who are receiving a coronal eyebrow and forehead lift [29–32] are asked to wash their hair with antibacterial shampoo the evening before surgery. Clothing that does not require removal over the head is worn on the day of surgery.

Surgical technique

In the preoperative holding area, the hair is parted and braided along the proposed coronal incision site with the help of water-based jelly (Fig. 24). Strips of aluminum foil or dental rubber bands may be used to braid the hair. The incision line extends from the superior point where the ear touches the scalp and proceeds along the coronal line from ear to ear. In the midline, the incision is placed 6 to 7 cm posterior to the hairline.

Step 1: In the operating room, the patient is prepared and draped. With a marking pen, a line is marked from the middle of the nose to the incision line. Another line is drawn from the lateral eyebrow just above the position of the lateral limbus to the incision line. This is generally 4 cm from the midline. A line is then drawn from the temporal portion of the

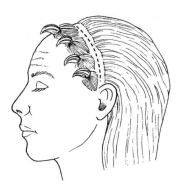

Fig. 24. The coronal incision extends from ear to ear. It is helpful to part and tie the hair with rubber bands or aluminum foil.

lateral canthus and ala of the nose, which intersects the incision line. This line generally intersects the incision line 10 cm from the midline (Fig. 25).

Step 2: I prefer performing the procedure under local anesthesia with intravenous sedation. General anesthesia causes vasodilatation and more bleeding. A solution of lactated Ringer's solution (1 L), 2% lidocaine (50 mL; without epinephrine), 1:1000 epinephrine (1 mL), and hyaluronidase (1500 U) is mixed together. This creates a (Klein's) solution of 0.1% Xylocaine, 1:1,000,000 epinephrine, and hyaluronidase at a rate of 1.5 U/mL. This dilute solution at a total rate of 100 to 150 mL is infiltrated throughout the scalp and forehead, along the eyebrows, and from the top of the ear along the zygomatic arch. Lidocaine 0.5% (20 mL) with 1:200,000 epinephrine and hyaluronidase is given as a "vascular tourniquet" along the incision line and across the eyebrows. Bupivacaine hydrochloride 0.5% (4 mL) with 1:200,000 epinephrine and hyaluronidase is given as a supraorbital block bilaterally. It is also helpful to give bupivacaine hydrochloride solution (1 mL) above each ear. Fifteen to 20 minutes are allowed to elapse for the epinephrine to have its hemodynamic effect. Excellent hemostasis is generally obtained, and the need for reinjection is rare. Raney clips are usually not necessary.

Step 3: A no. 15 Bard-Parker blade is used to make an incision through the galea aponeurosis to the level of the periosteum. Dissection

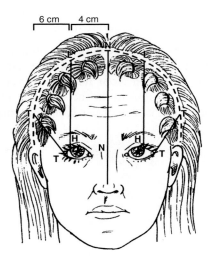

Fig. 25. Drawing illustrates the vectors of elevation used in a coronal lift. For the novice surgeon, it is helpful to draw these lines on the patient's face to determine the location of the incision and the vectors of pull. With a marking pen, a line is drawn from the middle of the nose (N) to the incision line. Another line is drawn from the lateral eyebrow just above the position of the lateral limbus to the incision line (H). This is generally 4 cm from the midline. A line is then drawn from the temporal portion of the lateral canthus and ala of the nose, which intersects the incision line (T). This line generally intersects the incision line 10 cm from the midline.

between the periosteum and loose aponeurotic tissue is performed with the fingers, a scalpel, or scissors. The forehead flap is elevated down to the level of the superior orbital rims. Because the temporal branch of the facial nerve lies within the flap, dissection is carefully performed along the deep temporalis fascia and blunt dissection with the finger wrapped in gauze is performed in these areas. Cautery is avoided in the temporal portion of the flap.

Step 4: The dissection plane is changed from the loose areolar plane to the subperiosteal plane at a point approximately 2 cm above the superior orbital rim (Fig. 26A). This allows for an easy continuation of the dissection to the superior orbital rims and inferior attachments of the procerus muscles, with easy preservation of the supraorbital neurovascular bundle. Once the superior orbital rims are exposed, the periosteum at the arcus marginalis is incised. The opening in the periosteum provides access to the corrugator and procerus muscles. This release and dissection is the most important aspect of the entire procedure. Remember that it is not creating a flap but rather what one does under the flap that determines the result of the surgery. The

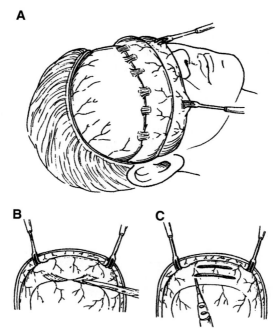

Fig. 26. (*A*) The subgaleal dissection is a rapid one and continues until approximately 2 cm above the orbital rims. (*B*) The procerus and corrugator muscles are identified and cut. Care must be taken to avoid damage to the supraorbital and supratrochlear neurovascular bundles. (*C*) Horizontal relaxing incisions are made in the frontalis muscle. This reduces the action of the muscle and thereby reduces the rhytids.

procerus and corrugator muscles that serve to pull the eyebrows down and closer together, creating vertical glabellar lines, are now dissected as appropriate. Care is taken to spare the supraorbital neurovascular bundle.

Step 5: At this point, superior traction of the scalp lifts the eyebrows but does not smooth the creases and furrows of the glabella or forehead. The procerus and corrugator muscle complex, if overacting and causing vertical lines, must be cut with scissors or dissected with electrocutting cautery (see Fig. 26B).

Step 6: To obliterate forehead furrows, one or more horizontal relaxing incisions may be made in the posterior muscle lamella of the forehead flap above the first forehead crease (see Fig. 26C). This allows the posterior lamella to relax and the anterior skin layer to be stretched. It also denervates motor movement to the frontalis muscle above the incision so that the forehead does not have horizontal lines. The cautery is carried through the frontalis muscle to subcutaneous tissue. Cautery is avoided in the hair-bearing scalp, however, to avoid follicle loss. Inferiorly, a thin strip of frontalis muscle is preserved between the first (most inferior) and second forehead creases to allow natural animation of the eyebrows.

Step 7: Using a D'Assumpcão clamp, the posterior scalp is advanced in the midline and marked with a no. 11 blade with a sentinel incision. This procedure is performed at the intersection between each of the "marionette" lines and the coronal line. Redundant scalp is then excised with scissors (Fig. 27A). The amount of scalp excised is gradually tapered as the excision proceeds laterally; little lift is gained, because less lift is desired lateral to the lateral eyebrow. Tension on the forehead flap can be adjusted to correct asymmetric eyebrow ptosis and to achieve the desired eyebrow arch.

Step 8: The galea is closed with multiple buried 3-0 PDS sutures. The skin is then closed with staples (see Fig. 27B).

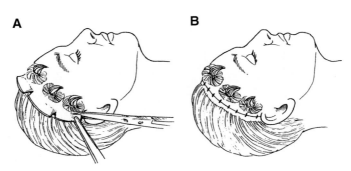

Fig. 27. (A) Redundant scalp is identified with the aid of the D'Assumpcão clamp. (B) The remaining redundant skin is excised, and the skin is closed with staples.

Step 9: The hair may be rinsed with 1.5% hydrogen peroxide to remove blood and is then rinsed with saline to avoid bleaching of the hair. The hair is dried with a towel, and antibiotic ointment is applied to the wound.

Step 10: Fluffs are placed across the flap, and a head wrap is made with gauze dressings, which is anchored with short pieces of tape. Ice compresses are applied to the eyes and forehead constantly for the first postoperative day and continued three or four times a day for the following 4 days to minimize edema. The head is kept elevated, and the head wrap is removed in 2 to 3 days. Patients are then instructed to shampoo the hair gently with their regular shampoo for several minutes a day to remove crusts. Staples are removed in 10 to 14 days.

Blepharoplasty may be performed after a coronal eyebrow lift at the same sitting. I perform coronal forehead lifts and blepharoplasties during the same session in approximately 50% of patients. When combining a forehead lift and upper blepharoplasty, I prefer to perform the forehead and eyebrow lift first. This allows a more accurate determination of the amount of redundant upper eyelid skin. It is noted that other authors advocate performing the blepharoplasty first and then performing the coronal forehead and eyebrow lift. Surgeons who use this sequence of procedures must be exceedingly conservative in the upper blepharoplasty or they may be forced to undercorrect the eyebrow lift or risk postoperative lagophthalmus. Overall, the open coronal eyebrow and forehead lift is an excellent procedure with the potential to maximize the structural, functional, and aesthetic forehead and eyebrow position (Fig. 28).

Pretrichial incision variation: open coronal forehead lift

The central portion of the open coronal forehead and eyebrow lift incision line may be brought anterior to the central hair line (pretrichial). This is called the pretrichial open coronal forehead lift. The excised

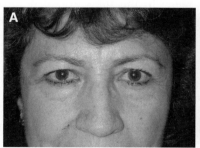
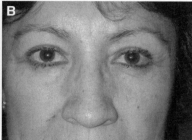

Fig. 28. Preoperative (*A*) and postoperative (*B*) photographs of a patient who underwent a coronal brow lift.

pretrichial tissue is forehead skin, and this procedure accomplishes the elevation of the eyebrows and the simultaneous lowering of the hair line. To maintain the aesthetically appropriate three equal vertical thirds of the face (aesthetic proportions), the forehead, in general, should be no more than 6 to 7 cm superior to the eyebrows. A standard open coronal forehead lift elevates the hairline as much as 1 to 2 cm. Thus, if the vertical forehead dimension is greater than 6 to 6.5 cm, consideration should be given to using the pretrichial incision coronal forehead lift variation.

All the geometric rules, and thus the geometric design, for the standard open forehead lift apply except that the central portion of the incision line is brought forward to pass anterior to the hairline. The surgery is performed exactly as described for the standard open coronal forehead lift. After surgery, the eyebrows have been lifted and the hairline has been brought down to shorten the forehead vertically.

Subperiosteal plane central dissection variation: open coronal forehead lift

Classically, the standard open coronal and pretrichial open coronal lifts have been performed temporally in the plane between the deep temporal fascia and the superficial temporal fascia and centrally in the loose areolar plane between the periosteum and the galea. Since the advent of the endoscopic forehead lift, surgeons have recognized the advantages of performing the central forehead zone dissection in the subperiosteal plane. With appropriate periosteal release along the superior orbital rim and appropriate release and dissection of the protractor muscles, the forehead and eyebrows may be lifted by the intact and nondistensible periosteum itself, providing a longer lasting lift. Additionally, the frontalis muscle and galea complex is not myotomized so that the frontalis muscle continues to act as an eyebrow elevator and is minimally opposed by the eyebrow protractor (depressor) muscles. Because the eyebrows depressors have now lost the tug of war that, along with gravity, held the eyebrows in the ptotic position, the eyebrows tend to move superiorly. I now favor the subperiosteal central zone dissection plane in the standard open coronal lift, pretrichial open coronal lift, and endoscopic eyebrow and forehead lift.

Endoscopic forehead lift

Patients who are receiving an endoscopic forehead lift [33–38] are asked to wash their hair with antibacterial shampoo the evening before surgery. Because the endoscopic forehead lift essentially accomplishes everything that the open coronal lift accomplishes, the goal is to have the forehead and eyebrows at the same position at the end of the small incision surgery as would be ideal at the end of the open coronal incision surgery.

Surgical technique

Step 1: Markings and incision sites. Five incision sites are demarcated (Fig. 29). One central vertical incision is placed at the hairline and extends 1.5 cm posteriorly. Two lateral vertical incisions of 1.5 cm are placed 0.5 cm posterior to the hairline at the level of the lateral canthus. Two 1.5-cm lateral vertical incisions are placed over the temporalis fossa. The incision sites can be modified according to the patient's forehead contour, degree of eyebrow ptosis, and hairline. The incisions can be made smaller in men with significant hair loss and closed meticulously with sutures in non–hair-bearing scalp. I prefer to make incisions anterior to any area of thinning hair to avoid the loss of hair follicles. As in the open coronal procedure, these incisions lie in appropriate traction lines for eyebrow lifting and afford the surgeon the opportunity to lift the eyebrow differentially. The hair is parted along the proposed incision sites with the help of water-based jelly. The incision lines are marked with a marking pen.

Step 2: Anesthesia. I prefer performing the procedure under modified local anesthesia with intravenous sedation. General anesthesia causes vasodilatation and more bleeding. Bupivacaine hydrochloride 0.25% with 1:100,000 epinephrine is used to provide dense supraorbital, supratrochlear, infratrochlear, and zygomaticofrontal nerve blocks. Tumescent solution (100–150 mL) is infiltrated throughout the scalp and forehead, along the eyebrows, and from the top of the ear along

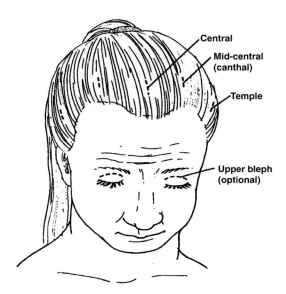

Fig. 29. Five vertical incisions are used for the endoscopic eyebrow lift. The positions of the incisions are similar to those of the open coronal approach (see Fig. 25), although the midcentral incisions are placed at the position of the lateral canthus.

the zygomatic arch. Lidocaine 0.5% (10 mL) with 1:200,000 epinephrine is given along the incision lines and across the eyebrows. Fifteen to 20 minutes are allowed to elapse for the epinephrine to have its hemodynamic effect. This technique creates a vascular tourniquet, and the large volume of fluid permits hydrodissection of all planes, especially the temporalis fascia plane.

Step 3: Visualization pocket (optical pocket). Attention is first focused on the safest region for dissection. This is the upper forehead between the temporal crests. A no. 15 Bard-Parker blade is used to make an incision along the previously demarcated lines. Through the central incision, blunt elevator dissection is performed in the subperiosteal plane. The dissection extends laterally to the lateral incision sites. Much of the subperiosteal dissection may be safely and quickly performed in a blind fashion, taking care to stay directly on the bone. Blind dissection is stopped 2 cm above the superior orbital rim to avoid the supraorbital and supratrochlear nerves. The temporal regions are then dissected. The dissection begins with an incision through the superficial temporalis fascia. Because of the ballooning effect of the tumescent solution, the superficial temporalis fascia may have several layers. The dissection continues until the shiny white temporal fascia is noted. A Senn retractor is then inserted, and a large blunt periosteal elevator is used to dissect along the deep temporalis fascia. The endoscope is then inserted into this temporal pocket.

Step 4: Conjoint fascia elevation. The conjoint fascia is approached with the dissector from the temporal incision. Under direct endoscopic visualization, the conjoint fascia is sharply elevated off the superior temporal line. Dissection from the central subperiosteal space toward the temporal zone creates the risk of entering too deep and disinserting the temporalis muscle or being too superficial and damaging the temporal branch of the facial nerve in the superficial temporal (temporoparietal) fascia. Therefore, it is best to dissect the temporal and central forehead spaces first and then to connect the two spaces by elevating the conjoint fascia. The release of the conjoint fascia proceeds inferiorly. The endoscope is then inserted through one of the paracentral incisions. Through the central incision, the dissection (in the subperiosteal plane) is carried inferiorly toward the superior orbital rims. There is now a continuous optical cavity involving the two temporal zones, the central forehead zone, and the posterior vertex zone. The flap is elevated along the orbital rim and glabellar region. I have found that elevators that are curved downward are most beneficial in this region. The periosteum and arcus marginalis are released with blunt dissection. Dissection is advanced onto the radix of the nose. The entire scalp is now mobile.

Step 5: Periosteal release. The periosteum and periorbita must be cut and separated. This incision facilitates repositioning of the forehead periosteum and also allows access to the eyebrow musculature for muscle modification. The periosteum is usually cut with a flat elevator. Alternatively, the periosteum can be cut with a long curved monopolar cautery, laser, or endoscopic scissors. Extreme care must be taken to avoid injury to the supraorbital and supratrochlear neurovascular bundles. In the temple region, the dissection proceeds along the deep temporalis fascia. A vein (sentinel) is encountered just lateral to the Yasergill's fat pad. This vein can be cauterized, but it is important to grasp the vein where it exits from the temporalis muscle. The frontal branch of the facial nerve lies anterior to the vein. The dissection then proceeds along the superior lateral orbital rim. A white dense ligamentous attachment is noted just superior to the lateral canthus. This represents the ligamentous attachment of the orbicularis muscle. This is often cut with endoscopic scissors.

Step 6: Procerus and corrugator resection. The procerus and corrugator muscle complex is identified at the bony rim. Separate the muscles with a hook, and cut with scissors or dissect with the laser or electrocutting cautery. Weakening these muscles relieves the deep rhytids in the glabellar region. Care must be taken to avoid overaggressive tissue removal, which results in a depression in the glabella region. There are several branches of the supratrochlear neurovascular bundle that lie within the corrugator muscle complex. It is best to preserve these branches to prevent postoperative hypesthesia.

Step 7: Elevation and fixation. Now, the scalp from the supraorbital region to the occiput is freed and "free floating," and the eyebrows can be advanced as necessary. There are numerous methods of fixation. It is my opinion that the key in obtaining successful brow lifting is not the method of fixation but the release of periosteum and ligamentous attachments along the lateral canthus. Through the lateral incision sites, the scalp is advanced superiorly with the aid of a single-pronged hook or forceps. When the proper eyebrow position is obtained, the bone underlying the inferior aspect of the central incision site is marked with a pen. In general, the central advancement is approximately 10 mm. Screw holes are made with a 4-mm drill bit on a manual screw driver handle. Alternatively, a power drill can be used. A 12-mm screw is placed in the drill hole and screwed into the skull to a depth of approximately 4 mm. Therefore, 8 mm of the 12-mm screw is left projecting from the skull. The scalp is pulled posteriorly, and a skin staple is placed behind the screw to support the scalp elevation. In the temple incisions, a 2-0 PDS mattress suture attaches the superficial temporalis fascia to the deep temporalis fascia. All incision sites are closed with staples. Alternatively, if the incisions are not covered by hair-bearing scalp, they should be meticulously sutured. The hair is washed and dressed in a similar manner to a standard coronal eyebrow lift. I do not use a head dressing or drain.

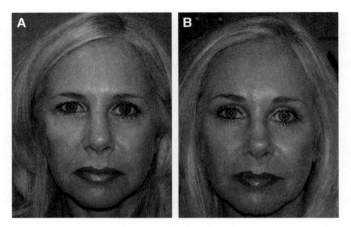

Fig. 30. Preoperative (*A*) and postoperative (*B*) photographs of a patient who underwent an endoscopic brow lift.

Step 8: The patient is seen 1 week to 10 days after surgery; at that time, the staples can be removed if the wound seems to be well healed. The screws are removed 14 days after surgery (Fig. 30).

A transblepharoplasty nonendoscopic subperiosteal lift can be performed and is the approach of choice if orbital rim augmentation is necessary. The scalp is prepared and anesthetized as in the endoscopic approach. The central and temporal pockets are dissected blindly in the safe zones. A blepharoplasty incision is made, and blunt dissection is performed to the orbital rim (Fig. 31). The arcus marginalis is incised, and a subperiosteal dissection is performed (Figs. 32 and 33). The dissection from above and below is joined. The bone can be thinned or burred down (Fig. 34). The brow is then pulled superiorly and fixated in a manner similar to the endoscopic approach. The eyelid is closed with a running 6-0 Prolene suture.

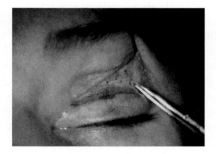

Fig. 31. An eyelid crease incision is used to gain access to the forehead. Blunt dissection is performed between the orbicularis and the orbital septum.

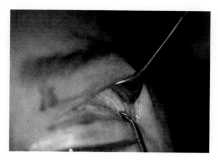

Fig. 32. An incision is made in the periosteum at the level of the superior arcus marginalis. Cottle elevators are used to elevate the periosteum superiorly.

Internal eyebrow pexy

Internal eyebrow pexy [39–43] is not a true eyebrow lifting procedure but an eyebrow stabilizing procedure. The eyebrow is fixated centrally and laterally, which prevents postblepharoplasty eyebrow descent.

Surgical technique

Step 1: The supraorbital notch is palpated and demarcated to localize the supraorbital nerve and vessels. The upper lid crease is then demarcated as in a standard upper blepharoplasty.

Step 2: After infiltration of 2% lidocaine with 1:100,000 epinephrine and hyaluronidase to the eyebrow and upper lid regions, a lid crease incision is made. A standard upper blepharoplasty is performed.

Step 3: Blunt dissection with scissors is extended superiorly in the submuscular plane toward the eyebrow. The dissection is carried 1 to 2.5 cm above the superior orbital rim. The dissection is limited to the central and lateral aspects of the eyebrow to avoid injury to the medial supraorbital neurovascular complex.

Step 4: A 4-0 Prolene suture is passed through periosteum approximately 1 to 2.0 cm above the orbital rim. The suture is then passed in the

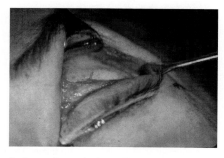

Fig. 33. The periosteum is elevated superiorly until it connects with superiorly based dissection.

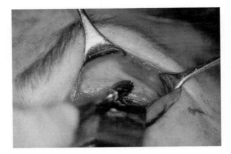

Fig. 34. The bone can be contoured using a high-speed drill and a 4-mm burr.

subeyebrow muscular tissue at the level of the lower edge of the eyebrow cilia. A needle can be inserted transcutaneously to facilitate identification of this level. Sutures are placed laterally and centrally. The eyebrow height and contour are adjusted by replacement of sutures until proper position and symmetry are achieved.

Orbicularis ROOF stabilization can also be performed through the blepharoplasty incision. The goal of this procedure is stabilization of the lateral brow and prevention of ROOF descent. Before closure of the blepharoplasty incision, cotton-tipped applicators are used to dissect the tissues off of the lateral portion of the arcus marginalis bluntly (Fig. 35). A 5-0 PDS suture is placed through the arcus marginalis and through the superior cut edge of the orbicularis muscle (Figs. 36 and 37). Two sutures are routinely placed. One suture is placed at the most superolateral aspect of the orbital rim, and the other is placed just superior to the lateral canthus. After the sutures are tied, it is difficult to displace the lateral brow inferiorly (Fig. 38). The upper eyelid skin is then closed as usual with 6-0 Prolene sutures (Fig. 39). Although the skin is taut in the lateral eyelid, closure is usually not effected (Fig. 40).

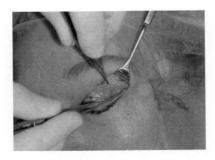

Fig. 35. Blunt dissection is performed to the superior orbital rim. The forceps demonstrate the superior arcus marginalis.

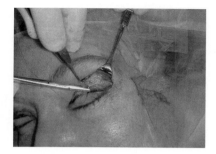

Fig. 36. 5-0 Vicryl suture is placed through the arcus marginalis.

Complications

Complications of eyebrow lifts are rare. Many of the complications are temporary and resolve over time. Preoperative consultation and discussion of the potential complications are imperative in avoidance of an unhappy and angry patient. The following is a list of the more common complications encountered:

1. Nerve damage: sensory and motor nerve damage can occur if the dissection is in the wrong surgical plane. Hypesthesia of the forehead can occur in the coronal and endoscopic lifts when cutting or removing the corrugator and procerus muscles. Overuse of cautery in the location of the nerves is the most common cause of nerve injury. Management of sensory nerve damage is conservative. As the sensory nerves regain function, the patient may have itching, hypesthesia, or other "funny feelings." These, fortunately, usually subside spontaneously over months or years. Damage to the frontal branch of the facial nerve is more worrisome. The lack of frontalis function on the paretic side, and the resultant eyebrow ptosis, is obvious to the patient and physician. Often, nerve function returns over time. A small amount of botulinum toxin to the functioning frontalis muscle can balance out the forehead and eyebrows while the nerve regenerates.

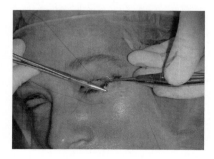

Fig. 37. 5-0 Vicryl suture is passed through the superior cut edge of the orbicularis muscle.

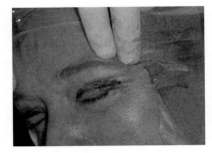

Fig. 38. Attempted downward displacement of the lateral brow is prevented by the browpexy sutures.

2. Scarring: techniques that involve direct incisions in the eyebrow or forehead result in scarring. The scar may be depressed because of improper closure and poor eversion of the wound edges. The patient must be aware of this potential complication before surgery. The forehead responds quite well to dermabrasion or laser resurfacing. I routinely perform dermabrasion on the patients who undergo direct or midforehead lifts 6 to 8 weeks after surgery.

3. Hematoma: if careful hemostasis is not achieved, large hematomas can accumulate under the temporal or coronal flaps and potentially lead to necrosis of the flap. If a scalp hematoma forms and continues to expand, the wound must be opened and the bleeding vessel cauterized.

4. Alopecia: hair loss can occur in endoscopic, coronal, or temporal brow lifts. Tension along incision lines or around external screws that are used for fixation in the endoscopic brow lifts is the main cause of alopecia. In most cases, the hair follicles go into shock and transition into a resting phase. This is known as telogen effluvium. Hair growth returns in several months. Occasionally, hair loss is permanent because of ischemic loss of the hair follicles. Overuse of cautery and a dissection

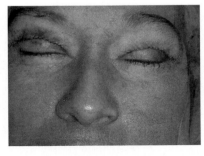

Fig. 39. The skin is closed in the usual manner. The browpexy sutures are only placed laterally to prevent lagophthalmus. At the termination of the case, the patient has complete eyelid closure.

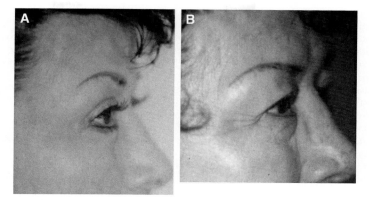

Fig. 40. Preoperative (*A*) and postoperative (*B*) photographs of a patient who underwent upper blepharoplasty and browpexy. Note the improvement in the lateral portion of the upper eyelid.

plane that is too superficial are the most common reasons for the ischemia. Permanent alopecia is most commonly seen with temple or coronal lifts.

References

[1] Shorr N, Enzer Y. Considerations in aesthetic surgery. J Dermatol Surg Oncol 1992;18: 1081–95.
[2] Shorr N, Cohen MS. Cosmetic blepharoplasty. Ophthalmol Clin North Am 1991;4(1): 17–33.
[3] Shorr N, Seiff S. Management of eyebrow ptosis. In: Hornblass A, editor. Oculoplastic, orbital and reconstructive surgery, vol. 1. Baltimore: Williams & Wilkins; 1988. p. 590–602.
[4] Shorr N, Green J, Shorr J. Eyebrow ptosis. Semin Ophthalmol 1996;11(2):138–56.
[5] Shorr N, Hoenig JA. Brow lift. In: Levine M, editor. Manual of oculoplastic surgery. Newton, MA: Butterworth-Heinemann; 1995. p. 47–62.
[6] Pitanguy I. Indications and treatment of frontal and glabellar wrinkles in an analysis of 3,404 consecutive cases of rhytidectomy. Plast Reconstr Surg 1981;67:157–66.
[7] Webster RC, Fanous N, Smith RC. Blepharoplasty: when to combine it with eyebrow, temple or coronal lift. J Otolaryngol 1979;8:339–43.
[8] Lemke BN, Stazior OG. The anatomy of eyebrow ptosis. Arch Ophthalmol 1982;100:981–6.
[9] Tolhurst DE, Carstens MH, Greco RJ, et al. The surgical anatomy of the scalp. Plast Reconstr Surg 1991;87(4):603–12.
[10] Gosain AK, Yousif NJ, Madiedo G, et al. Surgical anatomy of the SMAS: a reinvestigation. Plast Reconstr Surg 1994;92:1254–63.
[11] Furnas DW. Landmarks for the trunk and the temporofacial division of the facial nerve. Br J Surg 1965;52:694–6.
[12] Abul-Hassan HS, Draisek Ascher G, Ackland RD. Surgical anatomy and blood supply of the fascial layers of the temporal region. Plast Reconstr Surg 1986;77(1):17–24.
[13] Stuzin JM, Wagstrom L, Kawamoto HK, et al. Anatomy of the frontal branch of the facial nerve: the significance of the temporal fat pad. Plast Reconstr Surg 1989;83(2):265–71.
[14] Larrabee WF, Makielski KH, Cupp C. Facelift anatomy. Facial Plast Clin North Am 1993; 1(2):135–54.

[15] Correia P, Zani R. Surgical anatomy of the facial nerve, as related to ancillary operations and rhytidoplasty. Plast Reconstr Surg 1973;52:549–52.

[16] Loeb R. Technique for the preservation of the temporal branches of the facial nerve during facelift operations. Br J Plast Surg 1970;23:390–4.

[17] Pitanguay I, Ramos AS. The frontal branch of the facial nerve. The importance of its variations in facelifting. Plast Reconstr Surg 1966;38:352–6.

[18] Wassef M. Superficial fascial and muscular layers in the face and neck: a histological study. Aesthetic Plast Surg 1987;11:171–6.

[19] Pierce G. Useful procedures in plastic surgery. Plast Reconstr Surg 1947;2:361–8.

[20] Bames HO. Frown disfigurement and ptosis of eyebrows. Plast Reconstr Surg 1957;19:337–40.

[21] Castanares S. Forehead wrinkles, glabellar frown and ptosis of the eyebrows. Plast Reconstr Surg 1964;34:404–13.

[22] Tardy ME, Williams EF, Boyce RG. Rejuvenation of the aging eyebrow and forehead. In: Putternman AE, editor. Cosmetic oculoplastic surgery. Philadelphia: WB Saunders; 1994. p. 261–308.

[23] Tardy ME, Parras G, Schwartz M. Aesthetic surgery of the face. Dermatol Clin North Am 1991;9:169–87.

[24] Brennan HG, Rafarty FM. Mid forehead incisions in treatment of the aging face. Arch Otolaryngol 1982;108:732–4.

[25] Rafarty FM, Goode RL, Abramson NR. The eyebrow lift operation in a man. Arch Otolaryngol 1978;104:69–71.

[26] Ellenbogen R. Medial eyebrow lift. Ann Plast Surg 1980;5:151–2.

[27] Johnson CM, Waldman SR. Mid forehead lift. Arch Otolaryngol 1983;109:155–9.

[28] Gleason MC. Eyebrow lifting through a temporal scalp approach. Plast Reconstr Surg 1973; 52:141–4.

[29] Kaye BL. Forehead and eyebrow. In: Reed TD, editor. Aesthetic plastic surgery, vol. II. Philadelphia: WB Saunders; 1980. p. 731–48.

[30] Fett DR, Sutcliffe T, Baylis HI. The coronal eyebrow lift. Am J Ophthalmol 1983;96:751–4.

[31] Faivre J. The triple facelift. Current approach. Arch Otolaryngol Head Neck Surg 1991;117: 47–53.

[32] Ellenbogen R. Transcoronal eyebrow lift with concomitant blepharoplasty. Plast Reconstr Surg 1983;71:490–5.

[33] Toledo LS. Video-endoscopic facelift. Aesthetic Plast Surg 1994;18:149–52.

[34] Ramirez OM. Endoscopic techniques in facial rejuvenation: an overview. Aesthetic Plast Surg 1994;18:141–7.

[35] Maillard JF, Cornette de St. Cyr B, Scheflan M. The subperiosteal bicoronal approach to total facelifting: the DMAS—deep musculoaponeurotic system. Aesthetic Plast Surg 1991; 15:285–91.

[36] Chajchir A. Endoscopic subperiosteal forehead lift. Aesthetic Plast Surg 1994;18:269–74.

[37] Shorr N, Hoenig JA, Goldberg RA. Endoscopic forehead lift and facelift. A step by step surgical manual. Los Angeles, CA: UCLA Press; 1995.

[38] Steinsapir KD, Shorr N, Hoenig JA, et al. The endoscopic forehead lift. Ophthal Plast Reconstr Surg 1998;14:107–18.

[39] May JW, Fearson J, Zingarelli P. Retro-orbicularis oculus fat (ROOF) resection in aesthetic blepharoplasty: a 6 year study in 63 patients. Plast Reconstr Surg 1990;86:682–9.

[40] McCord CD, Doxanas MT. Eyebrowplasty and eyebrowpexy: an adjunct to blepharoplasty. Plast Reconstr Surg 1990;86:248–54.

[41] Sokol AB, Sokol TP. Transblepharoplasty eyebrow suspension. Plast Reconstr Surg 1982; 69:940–4.

[42] Owsley JQ Jr. Resection of the prominent lateral fat pad during upper lid blepharoplasty. Plast Reconstr Surg 1980;65:4–9.

[43] Stasior OG, Lemke BN. The posterior eyebrow fixation. Adv Ophthal Plast Reconstr Surg 1983;2:193–7.

ELSEVIER
SAUNDERS

Otolaryngol Clin N Am
38 (2005) 985–1007

OTOLARYNGOLOGIC
CLINICS
OF NORTH AMERICA

Reconstructive Blepharoplasty

Stephen L. Bosniak, MD[a],
Marian Cantisano-Zilkha, MD[b]

[a]*Manhattan Eye, Ear and Throat Hospital, 135 East 74th Street,
New York, NY 10021, USA*
[b]*Center for Clinical Studies, Oftalmoclinica Botafogo, Rio de Janeiro, Brazil*

With technologic advances and new anatomic concepts, the current approach to cosmetic eyelid procedures yields more natural-appearing, longer-lasting, and more physiologic results.

This procedure is no longer focused solely on fat and skin resections but on improving eyelid function as well as eyelid appearance—repositioning fat, tightening tendons, and repairing muscle disinsertions and lid margin malpositions. CO_2 laser–assisted techniques facilitate these procedures, providing a virtually bloodless field for skin and muscle resections, fat repositioning, and tendon and aponeurotic repairs [1–6].

Principles of upper eyelid repair

Accurate evaluation of the upper eyelid fold can be accomplished only after the brow level and contour have been established [7]. Palpating the superior orbital rim and observing its relationship with the eyebrow will show if brow ptosis (eyebrow level below the superior orbital rim) exists. Comparing the level and contour of the brow with old photographs will show if there has been a change in the level or configuration of the brow arch.

In general, the female brow is arched and sits superior to the superior orbital rim (Fig. 1), whereas the male brow is flat and is positioned just at the orbital rim (Figs. 2 and 3) [8]. Elevation of the brow reduces the amount of overlapping of the upper lid fold. In female patients, elevating the brow can recreate a pleasing arch and a deeper superior sulcus with a reduced lid fold. Elevation is not indicated in all female patients, however. Although the upper lid fold and superior sulcus may have a clean, sculpted look after an

E-mail address: info@eye-lift.com

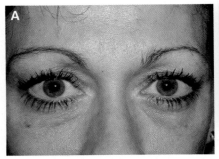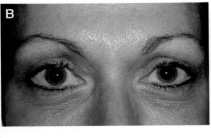

Fig. 1. (*A*) This patient had moderate redundancy of the upper lid fold and superior sulcus fullness with obscuration of upper lid crease but maintained a pleasing feminine brow arch. She had mild lower lid fatty prolapse with a mild tear trough depression and mild right lower lid inferior scleral show with mild lateral canthal angle rounding. (*B*) Her upper lids have been conservatively recontoured, exposing her upper lid crease and preserving her feminine brow arch. Her lower lids were recontoured through a transconjunctival approach. Her lateral canthal tendons were plicated. No laser resurfacing or fat transposition was performed.

effective brow elevation, brows positioned more than 5 mm above the superior orbital may give the patient a surprised, unnatural look.

Overelevation of the brow can feminize the appearance of male patients. Because of the short distance between the male brow and the upper lid margins, often only internal brow suspension and fixation with minimal elevation is required (Fig. 4). If the male brow can be manually moved more than 2 or 3 mm, internal fixation is indicated (Fig. 5) so a distance of at least 8 to 10 mm can be left between the upper edge of the lid fold resection and the brow.

Once the brow level and contour have been established, the amount of upper lid fold resection can be determined. Images from high school or college graduations and old wedding pictures are valuable for comparison of the superior sulcus contour, level of the upper lid crease, and degree of upper lid folding. Patients who have never had a deep superior sulcus will not recognize themselves if they are oversculpted. Conversely, patients who have ptosis, levator aponeurotic disinsertions, and retracted deep superior sulci must be informed that their lids will again fill their superior sulci when their ptosis is repaired and their levator aponeuroses are advanced (Fig. 6). The surgeon must be aware that, even though the superior sulcus appears deep, the upper lid folds will have to be trimmed when the levator aponeuroses are advanced.

"To resect or not to resect upper lid skin": that is the question. Again, evaluating the contour and extent of the upper lid folds in old photographs will help the surgeon decide if skin resection is appropriate. If there is a slight redundancy but an apparent change in texture, laser resurfacing alone may be an effective mode of treatment (Fig. 7). If there is moderate or

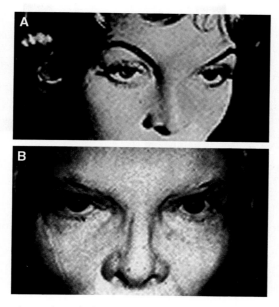

Fig. 2. (*A*) As a cabaret singer in Berlin in the 1930s, this patient maintained a stylized, exaggerated feminine brow arch. (*B*) Fifty years later, after too many upper eyelid skin resections and brow-supportive procedures, her brow arch has become ptotic and been transformed into a more masculine brow arch. When her brows were manually elevated to the level of the superior orbital rim, prominent lid lag and lagophthalmos were evident.

marked skin fold redundancy as well as changes in texture, resection and laser resurfacing are indicated (Fig. 8).

Diagnosing blepharoptosis preoperatively avoids an unwelcome surprise after blepharoplasty. A patient with a mild congenital ptosis or an acquired ptosis with levator aponeurotic disinsertion may compensate and obscure a narrowed palpebral aperture by unconsciously raising the brow. Unless the brow is held in its proper location just above the superior orbital rim when the vertical palpebral aperture is measured, blepharoptosis may be missed (Fig. 9). Other clues to diagnosing blepharoptosis include a raised brow, an elevated lid crease-fold complex, and a deep superior sulcus.

The contour of the upper lid must also be considered. There are central and nasal fat pockets in the upper lid. Often the nasal pocket is more visible and bothersome to patients. There is no lateral fat pocket in the upper lid. Any convex contours in the outer third of the upper lid are secondary to a prolapsed or enlarged palpebral lobe of the lacrimal gland (Fig. 10). Lacrimal gland prolapse is frequent in patients of African or Asian descent, in whom the bony orbit is shallow. Patients with thick, heavy brows and an ill-defined superior sulcus require CO_2 laser lipovaporization of the suborbicularis brow fat overlying the superior orbital rim as well as

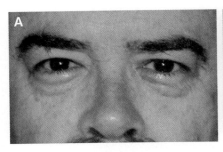
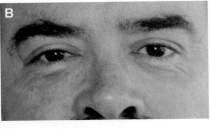

Fig. 3. (*A*) This patient exhibits a typical male brow contour, low and flat. (*B*) Internal brow suspension allows adequate lid crease exposure while maintaining an appropriate distance between the brow and the upper lid margin.

lipovaporization of the preaponeurotic fat to create a superior sulcus (Fig. 11).

Principles of lower eyelid repair

Perhaps the most critical factors in the evaluation the lower lid are the level and contour of the lower lid margin in relation to the inferior corneal limbus (Fig. 12) and any laxity of the lateral canthal tendon or the lower lid margin (Fig. 13). If there is any horizontal laxity of the lower lid margin or lateral canthal tendon, or if there is any lower lid retraction (inferior scleral show), even the most meticulous transcutaneous approach may cause a malposition of the lower lid margin. Retraction of the lower lid margin is common and may to secondary to an overactive thyroid, a shallow bony orbit, a highly myopic eye, a traumatic cicatricial deformity, or a previous transcutaneous blepharoplasty (Fig. 14). Avoiding the transcutaneous approach to the lower lid is the most efficient method of avoiding possible complications following lower lid surgery. All cosmetic procedures of the lower lid can be managed

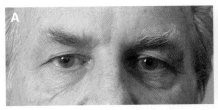
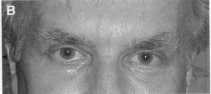

Fig. 4. (*A*) This patient's masculine brow level and contour had to be stabilized so that an effective upper lid blepharoplasty could be performed. To clear his visual axes, his brows were constantly elevated. (*B*) After internal brow suspension, upper lid myocutaneous resection, and laser resurfacing, he has a satisfactory upper eyelid contour. His lower eyelids were stabilized with lateral canthal tendon plications. They were recontoured with transconjunctival CO_2 laser lipovaporization and cutaneous resurfacing.

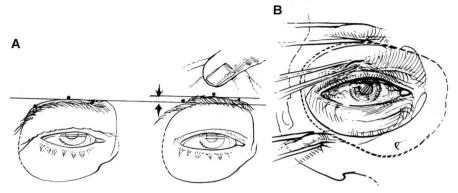

Fig. 5. (*A*) Preoperative mobility and level of the brow in relation to the superior orbital rim is determined manually. (*From* Bosniak S. Cosmetic blepharoplasty. New York: Raven Press; 1990.) (*B*) The thin eyelid skin is differentiated from the thicker skin external to the orbital rims. Over-resection of the upper lid will result in an inappropriate juxtaposition of the delicate eyelid skin with the thick brow skin. (*From* Bosniak S. Cosmetic blepharoplasty. New York: Raven Press; 1990. p. 15 and 30; with permission.)

using the transconjunctival approach. Lateral canthal support and cutaneous laser resurfacing can be performed simultaneously when necessary.

Lateral canthal tendon and lower lid margin laxity are gauged by the lid distraction test (how far the lid margin can be pulled away from the globe) and the snap test (how quickly the lid margin snaps back against the globe after it has been pulled away from it). A lid distraction test of more than 8 mm (Fig. 15) and a snap test of longer than 1 to 2 seconds indicate lid margin laxity. Lateral canthal laxity is also apparent when the normally acute lateral canthal angle is rounded (Fig. 16). Lateral canthal tightening re-establishes the lateral canthal angle, redrapes the lower lid skin, allows effective lower lid cutaneous laser resurfacing or chemical peel, and corrects lower lid retraction and lid margin malpositions (entropion and ectropion) secondary to lid margin laxity.

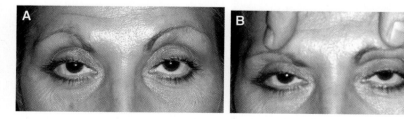

Fig. 6. (*A*) The hallmarks of upper lid blepharoptosis with aponeurotic disinsertions are compensatory brow elevation and a deep superior sulcus, with good to excellent upper lid margin excursions. (*B*) Manually fixating the brows at the level of the superior orbital rim accentuates the blepharoptosis.

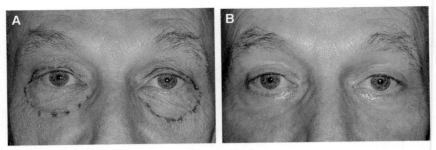

Fig. 7. (*A*) Apparent redundancy of the upper lid fold may be secondary to marked texture changes and rhytidosis. (*B*) Gratifying results can be achieved with cutaneous laser resurfacing without skin resection.

Lower lid contour adjustments can be addressed using a transconjunctival approach. Lower lid blepharoplasty, like upper lid blepharoplasty, is no longer a procedure limited to fat and skin resection. Prolapsing fat pockets can be vaporized, and depressions can be filled. There are three fat pockets in the lower lid—lateral, central, and medial—that can prolapse, giving convex contour irregularities. Traditionally the prolapsed lateral pocket has been problematic because a deeper component often was overlooked. The use of the CO_2 laser and the transconjunctival approach have facilitated effective sculpting of this pocket [11]. Concave contour defects such as tear trough deformities—medial depressions lateral to the anterior lacrimal crest—can be addressed with transconjunctival fat transposition (Fig. 17).

Lower eyelid skin resection is rarely indicated, except in patients with skin types IV, V, and VI. Mild dyspigmentation and rhytidosis can be

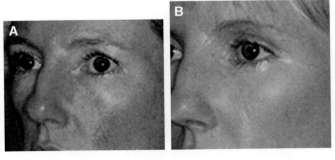

Fig. 8. (*A*) A full superior sulcus with true redundancy of the lid fold and skin texture changes responds best to skin resection and cutaneous laser resurfacing. (*B*) A CO_2 laser–assisted upper and lower lid blepharoplasty with eyelid and full face cutaneous laser resurfacing produced a dramatic improvement. (*From* Bosniak S, Cantisano-Zilkha M. Cosmetic blepharoplasty and facial rejuvenation. New York: Lippincott-Raven; 1999. p. 130; with permission.)

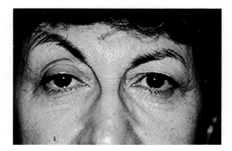

Fig. 9. This patient's right upper lid ptosis is manifested by a deep superior sulcus, a retracted lid crease, and a narrowed vertical palpebral aperture (partially camouflaged by compensatory brow elevation). Her left upper lid has a full superior sulcus and a normal brow contour and level. It is reasonable to assume that the full lid fold will need to be trimmed when the levator aponeurosis is repaired and the right upper lid crease is returned to its normal position.

managed with trichloroacetic acid (TCA) peels or Erbium:Yttrium aluminum garnet (YAG) laser resurfacing. Moderate and marked lower lid rhytidosis is managed with CO_2 laser resurfacing. Does excessive skin on the lower eyelid really exist? Lower lid rhytidosis may simply be the result of lost elasticity and lateral canthal laxity. Most cases of apparent excessive skin on the lower eyelid can be managed effectively with lateral canthal support and laser resurfacing (Fig. 18). This approach adequately corrects rhytidosis while allowing physiologic movement of the lower lid margin and avoiding lagophthalmos, lid retraction, and ectropion.

Principles of eyebrow and eyelash enhancement

To accentuate the benefits of a successful blepharoplasty—to create the frame for the eyes—attention must be directed to eyebrow and eyelash enhancement. Segmental or complete eyebrow or eyelash alopecia can be

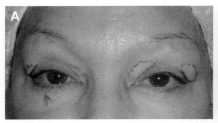 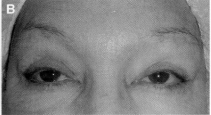

Fig. 10. (A) After an upper lid blepharoplasty, residual convexities are apparent in the temporal aspects of both upper lids. The prolapsed lacrimal glands are demarcated. (B) The upper lid contours are improved after suture suspensions of the palpebral lobes of the lacrimal gland to the periosteum of the lacrimal gland fossae within the superiolateral bony orbits.

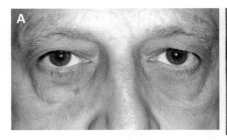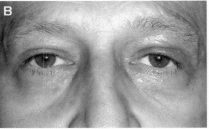

Fig. 11. (*A*) The patient presented with bilateral brow ptosis, redundant upper lid folds, and a narrowed distance between the brows and upper lid margins. He also had lower lid margin laxity, inferior scleral show, prolapsed inferior fat pockets, and malar festoons. (*B*) His appearance is markedly improved following internal brow suspension, upper lid myocutaneous resections, lipovaporization of the brow suborbicularis fat and upper lid preaponeurotic fat, transconjunctival lower lid lipovaporization, lateral canthal plication, and upper and lower lid cutaneous laser resurfacing. (*From* Bosniak S, Cantisano-Zilkha M. Minimally invasive techniques of oculo-facial rejuvenation. New York: Thieme; 2005. p. 79; with permission.)

camouflaged by micropigmentation or corrected with single-follicular-unit hair transplantation [1,12–16].

Upper eyelid blepharoplasty surgical techniques

Upper lid skin resection

If there is no levator aponeurotic disinsertion, the inferior aspect of the resection is delineated in the lid crease. If there is an aponeurotic disinsertion with lid crease retraction, the inferior aspect of the resection is delineated 8 to 10 mm above the lid margin or at the level of the contralateral lid crease. With the patient sitting in the upright position and facing the surgeon, the superior aspect of the resection is delineated, with care taken to maintain 8 to 10 mm between the superior aspect of the resection and the brow. If laser resurfacing is planned, the amount of skin resection is adjusted to compensate for 10% to 20% further skin contraction.

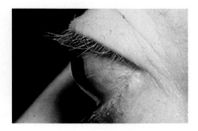

Fig. 12. Lower lid retraction may be evident in patients who are highly myopic (with large globes), have hyperactive thyroids, or have shallow bony orbits.

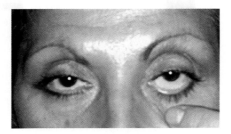

Fig. 13. Manual retraction of the lower lid margin narrows the horizontal palpebral aperture and causes rounding of the lateral canthal angle if there is lateral canthal tendon laxity.

If internal brow support is planned, the brow is held in position while the skin is demarcated. The medial extent of the resection is limited by the superior punctum. If upper lid skin redundancy is evident further medially, it can be managed with a W-plasty or laser resurfacing to avoid creating a medial canthal web (Fig. 19). The lateral extent of the resection is determined by the extent of temporal hooding not corrected by internal brow support. Ending the lateral aspect of the resection medial to the orbital rim is preferred, but more lateral resections can be extended in a smile line. Care is taken to keep these resections above the level of the lateral canthal angle to avoid postoperative lymphedema.

There are several choices of instrumentation for incising the skin: cold steel (#15 blade), fine-wire radiosurgical electrode (Vari-Tip, Ellman International, Oceanside, NY), cautery (Colorado needle), and CO_2 laser (0.2-mm hand piece, 5-μJ, Ultrapulse mode; Lumenus Ultrapulse 5000; Santa Ana, CA) [11]. For skin incision, all these modalities are about equally useful, providing that the surgeon is adept and can apply smooth, light, rapid strokes when using radiofrequency, cautery, or CO_2 laser. This

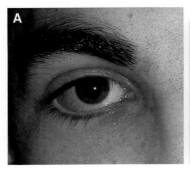
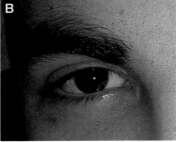

Fig. 14. (A) Cicatricial retraction of the lower lid margin creates 4 mm of inferior scleral show and a prominent rounding of the lateral canthal angle. (B) A normal palpebral aperture is restored after transconjunctival release of the cicatrix and lateral canthal suspension.

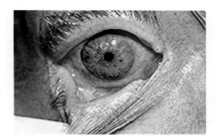

Fig. 15. Marked lower lid margin laxity is demonstrated by a positive lid distraction test. The lid margin is pulled more than 8 mm away from the globe.

technique will avoid prolonged tissue dwell time, increased lateral heat spread, and indurated would edges.

Lipovaporization

The most efficient technique for sculpting fat in a bloodless field uses CO_2 laser. Defocusing the 0.2-mm hand piece (5–8 watts in continuous wave [CW] mode) and moving it away from the tissue so that the aiming beam is not in focus increases lateral heat spread and vaporizes fat. This defocused beam also ablates larger-caliber blood vessels. Intermittent gentle pressure on the globe encourages further fatty prolapse so that it can be vaporized. In this manner, the volume of the fat pockets can be diminished and their anterior surfaces accurately recontoured. The alternatives are clamping, cutting, and cauterizing; open-sky resection with blood vessel cauterization when necessary; or radio-surgical resection with localized blood vessel ablation.

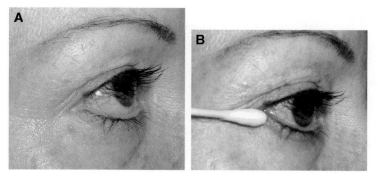

Fig. 16. (*A*) Mild lateral canthal laxity may present as a subtle loss of the acute lateral canthal angle and lower lid rhytidosis. (*B*) Lateral canthal tightening restores the acute lateral canthal angle and redrapes the lower lid skin.

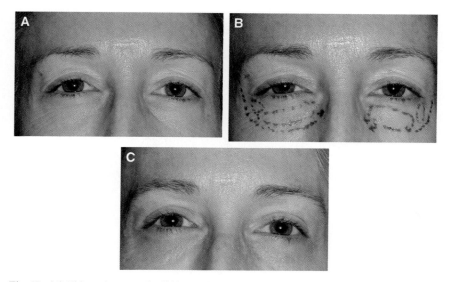

Fig. 17. (*A*) This patient noted mild lower lid fatty prolapse and mild tear trough depressions. (*B*) The areas of fatty prolapse, proposed fat transposition, and cutaneous laser resurfacing are demarcated. (*C*) Her eyelid skin texture and contours are improved following transconjunctival lower lid fat transposition and cutaneous resurfacing.

Lacrimal gland suspension

A prolapsed palpebral lobe of the lacrimal gland presents as a temporal bulge in the upper lid. After cutaneous or myocutaneous resection and central and medial fat pocket lipovaporization, the grayish lobular palpebral lobe is encountered. Its anterior surface can be tucked posterior to the lateral orbital rim with a mattress suture of 4-0 Prolene. Each arm of

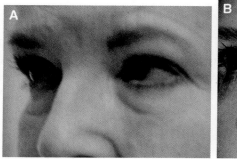
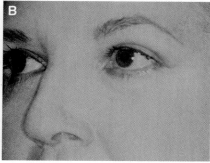

Fig. 18. (*A*) Mild-to-moderate lower lid fatty prolapse and rhytidosis create unpleasing shadows that are accentuated by lateral canthal laxity. (*B*) Marked improvement in lid contour and texture is evident following transconjunctival CO_2 laser lipovaporization, lateral canthal tendon plication, and eyelid and full-face CO_2 cutaneous laser resurfacing.

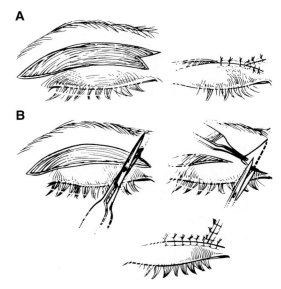

Fig. 19. (*A*) Upper lid skin excess medial to the superior punctum can be remedied with a W-plasty avoiding the formation of a medial canthal web. (*B*) An additional technique for resecting upper lid skin medial to the superior punctum is a Burrow's triangle. An incision perpendicular to the superior edge of the cutaneous resection is overlapped, and a base-down triangular skin resection is performed. (*From* Bosniak S. Cosmetic blepharoplasty. New York: Raven Press; 1990. p. 52; with permission.)

a double-armed suture is placed through the anterior surface of the gland (Fig. 20). The suture is passed into the periosteum of the lacrimal fossa (posterior and internal to the lateral orbital rim, superiorly at its junction with the superior orbital rim). When the suture is tied, the gland is pulled posterior behind the orbital rim.

Levator aponeurotic repair

When levator aponeurotic repair is planned, less than 1 cm^3 of local anesthetic is infiltrated subcutaneously under the demarcated lid crease incision. This dosage provides adequate anesthesia without akinesia so that the levator aponeurosis can be identified, its movement observed, and the palpebral aperture evaluated after the aponeurosis has been reattached to the tarsus. The lid crease is incised. A skin flap is developed inferiorly, exposing the pretarsal orbicularis muscles but avoiding the eyelash follicles. A 5-mm-wide strip of the superior pretarsal orbicularis muscle is resected, exposing the anterior surface of the superior tarsus. A myocutaneous flap is developed superiorly exposing the glistening white orbital septum. Gentle pressure on the globe causes preaponeurotic orbital fat to prolapse and the orbital septum to bulge. When the orbital septum is grasped and pulled

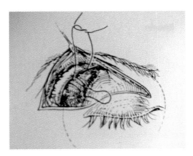

Fig. 20. A double-armed 4-0 Prolene suture suspends the prolapsed palpebral lobe of the lacrimal gland from the periosteum of the lacrimal fossa, retracting it into the orbit posterior to the superiolateral orbital rim. (*From* Bosniak S, Cantisano-Zilkha M. Cosmetic blepharoplasty and facial rejuvenation. New York: Raven-Lippincott; 1999. p. 67; with permission.)

inferiorly, it can be palpated at the arcus marginalis, just inferior to the superior orbital rim. The orbital septum is opened. The preaponeurotic fat is visualized and retracted. The diaphanous levator aponeurosis and its delicately rolled-up, disinserted inferior edge are now visible. Between the disinserted inferior edge of the aponeurosis and the superior border of the tarsus, the vascular Müller's muscle with its transverse arteriolar arcade is also clearly visible (Fig. 21). Three 6-0 black silk horizontal mattress sutures reapproximate the disinserted aponeurosis to the anterior surface of the tarsus (Fig. 22). These sutures are tied over a suture bolster so that the knots can be released when adjusting the lid margin level and contour. Patients open and close their eyes to confirm a pleasing arch of the upper lid margin (without segmental peaking) and a vertical palpebral that corresponds to

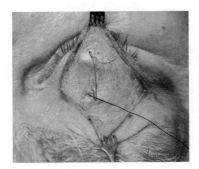

Fig. 21. The relevant eyelid anatomy is revealed during CO_2 laser–assisted levator aponeurotic surgery. The needle is in the superior tarsal margin. The suture loop is in the disinserted inferior edge of the rarefied levator aponeurosis. The intervening tissue is Müller's muscle (note its vascular arcade just superior to the superior tarsal border). The incised orbital septum is retracted, and the preaponeurotic fat is visible anterior to the levator muscle.

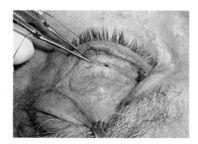

Fig. 22. One 6-0 black silk suture fixates the levator aponeurosis to the anterior tarsal surface. A second is being placed. Note that the rarefied levator aponeurosis appears very short (at least 10 mm is missing). This rarefaction may necessitate tying a loose suture loop to avoid inadvertent levator advancement and upper lid retraction.

the contralateral side (Fig. 23). If the orbital septum has been inadvertently included in the aponeurotic repair, lid lag on downgaze is apparent. After the upper lid level and contour have been secured, the superior myocutaneous flap is resected. The wound edges are closed, and the lid crease is recreated with interrupted sutures incorporating the advanced edge of the levator aponeurosis.

Müller's muscle resection and advancement plus tarsectomy (Fasanella–Servat procedure)

Patients with minimal ptosis (1–2 mm) whose eyelids after application of one drop of Neo-Synephrine 2.5% are candidates for this procedure.

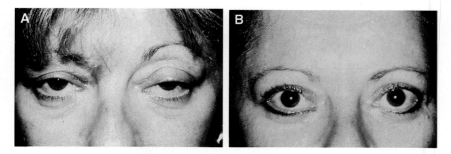

Fig. 23. (*A*) This patient had significant upper lid blepharoptosis with an obvious retraction of her left upper lid crease and compensatory brow elevation. She also had inferior scleral show and lower lid retraction. Correction of her upper lid ptosis without addressing the position of her lower lids would have resulted in an inappropriate widening of her vertical palpebral apertures. (*B*) After bilateral aponeurotic repair, upper lid myocutaneous trimming and lipovaporization, lateral canthal plication, and lower lid transconjunctival lipovaporization, her palpebral apertures improved markedly. (*From* Bosniak S, Cantisano-Zilkha M. Minimally invasive techniques of oculo-facial rejuvenation. New York: Thieme; 2005. p. 76; with permission.)

Performed through the posterior lamella, it can be easily performed in conjunction with skin and skin–muscle resections.

The upper eyelid is everted. The superior border of tarsus is retracted inferiorly while the eyelid skin is retracted superiorly, thus separating Müller's muscle from the levator aponeurosis. Two small curved hemostats are clamped (with their concave surfaces away from the lid margin) across superior tarsus (4 mm from the superior tarsal border), Müller's muscle, and conjunctiva (Fig. 24). Beginning at the nasal aspect of the upper lid crease, a running mattress suture of 5-0 nylon is passed through the skin, Müller's muscle, tarsus, and conjunctiva. It exits through the conjunctiva distal to the curved hemostat. It continues back and forth through conjunctiva, Müller's muscle, and tarsus until the lateral tarsus is reached. The final pass is through conjunctiva, Müller's muscle, tarsus, and skin, exiting at the lateral lid crease. The two external ends of the suture are pulled from side to side, nasally and temporally, to ensure smooth passage of the suture and ease of removal. The conjunctiva, Müller's muscle, and tarsus distal to the hemostats are resected. The clamps are released, the posterior lamella of the

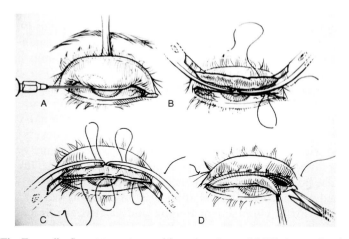

Fig. 24. The Fasanella–Servat tarsectomy with conjunctiva and Müller's muscle advancement and resection is a reliably predicable procedure for correction of 1 to 3 mm of ptosis in eyelids that respond to one drop of 2.5% Neo-Synephrine. (*A*) The upper lid is everted over a Desmarres retractor and subconjunctival infiltration is administered at the superior border of the tarsus. (*B*) Two curved hemostats are applied to the everted tarsus, conjunctiva, and Müller's muscle. Their concave surfaces are applied facing the superior border of the tarsus, but care is taken not to create an exaggerated arch centrally. (*C*) A 4-0 nylon suture is passed from lateral cutaneous lid crease, exiting distal to the hemostat on the conjunctival surface. It is continued in a running mattress fashion, angling the suture 45°, until the nasal extent of the tarsus is reached. (*From* Bosniak S. Cosmetic blepharoplasty. New York: Raven Press; 1990.) (*D*) The hemostats are released and the conjunctiva, tarsus, and Müller's muscle are resected in the crush marks, distal to the suture. (*From* Bosniak S. Cosmetic blepharoplasty. New York: Raven Press; 1990. p. 55; with permission.)

upper lid is smoothed, and the eyelid is returned to its normal anatomic position. The externalized ends of the suture are tied loosely to each other over the pretarsal skin. Care is taken not to tie them tightly, thus avoiding buckling of the tarsus. Skin and orbicularis muscle resections are then performed.

Lower eyelid blepharoplasty surgical techniques

Transconjunctival blepharoplasty

The lower lid is anesthetized with subconjunctival infiltration and a peribulbar block. If cutaneous resurfacing is planned, subcutaneous infiltration is also performed. The lid margin is everted with a toothed forceps, a small rake, a 4-0 black silk suture, or a Desmarres retractor. A 0.2-mm CO_2 laser hand piece (5 µJ, Ultrapulse mode; Lumenus Ultrapulse 5000) uses a focused beam to incise the conjunctiva 4 mm inferior to the inferior border of tarsus. Gentle pressure on the globe prolapses the orbital fat, and the incision is made over the most convex aspect of the bulge. The incision can also be made with a fine-wire Vari-Tip radiosurgical electrode, a Colorado needle #15 blade, or Wescott scissors. The conjunctival incision is widened, extending medially to within 2 mm of the caruncle and extending laterally until within 2 mm of the lateral border of the tarsus [9,10]. While the edges of the conjunctival incision are retracted with small rakes, the facial septae are divided with another pass using the 0.2-mm hand piece, allowing the fat pockets to prolapse. All three fat pockets (Fig. 25) and the inferior oblique muscle (nestled between the central and nasal pocket) are clearly visualized (Fig. 26). In a virtually bloodless field, they are vaporized and recontoured with a defocused beam, using the 0.2-mm hand piece (5–8 watts, CW mode). Large vessels on the surface of the fat pockets can also be obliterated with the defocused beam. Repeated gentle pressure on the globe and observation confirm the desired recontouring of the lower lid fat pockets. The lid is returned to its normal anatomic position, the conjunctiva is smoothed with a cotton-tipped applicator, and the lid margin is stretched superiorly to avoid conjunctival folding and cicatricial retraction. Gentle pressure on the globe while the lower lid is palpated gives final confirmation of the desired lower lid contour. The conjunctiva is not sutured.

Transconjunctival fat transposition

After the inferior palpebral conjunctiva is opened and the prolapsing fat pockets are exposed, a pedicle flap of fat can be transposed. Usually a central of medial pocket can be conveniently transposed into a medial tear trough depression. The anterior surface recontoured, allowing sufficient volume to fill the depression. The base of the flap is mobilized with a defocused 0.2-mm hand piece (Fig. 27A). A double-armed 6-0 plain catgut suture is passed through the apex of the flap (Fig. 27B). Each arm of the

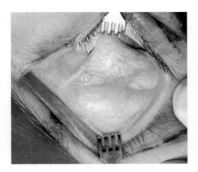

Fig. 25. The three distinct lower eyelid fat pockets—nasal, central, and lateral—are visible after the conjunctiva has been incised with a CO_2 laser.

double-armed suture is passed through the skin nasal to the depression. The suture ends are tied loosely to each other over the skin.

Lateral canthal tendon plication

Lateral canthal tendon plication is most effective for mild-to-moderate laxity of the lower lid margin and lateral canthal tendon or for rounding of the lateral canthal angle. A 2-mm lower lid subciliary incision is made at the extreme lateral aspect of the lid. A 4-mm lid crease incision is made in the lateral lid crease, straddling the lateral orbital rim. The periosteum of the lateral orbital rim is exposed, and a small myocutaneous flap is developed superiorly to ensure that the plication suture knot is buried. A double-armed 4-0 Prolene suture is passed from the lateral palpebral conjunctiva through the lateral subciliary incision. The sutures are then passed back into the subciliary incision but are directed laterally and superiorly, engaging the superior crus of the lateral canthal tendon posterior to the lateral orbital rim and exiting in the upper lid lateral lid crease incision (Figs. 28 and 29). The

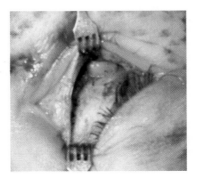

Fig. 26. The bulging inferior oblique muscle is identified between the central and nasal lower lid fat pockets. It is clearly visible after these fat pockets have been vaporized.

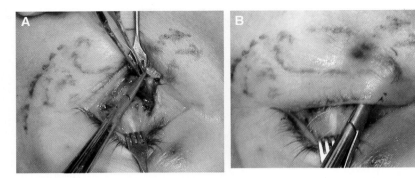

Fig. 27. (*A*) A 6-0 plain catgut horizontal mattress suture is placed into the nasal fat pocket before it is transposed. (*B*) The sutures are externalized through the skin at the medial orbital rim and tied loosely together.

lateral lid level and contour are determined by the suture placement. How tightly the suture is tied s the apposition of the lid margin and lateral canthal angle to the globe. The suture is then anchored to the periosteum of the superior aspect of the lateral orbital rim. The knot is buried under the myocutaneous flap.

Lateral tarsal strip suspension

Lateral canthal plication may be insufficient to correct the lower lid deformity in cases of extreme lower lid margin laxity or a lateral canthal cicatricial retraction. A lateral cantholysis is necessary to release the lateral canthal tendon and lateral aspect of the lower lid (Fig. 30). Creation of

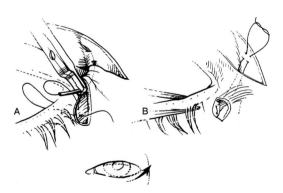

Fig. 28. (*A*) A lateral canthal plication is performed using a lower lid lateral conjunctiva entrance, a lateral cutaneous subciliary incision, and a lateral upper lid crease incision. (*B*) The vector of plication is customized depending on the desired angle of elevation, prominence of the lateral orbital rim, and degree of lower lid laxity. The suture is anchored to the periosteum of the superior aspect of the lateral orbital rim. (*From* Bosniak S, Cantisano-Zilkha M. Cosmetic blepharoplasty and facial rejuvenation. New York: Raven-Lippincott; 1999. p. 83; with permission.)

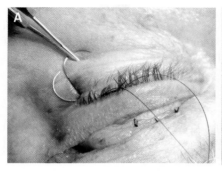
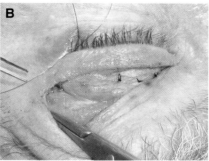

Fig. 29. (*A*) Lateral canthal plication. Step 1: both arms of a 4-0 Prolene suture are brought through a 2-mm lateral cutaneous subciliary incision from the palpebral conjunctival surface. (*B*) Step 2: each arm of the suture is passed posterior the lateral orbital rim to engage the deep arm of the lateral canthal tendon.

a lateral tarsal strip shortens the redundant lid margin, resuspends the lower lid, and reforms the lateral canthal angle. After the lateral cantholysis has been performed, the released lateral edge of the lower lid is pulled laterally, overlapping the lateral orbital rim. The lid margin is notched where it overlaps the orbital rim. The lid margin, the pretarsal myocutaneous flap, and palpebral conjunctiva lateral to the notch are resected . A 4-mm strip of tarsus is preserved. A 4-0 Prolene suture is used to suspend this tarsal strip from the superior crus of the lateral canthal tendon and periosteum of the

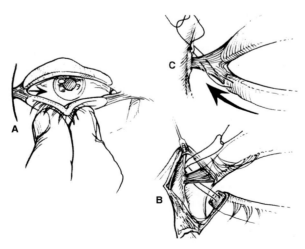

Fig. 30. (*A–C*) If there is marked laxity of the lower lid margin and lateral canthal tendon, a simple lateral canthal plication will not bring the lower eyelid margin into proper apposition with the globe. A folding of the lower lid margin may then be apparent. Under these circumstances, the creation of a lateral tarsal strip is indicated. (*From* Bosniak S. Cosmetic blepharoplasty. New York: Raven Press; 1990. p. 78; with permission.)

superior lateral orbital rim. The placement of this suture determines the level and contour of the lateral canthal angle. The lateral canthal angle itself is recreated by anastomosing the lash line and gray line of the lateral aspect of the upper and lower lids (Fig. 31). The suture ends are left long and are folded away from conjunctiva.

Ablative laser resurfacing

Eyelid laser resurfacing can be purely ablative (Erbium:YAG) with minimal thermal spread, or the epidermis can be vaporized in a controlled fashion with a CO_2 laser creating tissue tightening as a secondary thermal effect. The target chromophore for both Erbium (2940-nm) and CO_2 (10,600-nm) lasers is water. Because the Erbium laser's affinity for water is greater than that of the CO_2 laser, its effect is more superficial (5–20 μm of thermal injury) than that of the CO_2 laser (50–125 μm for each pass).

Minimal to mild rhytidosis can be ablated with Erbium:YAG laser resurfacing, using a small square pattern (pattern 3, size 4, 2 J) and one to three passes (Lumenis Ultra Fine). Three passes of the Erbium:YAG is equivalent to one pass of the CO_2 laser. Although more than three passes can be applied, the end point may be limited by punctate bleeding, and more intense resurfacing is better performed using a CO_2 laser. The recovery after three passes of Erbium resurfacing is rapid: 4 to 5 days for complete re-epithelialization. The erythema after re-epithelialization rarely persists longer than 3 to 4 weeks. Because there is little thermal effect following Erbium:YAG resurfacing, there is rhytid ablation without tissue tightening.

For mild rhytidosis one pass of the CO_2 laser using a lower power setting (Ultrapulse 150–200 μJ) and a small, square pattern (pattern 3, size 4, density 5) may be all that is necessary. For moderate to marked rhytidosis, 2 or 3 passes with Ultrapulse power settings from 200 to 300 μJ may be used. These treatments ablate rhytids, tighten the lower lid skin, and reduce malar festooning. To avoid postoperative malpositions of the lower lid margin,

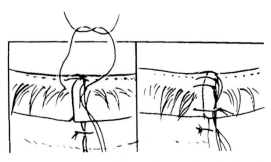

Fig. 31. Effective reapposition of the lid margin requires closing in three layers—the mucocutaneous junction (gray line), the meibomian line, and the lash line. (*From* Bosniak S. Cosmetic blepharoplasty. New York: Raven Press; 1990. p. 77; with permission.)

any lid margin or lateral canthal laxity must be corrected preoperatively. Re-epithelialization is usually complete within 7 days. This process is accelerated if occlusive dressings are applied to the lower lids at the conclusion of the procedure. The duration of the postoperative erythema is determined by the intensity of the treatment and may persist for several months. Camouflage make-up after re-epithelialization provides sun protection as well as improved cosmesis. This protection is critical, because sun exposure prolongs erythema and in some cases promotes postinflammatory hyperpigmentation.

Trichloroacetic acid peels

For lower eyelid pigment mottling and mild rhytidosis, 20% TCA is an effective superficial peeling agent requiring only 4 days or less of downtime. A thin layer is applied with a sterile cotton-tipped applicator. A light frosting appears within 5 minutes after application (Fig. 32A, B). After 5 to 10 minutes, the frosting disappears, and a mild erythema is apparent. Three to 4 days of mild, brownish crusting may follow (Fig. 32C). The regimen after peeling is frequent lubrication (CU3 copper peptide cream) and vinegar washes (1 tablespoon of white vinegar in 4 cups of tepid water) [1,17].

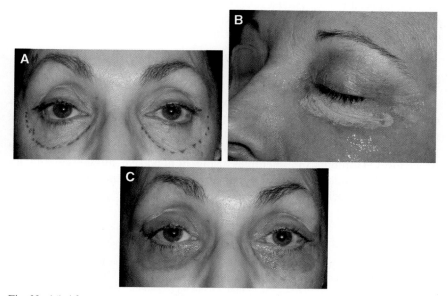

Fig. 32. (*A*) After a transcutaneous blepharoplasty, this patient was referred for correction of her lower lid retraction and rounded lateral canthal angles. (*B*) To improve her lower eyelid skin texture, a 20% trichloroacetic acid peel was performed. (*C*) On the fourth postoperative day, her lid levels and lateral canthal angles are improved. Mild lower lid discoloration persists.

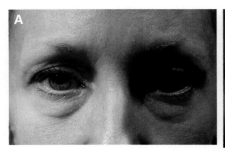 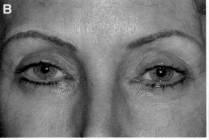

Fig. 33. (*A*) In addition to upper eyelid fold redundancy and lower lid fatty prolapse, this patient had segmental eyebrow alopecia and eyelash thinning. (*B*) After laser-assisted upper and lower blepharoplasty and cutaneous resurfacing, her final appearance was enhanced with eyebrow and eyelash micropigmentation and single-follicular-unit hair transplantation to the eyebrows. (*From* Bosniak S, Cantisano-Zilkha M. Minimally invasive techniques of oculo-facial rejuvenation. New York: Thieme; 2005. p. 85; with permission.)

Micropigmentation

Micropigmentation of the eyebrow and eyelashes, when performed in an understated, natural manner, yields long-lasting cosmetic enhancement (Fig. 33). It typically is performed using topical anesthetic cream, but anesthesia can be supplemented with local injections when necessary. Localized crusting may persist for several days and should be managed with frequent applications of bland ointment, with avoidance of water and skin-care products. Touch-ups may be performed in 3 to 4 weeks.

Summary

The current state of the art of cosmetic blepharoplasty transcends the concept of tissue removal and replaces it with a tissue-rejuvenating physiologic approach that treats and preserves tissues. This approach minimizes potential complications and enhances the longevity of these procedures. Combination therapies using noninvasive modalities and laser-assisted techniques further enhance the accuracy and effectiveness of blepharoplasty techniques.

References

[1] Bosniak S, Cantisano-Zilkha M. Minimally invasive techniques of oculo-facial rejuvenation. New York: Thieme Publishers; 2005.
[2] Bosniak S, Cantisano-Zilkha M. Total eyelid rejuvenation. Operative Techniques in Oculoplastic, Orbital, and Reconstructive Surgery 1999;2(4):198–203.
[3] Bosniak S. Cosmetic blepharoplasty. New York: Raven Press; 1990.
[4] Bosniak S, Cantisano-Zilkha M. Cosmetic blepharoplasty and facial rejuvenation. New York: Lippincott-Raven; 1999.

[5] Reifler DM. Upper eyelid blepharoplasty. In: Bosniak S, editor. Principles and practice of ophthalmic plastic and reconstructive surgery. Philadelphia: W.B. Saunders; 1996. p. 596–617.

[6] Wojno TH, Bosniak S. Cosmetic surgery. In: Bosniak S, editor. Principles and practice of ophthalmic plastic and reconstructive surgery. Philadelphia: W.B. Saunders; 1996. p. 543–5.

[7] Weiss RA. Brow ptosis. In: Bosniak S, editor. Principles and practice of ophthalmic plastic and reconstructive surgery. Philadelphia: W.B. Saunders; 1996. p. 578–89.

[8] Maries HM, Patrinely JR. Male blepharoplasty. In: Bosniak S, editor. Principles and practice of ophthalmic plastic and reconstructive surgery. Philadelphia: W.B. Saunders; 1996. p. 632–8.

[9] Custer PL. Lower eyelid blepharoplasty. In: Bosniak S, editor. Principles and practice of ophthalmic plastic and reconstructive surgery. Philadelphia: W.B. Saunders; 1996. p. 617–26.

[10] Goldberg RA, Baylis HI, Golden SH. Transconjunctival lower blepharoplasty. In: Bosniak S, editor. Principles and practice of ophthalmic plastic and reconstructive surgery. Philadelphia: W.B. Saunders; 1996. p. 626–32.

[11] Bosniak S, McDebitt T, Wojno TH. Alternative techniques of fat removal. In: Bosniak S, editor. Principles and practice of ophthalmic plastic and reconstructive surgery. Philadelphia: W.B. Saunders; 1996. p. 632–8.

[12] Bosniak S, Cantisano-Zilkha M, Ziering C, et al. Eyebrow rejuvenation: a multi-disciplinary approach. Operative Techniques in Oculoplastic, Orbital, and Reconstructive Surgery 2001;4(2):100–3.

[13] Gandelman M. Eyebrow and eyelash reconstruction. Operative Techniques in Oculoplastic, Orbital, and Reconstructive Surgery 2001;4(2):94–99.

[14] Mazza JF, Roger C. Blepharopigmentation: techniques, indications and comparison of modalities. In: Bosniak S, editor. Principles and practice of ophthalmic plastic and reconstructive surgery. Philadelphia: W.B. Saunders; 1996. p. 682–8.

[15] Meneuzes. The principles of permanent facial makeup. Operative Techniques in Oculoplastic, Orbital, and Reconstructive Surgery 1999;2(4):182–7.

[16] Ploof H. Electropigmentation and the cosmetic surgery patient. In: Bosniak S, editor. Principles and practice of ophthalmic plastic and reconstructive surgery. Philadelphia: W.B. Saunders; 1996. p. 676–81.

[17] Rubin MG. Manual of chemical peels—superficial and medium depth. Philadelphia: JB Lippincott Company; 1995.

ELSEVIER
SAUNDERS

Otolaryngol Clin N Am
38 (2005) 1009–1021

OTOLARYNGOLOGIC
CLINICS
OF NORTH AMERICA

The Diagnosis and Management of Blepharoplasty Complications

Ioannis P. Glavas, MD

Department of Ophthalmology, New York University Medical School,
Manhattan Eye, Ear and Throat Hospital,
210 East 64th Street, New York, NY 10021, USA

Blepharoplasty is the third most common cosmetic procedure performed by cosmetic surgeons according to the 2003 statistics of the American Society for Aesthetic Plastic Surgery. The number is growing each year, having increased by 17% from 2002 [1]. The procedure may involve removal of eyelid skin and orbital fat excision or repositioning. Occasionally needed complementary procedures are brow elevation, lateral canthal position adjustment, correction of lower eyelid laxity, and eyelid skin rejuvenation. Upper and lower lid blepharoplasty may be performed for cosmetic reasons. Upper lid blepharoplasty may also be performed for the functional correction of blepharochalasis and dermatochalasis.

Facial and especially eyelid appearance is scrutinized extensively by female and male patients. Increased acceptance of plastic surgery and easier access to medical information with the advent of the Internet and television have resulted in well-informed and demanding patients. Minute postoperative imperfections may be the source of unsatisfied patients and thus suggest an unsuccessful outcome.

Management of blepharoplasty complications should start before surgery. Building a strong and trusting relationship with the patient is as important as setting goals based on realistic expectations. Because eyelids are not all anatomically the same, the surgical plan should be individualized for each candidate. The possibility of real and perhaps debilitating complications should be clarified. Profound knowledge of eyelid and periocular anatomy and the performance of state-of-the-art surgery taking all standard precautions for proper healing is the physician's responsibility. Study of old photographs and photographic documentation at the preoperative and postoperative stages is necessary. They may prove useful in patient

E-mail address: iglavas@pol.net

education, evaluation of results, and, if necessary, to resolve unsubstanti-
ated claims of bad outcome.

Prevention of complications is the best approach to managing them. This
article briefly reviews the pertinent anatomy of the eyelids and the
preoperative planning to avoid complications before discussing their
management.

Anatomy

Detailed knowledge of the anatomy of the eyelids and surrounding
periocular tissues is of key importance. It allows the surgeon to plot a
preoperative plan based on his or her observations and to modify this plan
confidently and safely, if necessary, during the procedure.

The eyelids are located anterior to the orbital openings. They protect the
globe from external threats, contain the glands for the production of the
baseline tear film, and play an important role in the pump mechanism of
tear outflow into the nasolacrimal drainage system.

The average palpebral fissure measures 9 to 12 mm vertically and 28 to 30
mm horizontally with a slight upward slant toward the lateral side. The
lateral canthus is 1 to 2 mm higher than the medial canthus.

The lids are composed of anterior lamellae formed by the skin and
orbicularis muscle and posterior lamellae formed by tarsus and conjunctiva.
The tarsus is dense connective tissue measuring 10 mm and 4 mm vertically
in the upper and lower lids, respectively. The upper eyelid crease is formed
by the insertion of the levator muscle in the tarsus and skin. It is located 7 to
10 mm above the eyelid margin. The inferior lid crease is formed similarly by
the insertion of the lower lid retractors composed of the capsulopalpebral
fascia and inferior tarsal muscle. Cutaneous insertions of the orbitomalar
ligament form the malar and nasojugal folds. The position of eyelid folds
and the shape of the interpalpebral opening give the unique appearance that
characterizes persons of Far Eastern ancestry.

The medial and lateral canthal ligaments attach the eyelids to the orbital
rims medially at the anterior and posterior lacrimal crest and laterally on
Whitnall's tubercle. The orbital septum is a strong sheet of connective tissue
defining the anterior extent of the orbit. The septum creates a compartment.
Blood cannot escape from this compartment and forms the "raccoon eyes"
seen postoperatively. With aging, orbital fat may prolapse through thin
areas of the septum. The upper eyelid has two distinct fat pads, the
preaponeurotic lateral pad, which is more yellow in color, and the medial
pad, which is firmer and paler. The inferior lid has three distinct fat pads
separated by the inferior oblique muscle.

The upper lid is functionally and anatomically related to the eyebrow in
the protection of the globe and the facial expression of emotions [2]. The
eyebrow ideally is located at or above the superior orbital rim. A horizontal
T shape is more characteristic of the male face, and a superiorly convex

shape is more commonly observed in the female face. The lower border is usually located 1 cm above the lateral portion of the orbital rim. The skin of the eyebrows is thicker than that of the eyelids (a useful landmark for the uppermost line of incision). It is highly mobile because of its strong attachments to the subcutaneous muscles and the superficial galea aponeurotica. The retro-orbicularis oculi fat pad is located between the frontalis orbicularis and galea aponeurotica. With aging it may extend anterior to the septum and into the upper lid, falsely giving the impression of retroseptal fat. Neurogenic or involutional ptosis of the brow complex may give the impression of excess upper eyelid skin [3].

The lower lid is continuous with the suborbicularis oculi fat that extends posteriorly to the orbicularis and inferiorly to the midface. Ptosis of the midface tissues may contribute to the appearance of the tear-trough defect.

Blood supply of the eyelids is abundant from branches of the internal and external arteries forming vascular arcades in the eyelids. Venous drainage is from both facial and orbital veins.

Innervation of the eyelids is supplied by the seventh cranial facial nerve, the oculomotor third cranial nerve, the trigeminal nerve, and sympathetic nerves.

Prevention

As mentioned previously, management of blepharoplasty complications should start early in the preoperative period with proper patient evaluation and surgical planning.

Patient evaluation

Before any further action, establish a firm relationship with the patient. Are the expectations reasonable? What social and psychologic reasons led the patient to the consultation? What are the "deeper" changes sought from the surgical outcome—improved self-image or secondary gain?

Medical history should screen for specific conditions that may warrant additional medical consideration or negatively alter the outcome. Medical conditions that may affect the healing process or increase the risks for infection, such as diabetes and immunocompromised states, should be evaluated properly. Bleeding diathesis from disease or use of medicines, such as aspirin, nonsteroidal anti-inflammatory drugs, warfarin, and others, should be ruled out. Ask about use of over-the-counter medications (vitamin E) and homeopathic or other herbal medicines.

The quality of the skin should be evaluated. Does the patient have a tendency to form hypertrophic scars or keloids? Is there any known allergy to the suture materials used to close the wounds? Does the patient have any previous experience with surgery and anesthesia?

Surgical planning

Evaluation of the anatomy and marking of the patient should be done with the patient sitting in an upright position. Gravity is one of the most important culprits for the tissue changes that result in skin folding, connective tissue weakening, and fat pad prolapse. Notice asymmetry of eyelid crease and mark the new position. Outline the fat pads with the marker and identify the areas that may need fat repositioning rather than fat removal. All these tissue landmarks are lost when the patient is in supine position and local anesthetic is injected into the tissues.

Evaluation of old photographs is useful at this point to compare the former position of tissues with the present state and to plan surgery to match the appearance. The goal of surgery is to enhance and rejuvenate the eyelids without making a dramatic, overdone look. For example, it is not advisable to remove excess amounts of orbital fat and create a hollow look in a patient who always has had full-appearing upper lids.

Brow position

A ptotic brow decreases the vertical distance between the eyelashes and the brow and may give the false impression of excessive, hooding upper eyelid skin. Retro-orbicularis fat ptosis into the preseptal space of the upper eyelid may be mistaken for orbital fat prolapse. The brow may be repositioned at the time of the blepharoplasty procedure. Transblepharoplasty brow fixation using a nonabsorbable suture has been used successfully for small degrees of ptosis [3]. Endoscopic or coronal approaches may be used for more severe ptosis. Neuromodulating agents have been used successfully to elevate the lateral aspect of the brow and reduce the amount of skin hooding at the lateral aspect of the upper eyelid [4].

Upper eyelid crease

The position of the eyelid crease is probably the most important landmark for the upper lid blepharoplasty. The incision is usually hidden in the fold formed by the upper eyelid crease. A high crease may be the sign of levator aponeurosis dehiscence and involutional ptosis. In that case, the eyelid crease must be marked lower to the existing crease. After repair of ptosis, with advancement of the levator aponeurosis, the eyelid crease should be reformed at the desired level, taking small bites of the orbicularis muscle when closing the skin.

Lower lid

Evaluation of the lower lid is somewhat more complex than that of the upper lid. Canthal tendon laxity and tendency for postoperative lid malpositions should be addressed at this point. The snap test, which consists of pulling the lower lid inferiorly and observing the reaction of the tissues and the return to the anatomic position onto the globe, is an effective and easy method of evaluating lower lid laxity. Globe prominence must be evaluated in relation to the lid laxity or planed eyelid-tightening procedure. Tightening the lower canthal tendon over a prominent globe without addressing the vertical length of the eyelid may result in buckle (belt) effect and scleral show.

Hypertrophy of the orbicularis muscle should be differentiated from fat pad prolapse because surgical management is different. Evaluation of the midface tissues should be performed at the same time. Finally, attention should be given to the surgical technique planned. Is the patient candidate for a transcutaneous or transconjunctival approach? Even if skin is not removed, a transcutaneous approach will always result in vertical shortening of the lower lid because of scarring of the septum. With the transconjunctival approach, the septum is not injured at all. Skin rhytidosis can be addressed with laser resurfacing or chemical peels but with the disadvantage of longer recovery time.

Complications

Complications may arise even after the most meticulous preoperative evaluation and uneventful surgery. Box 1 lists all the possible adverse events. They can be categorized as tissue related or iatrogenic, but some may overlap into both groups.

Almost every patient experiences some degree of bleeding, skin edema, and ecchymosis. Conjunctival chemosis may be transient or take 2 to 5 months to resolve. It is believed to result from blockage of orbital or eyelid lymphatics and excessive cautery during surgery [5–7]. Gentle handling of tissues during surgery and preoperative discontinuation of medications that may increase the risk of bleeding minimize these events. The use of laser or radiofrequency incisional tools may further minimize ecchymosis and bleeding [8,9]. Application of ice compresses for the first 24 to 48 hours postoperatively helps minimize edema and inflammation and makes patients more comfortable.

Infection after blepharoplasty is uncommon because of the high vascularity of the eyelids. Topical application of antibiotic ointments is usually sufficient to avoid skin infection. The risk is slightly higher in patients who have adjunctive laser resurfacing [10]. The most common agents are skin flora, but unusual infections such as group A beta-hemolytic Streptococcus have been reported [11,12]. Surprisingly, infections from atypical mycobacteria seem to be common [13–17].

Orbital cellulitis and abscess formation have been reported [18–20]. Prompt recognition of the signs of cellulitis and treatment with antibiotics and other appropriate modalities may minimize scarring.

Retrobulbar hemorrhage and blindness are rare but severe complications with an incidence of approximately 0.04%. Retrobulbar hemorrhage occurs during the immediate postoperative period, but delayed incidents of

Box 1. Possible complications of blepharoplasty

Iatrogenic complications
- Lagophthalmos (may present after brow lift if not addressed first)
- Inferior scleral show
- Corneal exposure
- Astigmatism
- Corneal abrasion
- Corneal burn if using laser incision tool
- Strabismus
- Diplopia
- Oversculpting with superior sulcus defect
- Asymmetry of sides
- Misdiagnosis of ptosis
- Postoperative ptosis from levator injury
- Medial canthal webbing
- Dry eye
- Oversculpting of lower fat with tear trough defect and sunken appearance.
- Lower lid ectropion from anterior lamella shortening
- Lower lid retraction from middle lamellae shortening
- Entropion from posterior lamellae shortening
- Lower lid retraction from buckle effect over the globe
- Rounding of lateral canthus

Inherent tissue complications
- Infection
- Edema
- Chemosis of conjunctiva
- Ecchymosis
- Bleeding
- Orbital cellulitis
- Retrobulbar hemorrhage
- Blindness
- Wound dehiscence
- Hypertrophic scar formation
- Pyogenic granuloma
- Suture granuloma
- Suture allergy to plain gut
- Dry eye
- Loss of skin sensation in the eyelid

retrobulbar hematoma have been reported [21,22]. The clinical presentation is eye proptosis and increased intraocular pressure. The cause of blindness is unclear but is believed to be retinal ischemic changes or optic neuropathy or acute-angle closure glaucoma [23–25]. Measures to avoid this serious complication are observation of the patient for several hours after surgery and avoiding use of occlusive patches over the eyes [26]. Treatment of a retrobulbar hemorrhage is a true emergency. Medical treatment, which includes pharmacologic agents to reduce the intraocular pressure, is the first step. Surgical intervention performing lateral cantholysis and orbital decompression should be the immediate action when deterioration of vision is noted [27,28].

Several complications arise from poor healing of the skin or accidents. Wound dehiscence is almost always related to injury. Poor healing caused by systemic conditions such as diabetes may contribute to its occurrence. Débridement of the skin edges and closing of the wound is usually the only action needed. Hypertrophic scar formation has not been reported on the eyelid skin, even in individuals with diathesis, but it remains a theoretical possibility. Local injections of corticosteroids may prove useful in treating such a condition. In contrast, transient loss of skin sensation in the eyelid after incision blepharoplasty of the upper eyelid crease is relatively common and may take 2 to 6 months to resolve [29].

The transconjunctival approach offers the potential advantage of avoiding scar creation in the lower eyelid skin. Suture and pyogenic granulomas formation are possible complications with this approach. Pyogenic granulomas are vascular inflammatory lesions that represent an aberrant wound healing response [30–32]. A short course of topical corticosteroid application may result in complete resolution. If not, surgical resection is the treatment of choice. Lipogranuloma formation has been associated with use of topical antibiotic ointment postoperatively before conjunctival epithelialization has been completed [33].

Finally, allergic reactions to the suture material are an extremely rare but an unacceptable complication in the cosmetic patient. Treatment consists of removal of the suture material and use of local and systemic corticosteroids and antihistamines.

Exacerbation or new onset of dry eye may be transient or permanent. Preoperative evaluation of the lacrimal function, including tear composition, tear film stability, production rate, and drainage and eyelid position, is important. Management with use of topical lubricating agents is recommended initially. In addition, surgical correction of possible excessive vertical lid shortening or malpositioning may be necessary [34–37].

Cornea

The eyelids are in proximity to the globe, and minor changes in their anatomy or inadvertent intraoperative actions may result in corneal complications and vision changes [38]. Direct thermal injury or alteration of the lid position relative to the globe may lead to visually significant refractive astigmatism [39,40]. Corneal abrasions with conventional cold steel instruments or thermal burns from a CO_2 laser may result in significant scarring and stromal opacification [41–42].

Scleral and corneal exposure may result from causes related to upper and lower lid malpositions. Removal of excess skin from the upper lid results in lagophthalmos. Brow lift after upper blepharoplasty may create or exacerbate exposure [43]. Symptomatic scleral exposure may be tolerated and managed with frequent use of ophthalmic lubricants. Corneal exposure, especially when combined with a poor Bell's phenomenon, may result in persistent dry eye and eventually in cornea decompensation and even blindness. Graded full-thickness anterior blepharotomy, spreading the scar, or skin grafting are methods to reconstruct the upper eyelid with relatively acceptable aesthetic results [3,44–45]. Full-thickness skin grafts from the retroauricular area offer the best color match [46]. Full-thickness skin graft from the supraclavicular area may be used alternatively. Split-thickness grafts may be used, but they entail the risk of shrinkage and early failure [47,48].

Lower lid vertical shortening may also result in poor lid apposition during closure and corneal exposure. Preoperative evaluation of canthal tendon laxity with the distraction and snap test, of the prominence of the eye globe, and of the risk of inferior buckling of the eyelid is important. The transcutaneous approach entails the risk of anterior and middle lamellae scarring even if no skin is removed. Excessive electrocautery to the septum causes scarring and retraction, lateral canthus rounding, and temporal ectropion.

The severity of retraction and degree of lower lid laxity should be taken into consideration when repairing this type of defect. Small degrees of retraction may be adequately repaired with a canthoplication [3]. Non-absorbable suture is used to tighten the lateral canthus at the periosteum of the lateral orbital rim. For more severe retraction and rounding of the lateral canthus, a combined lateral tarsal strip procedure with grafting of the anterior and posterior lamellae is required. Free tarsal conjunctival graft from the upper lid and eyelid traction using a temporary Frost suture may correct the defect successfully [49]. Alternative graft areas are ear cartilage, chondromucosal palate graft, and commercially available spacers [50].

Upper lid

Oversculpting of excess amounts of orbital fat from the upper or lower lid may result in superior sulcus defect, with a hollow and unnatural appearance [51]. This effect may be especially undesirable effect in Asian patients. Free fat, composite fascia-fat and dermis-fascia grafts, and sclera with liquid collagen have been used to alleviate this complication [52–55].

Use of injectable collagen and hyaluronic acid for filling the supraorbital space has achieved promising but temporary results [56,57].

Ptosis is a frequently missed diagnosis in an elderly blepharoplasty patient. It usually presents as dermatochalasis or dehiscence of the levator aponeurosis. Other neurogenic or myogenic causes may be cause ptosis. Proper recognition of the symptoms is important to select the proper surgical procedure and to correct ptosis at the same time. Ptosis manifests with a high upper eyelid crease, decreased lid merging to corneal reflex distance, and superior visual field restriction. The patient looks oversculpted. Treatment consists of ptosis repair with levator advancement before or at the time of blepharoplasty.

Postoperative ptosis is infrequent complication. It may result from delayed resolution of edema, hematoma formation, local anesthetic toxic effects, adhesions of the septum, and levator injury [58]. It may result in asymmetric eyelid levels and visual symptoms from induced astigmatism or restriction of the superior visual field. Altered anatomy from scar tissue formation may make treatment of postoperative ptosis a challenge, because it usually is performed months after the causative event.

Lacrimal gland prolapse may result in lid asymmetry. Inability to recognize the gland and its injury during surgery may result in dry eye and postoperative hemorrhage. Lacrimal re-suspension using nonabsorbable suture is recommended in cases of prominent lacrimal glands [3,59].

Extension of the upper lid incision medially to the puncta or excessive removal of medial skin may result in webbing or prominent epicanthal folds. Massage, initially, or surgical correction using z or y-v plasty or other techniques used for the correction of epicanthal folds is recommended.

Lower lid

Ectropion may result from excessive excision of the anterior lamellae that disrupts the tear film meniscus and the lacrimal drainage apparatus, resulting in epiphora. Ectropion can be prevented by asking the patient to open the mouth while looking up to evaluate the amount of skin excision during surgery. Transcutaneous lower blepharoplasty with removal of excess skin in an attempt to minimize rhytidosis is the most common presenting scenario. Initial management is conservative with massage, temporary Frost sutures, or lid taping. Permanent solutions include correction of horizontal lid laxity through canthoplication or lateral tarsal strip or scar lysis and lid-lengthening procedures using lid spacers.

Entropion may result from posterior lamellae shortening. Postoperative management may be conservative at the early postoperative stages, but ultimately surgical correction is unavoidable. Entropion may present concurrently with lower lid retraction caused by septal scarring. Lysis of conjunctival adhesions and use of spacers is the treatment of choice. Available sources for grafts are oral mucosa, hard palate, ear cartilage, free tarsal conjunctival graft from the upper lid, or commercially available spacers.

Oversculpting of lower lid fat may result in tear-trough deformity or enophthalmos. Fat transposition may be necessary, but unpredictable localized resorption may result in partial or asymmetric correction. Treatment with injectable fillers (Restylane, Medicis Aesthetics, Inc., Scottsdale, AZ; Sculptra, Dermik Laboratories, Berwyn, PA) placed in the subperiosteal space may be used, but their long-term effect has not been studied. Suborbicularis oculi fat lift or subperiosteal midface elevation may alleviate the problem.

Finally, diplopia is a rare but severe complication. It can be temporary or permanent. Causes of temporary diplopia are hematomas, ischemic contractures of the extraocular muscles, and toxicity of local anesthetics [60]. Permanent diplopia from strabismus may result from structural damage of the extraocular muscles. Injury may be direct from excessive dissection or indirect from hemorrhage and deep orbital cautery.

The inferior oblique muscle is the most commonly injured because of its anatomic relationship with the lower lid fat pads. This muscle should be identified and protected during fat excision. The superior oblique may be injured as well and cause strabismus and diplopia. Mechanisms can be restrictive (eg, incarceration of the tendon in the septum resulting in Brown's syndrome) or paretic (eg, excessive use of electrocautery resulting in superior oblique palsy) [61]. Restrictive strabismus and diplopia may be the result of conjunctiva and Tenon's capsule scarring and retraction after transconjunctival lower blepharoplasty.

Summary

Upper and lower lid blepharoplasty seem to be technically simple procedures, but the unique anatomy of the eyelids and their close relationship to the eyebrows, forehead, and midface hide serious surgical pitfalls. Evaluation and concomitant correction of brow position, eyelid ptosis, lower lid laxity, and midface ptosis should be addressed before at the time of blepharoplasty. Several adverse events may arise from improper handling of the orbital fat, which is located posterior to the orbital septum and around the extraocular muscles. Minimally invasive procedures such as use of a neuromodulating agent, filler injections, and skin rejuvenating procedures may be performed before surgery to provide a healthier framework for better healing of the tissues.

Management of blepharoplasty complications should begin at the preoperative period. Proper patient evaluation, establishment of realistic expectations, and meticulous surgical planning and execution are important steps to minimize adverse outcomes.

Postoperative care is equally important for the avoidance, early recognition, and management of complications.

References

[1] American Society for Aesthetic Plastic Surgery (ASAPS). 2003 statistics. New York: ASAPS, 2004.

[2] Aguilar GL, Nelson C. Eyelid and anterior orbital anatomy. In: Hornblass A, editor. Oculoplastic, orbital, and reconstructive surgery. Baltimore: Williams & Wilkins; 1988. p. 3–14.

[3] Bosniak M, Cantisano-Zilkha M. Cosmetic blepharoplasty and facial rejuvenation. 2nd edition. Philadelphia: Lippincott-Raven; 1999.

[4] Bosniak S. Neuromodulation and management of facial rhytidosis. In: Bozniak SL, Cantisano-Zilkha M, editors. Minimally invasive techniques of oculo-facial rejuvenation. New York: Thieme, 2005. p. 30–40.

[5] Levine MR, Davies R, Ross J. Chemosis following blepharoplasty: an unusual complication. Ophthalmic Surg 1994;25(9):593–6.

[6] Honrado CP, Pastorek NJ. Long-term results of lower-lid suspension blepharoplasty: a 30-year experience. Arch Facial Plast Surg 2004;6(3):150–4.

[7] Enzer YR, Shorr N. Medical and surgical management of chemosis after blepharoplasty. Ophthal Plast Reconstr Surg 1994;10(1):57–63.

[8] David LM, Sanders G. CO2 laser blepharoplasty: a comparison to cold steel and electrocautery. J Dermatol Surg Oncol 1987;13(2):110–4.

[9] Nicolle FV, Bentall RM. Use of radio-frequency pulsed energy in the control of postoperative reaction in blepharoplasty. Aesthetic Plast Surg 1982;6(3):169–71.

[10] Carter SR, Stewart JM, Khan J, et al. Infection after blepharoplasty with and without carbon dioxide laser resurfacing. Ophthalmology 2003;110(7):1430–2.

[11] Goldberg RA, Li TG. Postoperative infection with group A beta-hemolytic Streptococcus after blepharoplasty. Am J Ophthalmol 2002;134(6):908–10.

[12] Suñer IJ, Meldrum ML, Johnson TE, et al. Necrotizing fasciitis after cosmetic blepharoplasty. Am J Ophthalmol 1999;128(3):367–8.

[13] Rao J, Golden TA, Fitzpatrick RE. Atypical mycobacterial infection following blepharoplasty and full-face skin resurfacing with CO2 laser. Dermatol Surg 2002;28(8):768–71 [discussion: 771].

[14] Chen SH, Wang CH, Chen HC, et al. Upper eyelid mycobacterial infection following Oriental blepharoplasty in a pulmonary tuberculosis patient. Aesthetic Plast Surg 2001; 25(4):295–8.

[15] Yang JW, Kim YD. A case of primary lid tuberculosis after upper lid blepharoplasty. Korean J Ophthalmol 2004;18(2):190–5.

[16] Moorthy RS, Rao NA. Atypical mycobacterial wound infection after blepharoplasty. Br J Ophthalmol 1995;79(1):93.

[17] Kevitch R, Guyuron B. Mycobacterial infection following blepharoplasty. Aesthetic Plast Surg 1991;15(3):229–32.

[18] Allen MV, Cohen KL, Grimson BS. Orbital cellulitis secondary to dacryocystitis following blepharoplasty. Ann Ophthalmol 1985;17(8):498–9.

[19] Rees TD, Craig SM, Fisher Y. Orbital abscess following blepharoplasty. Plast Reconstr Surg 1984;73(1):126–7.

[20] Morgan SC. Orbital cellulitis and blindness following a blepharoplasty. Plast Reconstr Surg 1979;64(6):823–6.

[21] Anderson LG. A perplexing intra-operative complication case study: retrobulbar hemorrhage during blepharoplasty. Plast Surg Nurs 2001;21(1):35–6.

[22] Cruz AA, Ando A, Monteiro CA, et al. Delayed retrobulbar hematoma after blepharoplasty. Ophthal Plast Reconstr Surg 2001;17(2):126–30.

[23] Wride NK, Sanders R. Blindness from acute angle-closure glaucoma after blepharoplasty. Ophthal Plast Reconstr Surg 2004;20(6):476–8.

[24] Good CD, Cassidy LM, Moseley IF, et al. Posterior optic nerve infarction after lower lid blepharoplasty. J Neuroophthalmol 1999;19(3):176–9.

[25] Goldberg RA, Marmor MF, Shorr N, et al. Blindness following blepharoplasty: two case reports, and a discussion of management. Ophthalmic Surg 1990;21(2):85–9.

[26] Callahan MA. Prevention of blindness after blepharoplasty. Ophthalmology 1983;90:1047–51.

[27] Goldberg RA, Markowitz B. Blindness after blepharoplasty. Plast Reconstr Surg 1992;90(5):929–30.

[28] Hepler RS, Sugimura GI, Straatsma BR. On the occurrence of blindness in association with blepharoplasty. Plast Reconstr Surg 1976;57(2):233–5.

[29] Black EH, Gladstone GJ, Nesi FA. Eyelid sensation after supratarsal lid crease incision. Ophthal Plast Reconstr Surg 2002;18(1):45–9.

[30] Fryer RH, Reinke KR. Pyogenic granuloma: a complication of transconjunctival incisions. Plast Reconstr Surg 2000;105(4):1565–6.

[31] Soll SM, Lisman RD, Charles NC, et al. Pyogenic granuloma after transconjunctival blepharoplasty: a case report. Ophthal Plast Reconstr Surg 1993;9(4):298–301.

[32] Goldberg RA, Lessner AM, Shorr N, et al. The transconjunctival approach to the orbital floor and orbital fat. A prospective study. Ophthal Plast Reconstr Surg 1990;6(4):241–6.

[33] Heltzer JM, Ellis DS, Stewart WB, et al. Diffuse nodular eyelid lipogranuloma following sutureless transconjunctival blepharoplasty dressed with topical ointment. Ophthal Plast Reconstr Surg 1999;15(6):438–41.

[34] Saadat D, Dresner SC. Safety of blepharoplasty in patients with preoperative dry eyes. Arch Facial Plast Surg 2004;6(2):101–4.

[35] Floegel I, Horwath-Winter J, Muellner K, et al. A conservative blepharoplasty may be a means of alleviating dry eye symptoms. Acta Ophthalmol Scand 2003;81(3):230–2.

[36] Vold SD, Carroll RP, Nelson JD. Dermatochalasis and dry eye. Am J Ophthalmol 1993;115(2):216–20.

[37] Rees TD. The "dry eye" complication after a blepharoplasty. Plast Reconstr Surg 1975;56(4):375–80.

[38] Pessa JE, Desvigne LD, Lambros VS, et al. Changes in ocular globe-to-orbital rim position with age: implications for aesthetic blepharoplasty of the lower eyelids. Aesthetic Plast Surg 1999;23(5):337–42.

[39] Chou B, Boxer Wachler BS. Astigmatism after corneal thermal injury. J Cataract Refract Surg 2001;27(5):784–6.

[40] Brown MS, Siegel IM, Lisman RD. Prospective analysis of changes in corneal topography after upper eyelid surgery. Ophthal Plast Reconstr Surg 1999;15(6):378–83.

[41] Christian MM, Cox DO, Smith CV, et al. Ocular damage due to chlorhexidine versus eyeshield thermal injury. Dermatol Surg 2001;27(2):153–7.

[42] Schomacker KT, Walsh JT Jr, Flotte TJ, et al. Thermal damage produced by high-irradiance continuous wave CO2 laser cutting of tissue. Lasers Surg Med 1990;10(1):74–84.

[43] McKinney P, Zuckerbraun BS. An alternative to a graft of skin in the treatment of lagophthalmos. Plast Reconstr Surg 1995;96(6):1448–50.

[44] Elner VM, Hassan AS, Frueh BR. Graded full-thickness anterior blepharotomy for upper eyelid retraction. Arch Ophthalmol 2004;122(1):55–60.

[45] Shorr N, Goldberg RA, McCann JD, et al. Upper eyelid skin grafting: an effective treatment for lagophthalmos following blepharoplasty. Plast Reconstr Surg 2003;112(5):1444–8.

[46] Brown BZ, Beard C. Split-level full-thickness eyelid graft. Am J Ophthalmol 1979;87(3):388–92.

[47] Small RG, Sahl WJ. The use of split-thickness skin grafts for eyelid and facial reconstruction after Mohs' fresh-tissue surgery. Ophthal Plast Reconstr Surg 1989;5(4):266–70.

[48] McCord CD. Complications of upper lid blepharoplasty. In: Putterman A, editor. Cosmetic oculoplastic surgery. New York: Grune & Statton; 1982. p. 250–74.

[49] Glavas IP, Cantisano-Zilkha M, Bozniak SL. Free tarsal conjunctival grafting for management of post blepharoplasty lower lid retraction. Presented at the annual meeting

of the American Society of Ophthalmic Plastic and Reconstructive Surgery, New Orleans, LA. October 22–23, 2004.

[50] Taban M, Douglas R, Li T, et al. Efficacy of "thick" acellular human dermis (AlloDerm) for lower eyelid reconstruction: comparison with hard palate and thin AlloDerm grafts. Arch Facial Plast Surg 2005;7(1):38–44.

[51] Schiller JD, Lin S, Neigel JM. Deepening of the superior sulcus after isolated lower transconjunctival blepharoplasty. Ophthal Plast Reconstr Surg 2004;20(6):433–5.

[52] Lee Y, Kwon S, Hwang K. Correction of sunken and/or multiply folded upper eyelid by fascia-fat graft. Plast Reconstr Surg 2001;107(1):15–9.

[53] Rubin PA, Fay AM, Remulla HD, et al. Ophthalmic plastic applications of acellular dermal allografts. Ophthalmology 1999;106(11):2091–7.

[54] Van Gemert JV, Leone CR Jr. Correction of a deep superior sulcus with dermis-fat implantation. Arch Ophthalmol 1986;104(4):604–7.

[55] Smith B, Lisman RD. Use of sclera and liquid collagen in the camouflage of superior sulcus deformities. Ophthalmology 1983;90(3):230–5.

[56] Cahill KV, Burns JA. Volume augmentation of the anophthalmic orbit with cross-linked collagen (Zyplast). Arch Ophthalmol 1989;107(11):1684–6.

[57] I.P Glavas, Cantisano-Zilkha M, Bosniak S. Injectable non-animal derived hyaluronic acid gel as orbital implant. Presented at the annual meeting of the American Society of Ocularists, Medical Advisory Seminar. Anaheim, CA, November 15–19, 2003.

[58] Baylis HI, Sutcliffe T, Fett DR. Levator injury during blepharoplasty. Arch Ophthalmol 1984;102(4):570–1.

[59] Smith B, Lisman RD. Dacryoadenopexy as a recognized factor in upper lid blepharoplasty. Plast Reconstr Surg 1983;71(5):629–32.

[60] Smith B, Lisman RD, Simonton J, et al. Volkmann's contracture of the extraocular muscles following blowout fracture. Plast Reconstr Surg 1984;74:200–9.

[61] Neely KA, Ernest JT, Mottier M. Combined superior oblique paresis and Brown's syndrome after blepharoplasty. Am J Ophthalmol 1990;109(3):347–9.

ELSEVIER
SAUNDERS

Otolaryngol Clin N Am
38 (2005) 1023–1032

OTOLARYNGOLOGIC
CLINICS
OF NORTH AMERICA

Reconstruction of the Upper Eyelid

Randal T. Pham, MD[a,b]

[a]*Division of Ophthalmic Plastic & Reconstructive Surgery, Department of Ophthalmology,
Stanford University, Stanford, CA, USA*
[b]*Aesthetic & Refractive Surgery Medical Center, San Jose, CA*

Reconstruction of the upper eyelid can be achieved by an array of procedures. Defects of the upper eyelid are categorized by size. This article describes a basic approach to repair the upper eyelid and a method of repair for each defect.

Goals and principles

The objectives of repairing the upper eyelid are to preserve function and to restore a cosmetically acceptable appearance. To achieve these goals, a surgeon must be able to select the appropriate procedure for a given defect. Size, location, and configuration of the defect should be considered in this selection process. The size of the defect determines how much tissue is needed to reconstruct the eyelid. The availability of tissue in turn determines the type of procedure to be performed. In terms of location, for example, the lacrimal system should be thoroughly evaluated if the medial canthal area is involved. Irregularly shaped defects may require trimming so that a good approximation of tissues can be achieved. The patient's age is also important because the skin of older patients is more lax than that of younger patients. Thus, in an elderly patient, it is possible to close moderately larger defects by direct closure. Finally, levator function must be assessed to determine whether concurrent ptosis repair is indicated. Approaches to repair ptosis are, however, beyond the scope of this article.

Surgical techniques

Repair of defects involving fifty percent of the eyelid or less

The eyelid is generously vascularized, and tissue ischemia rarely is a concern in the reconstruction of eyelid defects. Rapid tissue healing is also

E-mail address: randalpham@lasernews.com

oto.theclinics.com

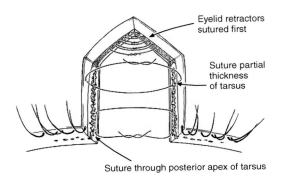

Eyelid retractors
sutured first

Suture partial
thickness
of tarsus

Suture through posterior apex of tarsus

Fig. 1. Approximation of the posterior lamella.

expected with good apposition of wound edges. With good sterile technique infection is rare even in cases of trauma with dirty wounds.

Alignment of the lid margin is crucial in obtaining a satisfactory result. If the upper eyelid defect is extremely irregular, it may be trimmed with a blade or scissor [1].

Approximation of the posterior lamella is achieved by placing simple interrupted sutures, using 6-0 polyglactin sutures, starting from the superior edge in the upper eyelid (Fig. 1). The suture should enter the tarsal plate anteriorly (1.5 mm from the lacerated edge) and exit only in partial thickness to the wound edge. The suture is then directed to the opposite edge of the wound and allowed to exit anteriorly, 1.5 mm from this edge. Care should be taken to avoid misalignment of the wound edges. Penetration of the tarsal plate must be avoided, or corneal irritation may ensue.

Anchoring of the edge of the lid margin is performed by placing a double-armed 6-0 silk suture 3 mm into the depth of the lid and exiting 3 mm from the wound edge (Fig. 2) [2]. The opposite end of the suture is placed in the same manner in the other side. A second suture is passed through the tarsal

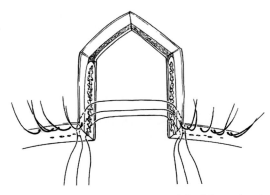

Fig. 2. Anchoring of the edge of the lid margin.

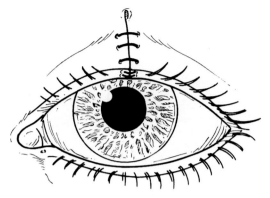

Fig. 3. The lid margin sutures are tied. The two posterior sutures are cut and left long enough to be buried under the anterior-most suture.

layer in the same manner. Similarly, a third suture is then passed anteriorly at the level of the base of the lashes.

At this point, the lid margin sutures are tied. The two posterior sutures are cut and left long enough to be buried under the most anterior suture. This maneuver helps prevent the rubbing of these sutures against the cornea (Fig. 3).

Closure of the anterior lamella is achieved with simple interrupted sutures, using 6-0 silk. Selective suturing of the orbicularis is not necessary because the thin eyelid skin adheres well to the muscular layer beneath it.

Repair of defects involving fifty to seventy-five percent of the eyelid

In cases of moderate tissue loss, a lateral cantholysis should be performed [2]. A hemostat is placed over the lateral canthus for 1 minute. Sharp, straight scissors are then used to make an 8-mm horizontal cut into the common crus of the lateral canthal tendon (Fig. 4). If mobilization of tissue cannot be adequately achieved with canthotomy, cantholysis should be performed, in which the superior limb of the lateral palpebral tendon is severed. After identifying this tendon by palpation, the tendon is cut with the scissors pointing superolaterally with one blade of the scissors behind the skin and orbicularis and the other blade in front of the conjunctiva (Fig. 5).

If a greater length of tissue is needed to fill the lid defect, a semicircular flap may be created at this time [3]. An inferior, arching line is drawn, starting at the lateral canthus. An incision is made along the line, and a flap of cutaneous tissue is dissected out (Fig. 6). The flap is advanced medially and placed over the defect. Reapproximation of the mucocutaneous junction is performed using 6-0 polyglactin sutures. The lateral canthal angle is reconstructed by attaching the dermis of the new lateral canthus to the periosteum of the lateral orbital rim using a double-armed 6-0 Prolene suture. A running 6-0 silk suture is used to fix the conjunctiva to the new lid

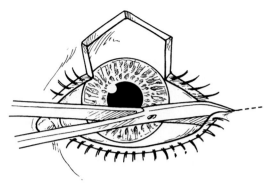

Fig. 4. Sharp, straight scissors are used to make an 8-mm horizontal cut into the common crus of the lateral canthal tendon.

margin. Skin closure of the lateral canthal angle is performed with interrupted sutures, using 6-0 silk.

Ophthalmic antibiotic ointment should be applied to the wound three times each day for 1 week and into the eye the night of surgery. Lid margin sutures should be removed approximately 10 days postoperatively. All other cutaneous sutures may be removed 4 to 5 days after repair.

Repair of defects involving seventy-five percent of the eyelid or more

Cutler–Beard technique

The Cutler–Beard procedure is reserved for defects that include 70% or more of the upper eyelid [4]. Skin, muscle, and conjunctiva from the lower

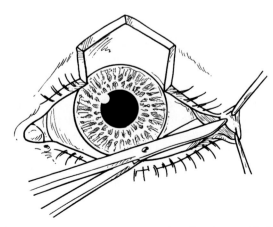

Fig. 5. To perform cantholysis, the lateral palpebral tendon is cut with the scissors pointing superolaterally with one blade of the scissors behind the skin and orbicularis and the other blade in front of the conjunctiva.

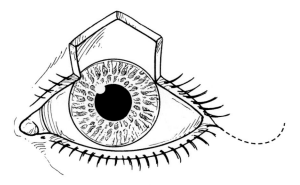

Fig. 6. To create a semicircular flap, an inferior, arching line is drawn, starting at the lateral canthus. An incision is made along the line, and a flap of cutaneous tissue is dissected out.

lid are used to fill the upper eyelid defect. The flap of tissue from the lower lid is outlined. The size of this flap should be compatible with the defect in the upper eyelid. With a globe protector in place and using a #15 Bard-Parker blade, a horizontal incision is made 5 mm below the lid margin along the marked portion of the lower lid that is used to fill the defect. This incision should be at least 5 mm below the lid margin to preserve the marginal artery. Two posteriorly directed vertical incisions 10 to 15 mm long are made in the lower lid. A through-and-through incision along the previous horizontal incision is made with straight Stevens scissors, leaving the conjunctival edge slightly longer than the skin edge. This incision is then extended in the vertical direction along the previous incisions and may be lengthened toward the inferior orbital rim. The flap is advanced superiorly beneath the 5-mm lid margin left on the lower lid (Fig. 7). The conjunctiva is sutured to any conjunctiva remaining in the upper lid, using either

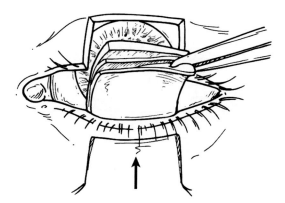

Fig. 7. The flap is advanced superiorly beneath the 5-mm lid margin left on the lower lid.

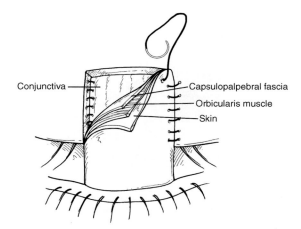

Conjunctiva ——
Capsulopalpebral fascia
Orbicularis muscle
Skin

Fig. 8. The medial and lateral edges of the flap are sutured to the corresponding layers of the upper eyelid.

interrupted or continuous 6-0 plain or chromic sutures. The capsulopalpe-bral fascia of the advanced flap is sutured to the levator or its aponeurosis using 6-0 Vicryl suture. Skin is closed using continuous 6-0 nylon sutures. The medial and lateral edges of the flap are sutured to the corresponding layers of the upper eyelid as described previously (Fig. 8). This flap is allowed to stretch over a period of 3 to 8 weeks (Fig. 9).

When the advanced flap becomes adequately lengthened and well vascularized with blood supplied from the adjacent upper eyelid tissue, it can be severed to create a new upper eyelid margin. With downward traction of the flap using a skin hook, a groove director is inserted beneath the flap.

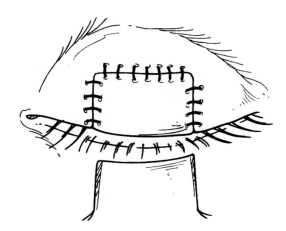

Fig. 9. The flap is allowed to stretch over a period of 3 to 8 weeks.

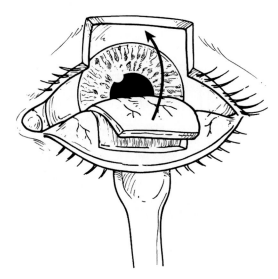

Fig. 10. The lower eyelid is everted with a Desmarres retractor, and the tarsoconjunctival flap is created with a horizontal incision 5 to 6 mm from the lid margin.

The new upper eyelid margin is outlined. Ample tissue should be left on the upper eyelid because later retraction may result in exposure keratitis. A superficial incision is made straight across the flap using a #15 Bard-Parker blade. A deep incision along the superficial incision is made with sharp

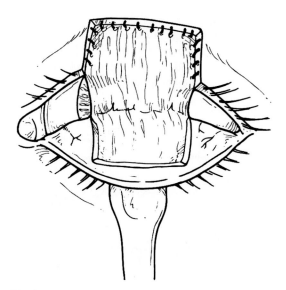

Fig. 11. The combined tarsoconjunctival flap is advanced into the upper eyelid defect and sutured with 6-0 polyglactin sutures.

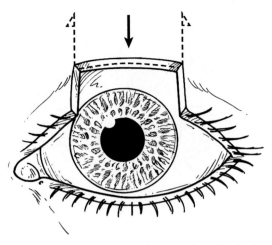

Fig. 12. A skin flap is created from tissue above the defect in the upper lid.

blepharoplasty scissors. The conjunctival edge should be made slightly longer than the skin edge to prevent trichiasis.

Modified Hughes tarsoconjunctival repair

Advancement technique

The advancement technique is used as an alternative to the Cutler–Beard technique for closing a defect that involves 70% or more of the upper eyelid when there is adequate skin to fill the defect [5]. Tarsus and conjunctiva from the lower eyelid are used to fill the defect in the upper eyelid. A marking pen is used to outline the portion of the lower eyelid that will be

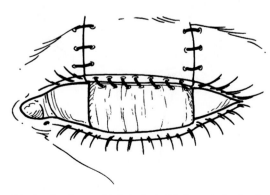

Fig. 13. The skin flap is advanced inferiorly to fill the anterior lamina of the defect.

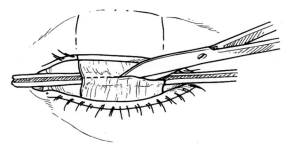

Fig. 14. After 6 to 12 weeks, the flap is divided to create a new lid margin.

used to compensate for the upper eyelid defect. The lower eyelid is everted with a Desmarres retractor, and the tarsoconjunctival flap is created with a horizontal incision 5 to 6 mm from the lid margin (Fig. 10). The capsulopalpebral fascia is separated from the tarsus. The palpebral conjunctiva is undermined from the capsulopalpebral fascia using blunt scissors directed toward the lower fornix. The combined tarsoconjunctival flap is then advanced into the upper eyelid defect and sutured with 6-0 polyglactin sutures (Fig. 11). Sutures should first be placed at the four corners. A skin flap is created from tissue above the defect in the upper lid (Fig. 12) and advanced inferiorly to fill the anterior lamina of the defect (Fig. 13). In young patients, a skin graft may be necessary to fill the anterior lamina because the skin is not lax enough to be advanced adequately [6].

After 6 to 12 weeks, the flap is divided to create a new lid margin (Fig. 14). Sufficient stretching and vascularization of the flap must be secured before dividing the flap. The procedure is similar to the division of the Cutler–Beard flap described previously, except that the conjunctiva is left 1 to 2 mm higher than the anterior lamella and is sutured to the skin using 6-0 chromic horizontal mattress sutures to prevent entropion caused by conjunctival retraction.

Summary

Repair of the upper eyelid can be achieved by an array of procedures. By selecting the proper method of repair, with due consideration of the size, location, and configuration of the defect, the surgeon can repair the upper eyelid while maintaining the best possible function and cosmetic appearance.

This article has described the basic approaches to repairing the upper eyelid. The author has categorized these approaches by the size of the defect of the upper eyelid. The method of repair for each type of defect has been described accordingly. Where appropriate, the merit of a given method has been discussed.

References

[1] Phelps CD. Manual of common ophthalmic surgical procedures. Edinburgh (UK): Churchill Livingstone; 1986. p. 23.
[2] Levine MR. Manual of oculoplastic surgery. Philadelphia: Butterworth Heinemann; 2003. p. 29.
[3] Tenzel RR. Reconstruction of the central one half of an eyelid. Arch Ophthalmol 1975;93: 125–6.
[4] Cutler N, Beard C. A method for partial and total upper lid reconstruction. Am J Ophthalmol 1955;39:1–7.
[5] Mauriello JA Jr, Antonacci R. Single tarsoconjunctival flap (lower eyelid) for upper eyelid reconstruction ("reverse" modified Hughes procedure). Ophthalmic Surg 1994;25(6):374–8.
[6] Hornblass A. Oculoplastic, orbital, and reconstructive surgery, vol. 1. Baltimore (MD): Williams and Wilkins; 1988. p. 630–42.

ELSEVIER
SAUNDERS

Otolaryngol Clin N Am
38 (2005) 1033–1042

OTOLARYNGOLOGIC
CLINICS
OF NORTH AMERICA

Lower Eyelid Reconstruction

Damon B. Chandler, MD*, Roberta E. Gausas, MD

Division of Oculoplastic and Orbital Surgery, Scheie Eye Institute, University of Pennsylvania, 51 N. 39th Street, Philadelphia, PA 19104-2689, USA

Reconstruction of the lower eyelid seeks to restore both anatomic function and prereconstructive lid aesthetics. A sound understanding of the nature of lower eyelid anatomy and function is required to acheive these goals. The lower eyelid differs in several crucial ways from the upper eyelid, and only by appreciating these differences can optimal lower eyelid surgery be achieved. A multitude of approaches to lower eyelid reconstruction exist. The proper choice of technique is guided by two major factors: size of defect and involvement of anterior or posterior lamellae.

Lower eyelid anatomy and function

Medial and lateral canthal tendons

The lower eyelid has a number of unique anatomic features. The height of the tarsus of the lower eyelid is approximately 3 to 4 mm, far shorter than the 10 to 12 mm found in the upper lid [1]. The lower eyelid is in apposition with the globe for the full length of the eyelid and is suspended on either side by tendinous attachments to the orbital rim. The inferior crus of the lateral canthal tendon inserts just inside the lateral orbital rim at a bony protuberance named Whitnall's tubercle [2]. The medial canthal tendon attaches to the lacrimal crest both anteriorly and posteriorly. These two portions of the medial canthal tendon envelop the lacrimal sac, which rests in the lacrimal sac fossa [3]. Importantly, it is the posterior portion of the medial canthal tendon that maintains the integrity of medial eyelid support. Functionally, the tarsal plate and its canthal tendon insertions act as a sling for the lower eyelid, referred to as a *tarsoligamentous band* [4]. This band not only maintains the eyelid in a normal anatomic position, but also supports the globe and orbital contents. The lower eyelid also is subject to the vertical

* Corresponding author.
  E-mail address: damon_chandler@yahoo.com (D.B. Chandler).

0030-6665/05/$ - see front matter © 2005 Elsevier Inc. All rights reserved.
doi:10.1016/j.otc.2005.03.006

force of gravity that acts to pull the lid out of position. The lower eyelid exists in continuum with the cheek and the midface, which exert forces on the eyelid. Scarring, contraction, or descent of the cheek or midface may contribute substantial additional vertical forces influencing lower eyelid position.

Anterior and posterior lamella

The eyelid is comprised of two major structural divisions: an anterior lamella and a posterior lamella [3]. The anterior lamella consists of the eyelid skin and the underlying orbicularis oculi muscle. Recall that the eyelid skin has virtually no subcutaneous tissue. The posterior lamella refers to the tarsal plate and the conjunctiva. Eyelid reconstruction must address both structural divisions of the lid to be successful.

Reconstructive techniques

Laissez faire

One initial decision that must be made for all defects of the eyelids is whether or not reconstruction is in fact necessary. Allowing a wound to heal secondarily by granulation may avoid the time, morbidity, and cost of reconstruction. Wounds that are small (<25% of the lid), superficial, and do not involve exposed bone or cartilage are intuitively good candidates for a laissez faire approach. Properly chosen wounds may heal with minimal scarring and acceptable cosmesis. Older patients tend to have more skin laxity and irregular skin pigmentation and therefore tend to develop more camouflaged scars than young patients. Wound care during the granulation process requires the wound to be kept clean and the application of topical antibiotic ointment several times a day. The healing process can be expected to range from 2 to 6 weeks in length, depending on the patient and the size and depth of the wound. Pain, infection, or excessive bleeding is not commonly experienced. The negative aspects of second-intention healing include the inability to predict precise wound healing, scar contracture, tissue distortion or lid malposition, and acceptable cosmesis. It is for these reasons that healing by secondary intention is often chosen only when other reconstructive options are not feasible. However, carefully selected patients with appropriate defects may have satisfactory outcomes without the need for periocular reconstruction [5].

Direct closure

Once eyelid reconstruction has been selected, the first point to consider is whether or not the defect can be closed directly. It is most desirable to close a wound without the need for a graft or flap if possible. In general, defects comprising 25% or less of the lid are suitable for direct closure [6]. First the tissues must be grasped and tested to ensure that the tissues reapproximate without undue tension, because many wounds may appear deceptively easy to close. Avoiding vertical tension on the lower eyelid is critical for prevention of postreconstruction sequelae such as lid retraction, ectropion, or lagophthalmos [7]. For this reason, lower eyelid defects may be closed with vertical scars, despite the cosmetic dictum to close wounds along relaxed skin tension lines. In general, lower eyelid defects that are marginal or juxtamarginal are more readily closed directly. Young patients with taut skin will require extensive undermining of tissue if direct closure is to be successful. Even older patients frequently have far less excess skin than appears to be the case despite age-related changes. Experience is an invaluable guide when working around the lower eyelid, because eyelid retraction or ectropion must be avoided.

Full-thickness defects of the margin that are small (<25% of the lower lid) can be closed directly by converting the defect to a pentagonal shape [8]. The principles that are employed in this closure are those used in repairing a full-thickness laceration of the eyelid. The lid margin should be reapproximated with a primary fixation suture (6-0 silk) placed through the gray line of the lid margin in a vertical mattress fashion and left with a long tail. The tarsal plate should be closed, partial thickness, with interrupted 6-0 vicryl sutures (two or three usually suffice). Full-thickness tarsal sutures risk exposing the cornea to irritation by sutures exposed through the inside of the lid. It is advisable not to tie any of the tarsal sutures until all are placed. If the initial tarsal suture is tied, it may become challenging to close the rest of the tarsus adequately in such a confined space. The lid margin is further secured with one suture placed anteriorly and one placed posteriorly to the gray line suture. The edge of the margin should be slightly everted to avoid unsightly notching, which may occur when a poorly closed lid margin contracts during healing. Finally, the orbicularis muscle and skin are closed in two layers. The skin may be closed with either permanent or dissolving sutures.

Lid defects involving the lateral or medial canthi pose additional complexity. Lateral canthal defects should be repaired with care to support the tarsus of the lower lid to the lateral orbital rim. A lateral tarsal strip can be fashioned to anchor the tarsus, or a periosteal strip can be rotated and used as a bridge. Medial canthal defects may involve the canalicular system, and care must be taken to preserve delicate canalicular structures if possible [9].

Tissue advancement

Direct closure combined with canthal release

If direct closure is insufficient to close a lower lid defect, tissue advancement or rotation should be used. Approaches for intermediate sized defects (25–50% of the lower eyelid) include releasing the lateral canthus via canthotomy and cantholysis, and the semicircular advancement flap procedure [7,8]. In fact, closure of more complex eyelid defects often relies on combinations of approaches rather than one single procedure. For example, if a full-thickness defect involving half of the lower lid is too large to close directly, a canthotomy and cantholysis may mobilize sufficient tissue to allow a standard pentagonal closure as described above (Fig. 1) [8].

The lateral and medial canthal tendons inhibit horizontal movement of the lower eyelid tissues during reconstruction. For this reason, the lateral canthal tendon is often severed to allow movement of the lid tissues medially and can be reconstituted following reconstruction [6]. If these supporting tendons have been violated by the creation of an anatomic defect, support must once again be provided. Care must be taken to contour the lower eyelid properly to the globe. Anterior lamella repair without attention to correction of horizontal lid laxity may result in lid malposition such as ectropion, lid retraction, or epiphora [7]. In cases of medial canthal tendon laxity, plication of the tendon helps to reestablish a normal tear pump mechanism and to prevent punctal eversion.

An essential technique for lower eyelid surgery is the mobilization of the lower lid by releasing the lateral canthal tendon [10]. The initial step—the canthotomy—is to incise the lateral canthus in a horizontal fashion using

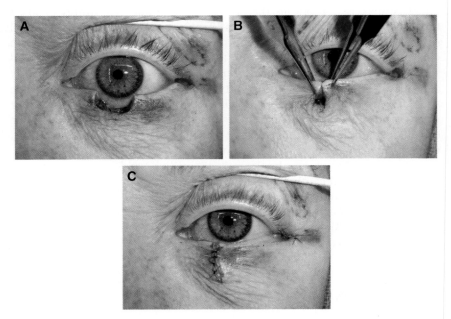

Fig. 1. Direct closure. (A) Left lower eyelid status after skin cancer resection reveals a 25% full-thickness defect. (B) Tissue forceps demonstrate that direct closure is feasible after lateral canthal release. (C) Final intraoperative result reveals proper lid to globe apposition and reformed lateral canthal angle.

a scissors to divide the lower eyelid from the upper eyelid. Recall that the lateral canthal tendon has a superior and an inferior crus and that these fuse and insert on the inner aspect of the lateral orbital rim [2,3]. After the canthotomy, the insertion of the inferior crus of the tendon remains firmly adherent to the orbital rim, and complete release of the lower lid has not yet occurred. The critical step—the cantholysis—releases the lower eyelid from the orbital rim by severing its attachment. Scissors are directed inferiorly with the blades placed across the canthal tendon, but with care to avoid incising any skin or precious conjunctiva. A forcep is used to grasp the edge of the lower eyelid and is pulled to create countertraction from the canthal angle. The scissors are then used to cut into the tendon and divide it completely. With each proper cut of the scissors, the lower eyelid will move further away from the orbital rim until it is completely mobilized. The lower eyelid can be shifted into position to close many small to moderately sized defects. Mastery of this technique comes with experience and is of great use in lower eyelid reconstructive surgery.

Semicircular advancement combined with canthal release

A semicircular advancement flap, first described in 1975 by Richard Tenzel, is useful for moderately sized defects (25%–50%) [11,12]. This myocutaneous advancement flap allows for direct closure of the lid once the proper tissue mobilization via lateral canthal release has occurred. The eyelid defect size is estimated, and this is used to create an appropriately sized semicircle arching outward from the lateral canthal angle. Tissue undermining is performed until the flap can be advanced into the lower lid defect without undue tension. Once the tissue is advanced into position, the flap should be supported at the level of the lateral canthal angle to the periosteum of the lateral orbital rim. For some larger defects, further lateral support is required in the form of a periosteal flap [13]. Adequate exposure of the periosteum of the lateral orbital rim is required to elevate a rectangular flap based medially at the anterior crest of the orbital rim. The flap is then reflected 180° into the lower lid defect and anchored to the lateral aspect of residual tarsus. The periosteal flap thus serves as a posterior lamellar substitute. The semicircular advancement flap then acts as the anterior lamella with an appropriate blood supply. The eyelid margin and remaining vertical defect in the lower eyelid is now repaired in the manner of direct eyelid defect closure. The lateral canthal angle should be properly reformed, and the skin of the semicircle should be closed with interrupted sutures (Fig. 2).

Transpositional Flap (Hughes Procedure)

For defects that comprise more than 50% of the lower eyelid, a transpositional flap is the most appropriate step. The best available technique to rebuild the lower eyelid posterior lamella is to borrow the

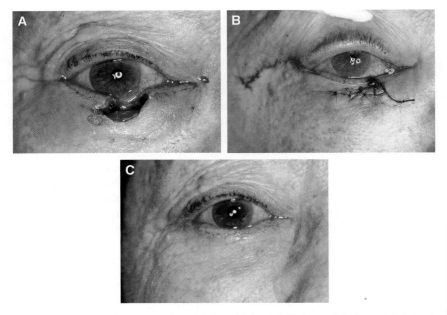

Fig. 2. Semicircular advancement flap. (*A*) Post-Mohs full-thickness right lower lid defect in which direct closure was inadequate. (*B*) Defect was closed using a semicircular (Tenzel) advancement flap. (*C*) Six-month postoperative result reveals good cosmesis.

tarsus and its conjunctival blood supply from the ipsilateral upper eyelid. This is known as a *tarsoconjunctival flap*, or *Hughes procedure*, which is named for Wendell Hughes, who first described this method in 1937 [14,15]. A 6-0 silk traction suture is placed at the gray line of the upper eyelid, and the lid is everted on a Desmarres retractor. The palpebral conjunctival surface of the upper lid is marked 3 to 4 mm from the lid margin for a length based on the horizontal defect size to be repaired. This incision location avoids destabilizing the upper lid, avoids lid retraction, and prevents lash loss from injury to the lash bed. A blade is used to incise the conjunctiva and full-thickness tarsal plate until the underlying levator is revealed. Two vertical incisions are extended from the most lateral edges of the horizontal tarsal incision and carried just past the superior border of tarsus. A blade is then used first to isolate the tarsoconjunctival flap from the underlying levator muscle. As the superior tarsal border is reached, blunt dissection is used to separate the conjunctiva from the overlying Mueller's muscle. Care is taken to avoid the marginal arcade at this location. Relaxing incisions in the conjunctiva laterally allows full mobilization of the tarsoconjunctival flap and avoids late upper eyelid retraction. The flap is then reflected 180°, placed into the lower eyelid defect, and anchored medially and laterally onto the residual tarsus. The inferior edge of the flap is then fixed to the conjunctiva and lower lid retractors. A substitute, reconstructed anterior lamella must now be selected to be placed onto this posterior lamellar base. A myocutaneous flap can be advanced from the lower eyelid/cheek complex if enough tissue is available. As mentioned above, a lateral canthal release or semicircular flap may aid in mobilizing anterior lamella. Alternatively, a full-thickness skin graft may be harvested from the upper lid, pre-auricular, post-auricular, or supraclavicular region. The graft can be anchored wth interrupted 6-0 prolene suture and fixed with a running 6-0 fast absorbing gut suture (Fig. 3A–C).

The Hughes procedure effectively sutures the lid shut and obstructs the central visual axis. This requires that a second stage severing of the flap be performed. This procedure is performed under local anesthesia in the office approximately 4 to 6 weeks after the initial operation. Proparacaine is placed onto the ocular surface and the lid is anesthetized with lidocaine 1% with epinephrine 1:100,000. A Westcott scissors is then used to sever the flap, with care taken to transect slightly higher than the eventual intended lower eyelid margin. This is important, because some of the flap will regress after it is severed, and this technique helps form a natural appearing level for the mucocutaneous junction [8]. The residual tarsoconjunctival flap is then severed from the upper eyelid, and a hand-held cautery is used for hemostasis (Fig. 3D–F).

Grafts

Though the authors prefer the Hughes tarsoconjunctival flap whenever possible, there are numerous substitute graft materials that are available for posterior lamellar reconstruction. These include autogenous tissue, preserved human tissues, and synthetic implant material. Posterior lamellar grafts for the lower eyelid need to be sturdy enough to support the horizontal and vertical forces that act on the lower eyelid [16]. All posterior lamellar grafts must provide a nonkeratinized posterior surface, because they will be in contact with the cornea and globe. Most importantly, all free graft materials require an adequate blood supply that can be provided by a myocutaneous flap. For that reason, a free anterior graft such as full-thickness skin should not be placed on a free posterior lamellar graft, because there will not be sufficient blood supply for graft survival [7,17].

Autogenous grafts avoid the risks of infection, including HIV, hepatitis, or Creutzfeld-Jacob disease. However, donor site morbidity can be a disadvantage. The variety of autogenous tissues that can be selected include free tarsal grafts, ear cartilage, nasal septal cartilage, or hard palate mucosa [16,18]. Free tarsal grafts are harvested from the ipsilateral or contralateral upper eyelid and have similar reconstructive characteristics as tarsus used in a Hughes flap, without the blood supply. Donor site complications may include eyelid notching, contour peaking, lid retraction, and lash ptosis, although Leibovitch and colleagues [19] found in a review of 91 eyelids that these complications are often minimal. Ear cartilage and

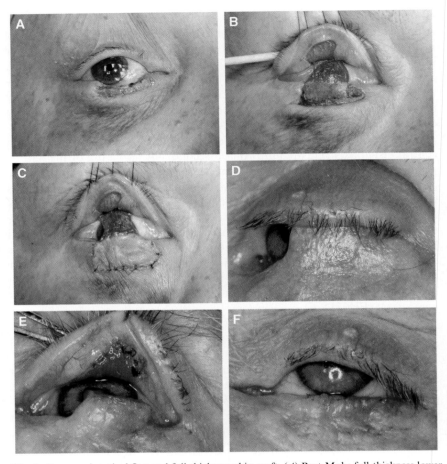

Fig. 3. Tarsoconjunctival flap and full-thickness skin graft. (*A*) Post-Mohs full-thickness lower lid defect measuring more than 50%. (*B*) Tarsoconjunctival flap reflected 180° into lower lid defect acts as posterior lamellar replacement. (*C*) Full-thickness skin graft harvested from left upper eyelid acts as anterior lamellar replacement. (*D*) A second example of tarsoconjunctival flap after 4 weeks in preparation for second stage of reconstruction. (*E*) The flap is divided superiorly at the upper lid and inferiorly along the lid margin. (*F*) Postoperative result after severing of flap.

nasal septal cartilage may be used, but these tissues are rigid and must be molded with great care to achieve a natural-appearing lid contour. Hard palate mucosa is more suitable because it is readily harvested, provides an appropriate mucosal surface, contracts minimally, and provides good contour and support for the lower eyelid [20]. Homologous tissue such as preserved human sclera is readily available and avoids a second operative site. However, banked sclera is limited by graft shrinkage and absorption, possible tissue reactions, and risk of infection or exposure. Finally, synthetic materials are available, such as polytetrafluoroethylene (Goretex) and porous polyethylene (Medpor) [21,22]. These materials have the risk of extrusion, shifting of the implant material, bulkiness of the eyelid, and the reported frequent need for surgical revisions [21]. The authors prefer autogenous tissue whenever possible because of these limitations.

Summary

Lower eyelid reconstruction requires an understanding of functional anatomy along with a logical approach tailored to each particular defect. The lower eyelid has key anatomic features that should be recognized to avoid late complications of repair, such as ectropion, exposure keratopathy, or chronic epiphora. A full complement of strategies exists, ranging from laissez faire healing for small defects to complex lid sharing reconstruction with full-thickness skin grafts for large defects. No one approach to lower eyelid reconstruction is always best, and each patient and each defect must be evaluated independently.

References

[1] Zide BM, Jelks GW. The eyelids. In: Surgical anatomy of the orbit. New York: Raven Press; 1985. p. 21–32.
[2] Jordan DR, Anderson RL. Eyebrows, eyelids and canthi. In: Surgical anatomy of the ocular adnexa: a clinical approach (Ophthalmology Monographs, Volume 9). San Francisco: Palace Press; 1996. p. 1–30.
[3] Nerad JA. Clinical anatomy. In: Oculoplastic surgery: the requisites in ophthalmology. St. Louis: Mosby; 2001. p. 25–70.
[4] Jelks GW, Jelks EB. The influence of orbital and eyelid anatomy on the palpebral aperture. Clin Plast Surg 1991;18:183–95.
[5] Lowry JC, Bartley GB, Garrity JA. The role of second-intention healing in periocular reconstruction. Ophthal Plast Reconstr Surg 1997;13:174–88.
[6] Brown BZ. Reconstruction of the lower eyelid: moderate defects. In: Hornblass AC, Hanig CJ, editors. Oculoplastic, orbital, and reconstructive surgery. Volume 1. Baltimore: Williams & Wilkins; 1988. p. 624–9.
[7] Nerad JA. Eyelid reconstruction. In: Oculoplastic surgery: the requisites in ophthalmology. St. Louis: Mosby; 2001. p. 282–311.
[8] Dryden RM, Wulc AE. Reconstruction of the lower eyelid: major defects. In: Hornblass AC, Hanig CJ, editors. Oculoplastic, orbital, and reconstructive surgery. Volume 1. Baltimore: Williams & Wilkins; 1988. p. 630–42.
[9] Holds JB, Anderson RL. Medial canthotomy and cantholysis in eyelid reconstruction. Am J Ophthalmol 1993;116:218–23.
[10] Anderson RL. The tarsal strip procedure. Arch Ophthalmol 1979;97:2192–6.
[11] Tenzel RR. Reconstruction of the central one half of an eyelid. Arch Ophthalmol 1975;93: 125–6.
[12] Tenzel RR, Stewart WB. Eyelid reconstruction by the semicircle flap technique. Ophthalmology 1978;85:1164–9.
[13] Leone CR Jr. Periosteal flap for lower eyelid reconstruction. Am J Ophthalmol 1992;114: 513–4.

[14] Hughes WL. A new method for rebuilding a lower lid: Report of a case. Arch Ophthalmol 1937;17:1008–17.

[15] Hughes WL. Total lower lid reconstruction: technical details. Trans Am Ophthalmol Soc 1976;74:321–9.

[16] Bartley GB, Kay PP. Posterior lamellar eyelid reconstruction with a hard palate mucosal graft. Am J Ophthalmol 1989;107:609–12.

[17] Putterman AM. Viable composite grafting in eyelid reconstruction. Am J Ophthalmol 1978; 85:237–41.

[18] Stephenson CM, Brown BZ. The use of tarsus as a free autogenous graft in eyelid surgery. Ophthal Plast Reconstr Surg 1985;1:43–50.

[19] Leibovitch I, Selva D, Davis G, et al. Donor site morbidity in free tarsal grafts. Am J Ophthalmol 2004;138:430–3.

[20] Wearne MJ, Sandy C, Rose GE, et al. Autogenous hard palate mucosa: the ideal lower eyelid spacer? Br J Ophthalmol 2001;85:1183–7.

[21] Tan J, Olver J, Wright M, et al. The use of porous polyethylene (Medpor) lower eyelid spacers in lid heightening and stabilisation. Br J Ophthalmol 2004;88:1197–200.

[22] Walton WT, Gardner TA, Pernelli DR, et al. Repair of the tarsoligamentous sling in New Zealand white rabbits using polytetrafluoroethylene graft material. Ophthal Plast Reconstr Surg 1993;9:254–9.

ELSEVIER
SAUNDERS

Otolaryngol Clin N Am
38 (2005) 1043–1074

OTOLARYNGOLOGIC
CLINICS
OF NORTH AMERICA

Diagnosis and Management of Thyroid Orbitopathy

John G. Rose Jr, MD[a,b], Cat Nguyen Burkat, MD[b], Cynthia A. Boxrud, MD, FACS[c,*]

[a]*Oculofacial and Facial Cosmetic Surgery, Davis Duehr Dean, Madison, WI, USA*
[b]*Oculoplastics Service, Department of Ophthalmology and Visual Sciences,*
University of Wisconsin-Madison, Madison, WI, USA
[c]*Department of Ophthalmology, Division of Ophthalmic Plastic and Reconstructive Surgery,*
University of California-Los Angeles, Jules Stein Eye Institute, 2021 Santa Monica Blvd,
Suite 700E, Santa Monica, CA 09404, USA

Pathophysiology

Thyroid orbitopathy, also known as Graves' orbitopathy, is an autoimmune orbital disease characterized by abnormal percentages of peripheral blood suppressor/cytotoxic T8+ lymphocytes, and a depressed T4/T8 ratio [1]. Environmental and genetic factors, such as HLA-DR histocompatibility loci, may play a role in developing thyroid orbitopathy, although a specific cause has not yet been undetermined. Both cellular and humoral immune mechanisms contribute to the disorder.

A variety of antibodies to thyroid antigens have been identified over the years, including antimicrosomal antibodies directed against microsomal cell surface antigen (thyroid peroxidase) and antibodies directed against thyroglobulin and the thyroid-stimulating hormone (TSH) receptor. These antibodies, originally classified as thyroid-stimulating immunoglobulin and TSH-binding inhibiting immunoglobulin, are now referred to collectively as thyrotropin receptor antibodies. Whether the antibodies actually play a major role in the pathogenesis of the orbitopathy or are simply markers of the orbital autoimmune process is unknown. Furthermore, antibodies are not present in all patients with thyroid orbitopathy, and there is often no correlation between the antibody level and the clinical progression or severity of the orbitopathy [2].

* Corresponding author.
E-mail address: cboxrudmd@aol.com (C.A. Boxrud).

0030-6665/05/$ - see front matter © 2005 Elsevier Inc. All rights reserved.
doi:10.1016/j.otc.2005.03.015

The targets of the lymphocytes are the orbital connective tissues, lipocytes, and extraocular muscles. Activated T cells, accompanied by macrophages, B lymphocytes, plasma cells, and mast cells, infiltrate the orbital tissues. Release of cytokines and oxygen-free radicals results in significant local inflammation. Subsequent fibroblast stimulation results in increased production and deposition of glycosaminoglycans between the extraocular muscle fibers [3]. These hydrophilic glycosaminoglycans then lead to more inflammatory edema, increased muscle and fat volumes, and muscle injury and scarring.

The active inflammatory stage with muscle and soft tissue swelling manifests as tearing, conjunctival injection, and periorbital edema with eyelid retraction, lagophthalmos, and corneal exposure. As the orbital fat and muscle volumes increase, a mass effect occurs, with increasing proptosis, retrobulbar pressure, and risk of optic nerve compromise. Decreased compliance within the orbit leads to venous congestion, which further exacerbates the orbital and periorbital edema. Enlargement of the superior rectus muscle may compress the superior ophthalmic vein and further reduce venous outflow. With disease of longer duration, increased collagen and fat deposition may replace degenerated extraocular muscles in the quiescent stage of thyroid orbitopathy.

Histopathology

The predominant orbital pathology is inflammation of the orbital soft tissues and extraocular muscles. The earliest changes consist of a light infiltration of lymphocytes and plasma cells within the connective tissues spaces of the extraocular muscles. Each extraocular muscle is composed of many fascicles or myofibers surrounded by connective tissue called perimysium. Each fascicle of muscle fiber is surrounded by endomysium. The perimysium and endomysium of the extraocular muscles are affected in Graves' orbitopathy.

This early phase is followed by activation of endomysial fibroblasts that produce extracellular glycosaminoglycans and collagen. The glycosaminoglycans, hyaluronic acid in particular, are hydrophilic macromolecules that result in increased orbital volume. The extraocular muscle fibers may become distended, embedded in a loose stroma rich in extracellular glycosaminoglycans [3]. These molecules are long, unbranched polysaccharides containing a repeating disaccharide unit. The disaccharide units contain either of two modified sugars, N-acetylgalactosamine or N-acetylglucosamine, and a uronic acid such asglucuronate or iduronate. Glycosaminoglycans are highly negatively charged molecules located primarily in the extracellular matrix. Hyaluronic acid is a specific glycosaminoglycan deposited in thyroid orbitopathy. With fibroblast proliferation and continued deposition of glycosaminoglycans, hyaluronic acid, and collagen, eventual restriction of orbital tissues may occur [4].

The lacrimal gland, which is composed of saclike structures called acini, has no definite capsule and is thought to be enclosed by periorbita. These structures may demonstrate a mild degree of mononuclear cell infiltration and interstitial edema without fibrosis or obliteration of acinar components of the gland.

In thyroid orbitopathy, the orbital fat compartments may also demonstrate a mild degree of inflammation [5], whereas the tendinous muscle insertions on the globe and the optic nerve sheath generally show no inflammation. In contrast, more prominent lymphocytic infiltration of the orbital fat and muscles is seen in idiopathic orbital inflammatory disease [4]. Eosinophils and germinal centers with follicles may be found in other noninfectious orbital inflammations but are typically absent in thyroid orbitopathy.

Lipomatosis within the muscles occurs later in the disease [4,6]. Intracellular and extracellular lipids, rather than mucopolysaccharides, are deposited within the extraocular muscle tissues. CT thus shows enlarged recti with radiolucent centers [6]. Lipid deposition replacing degenerated muscle represents a degenerative change indicative of longstanding thyroid orbitopathy.

Incidence and patient demographics

Thyroid orbitopathy is usually a slowly progressive disease that may have a fluctuating course before stabilizing and eventually resolving. Clinically significant orbitopathy affects 10% to 15% of patients with thyroid dysfunction; 5% to 7% develop severe disease such as progressive proptosis, myopathy, and optic neuropathy [3]. Up to 50% of patients have mild or subclinical evidence of orbitopathy on radiologic imaging [7].

Thyroid orbitopathy typically affects females four to five times more often than males [3,8]. The mean age of onset of orbitopathy is 43 to 45 years [9,10]. Males tend to have a later onset and more severe disease. Younger patients have milder disease than patients over age 50 years [9]. Greater increases in intraocular pressure during upgaze are found in men and in patients older than 50 years [9]. Asians may have less severe disease than whites, with fewer extraocular muscles involved and less muscle enlargement [3].

The onset of orbitopathy is typically insidious, with gradual progression over months. Patients who present with an acute history of symptoms and rapid progression over several weeks are more likely to develop severe orbitopathy. Bartley [11] demonstrated that in patients with clinical orbitopathy, 90% were found to be hyperthyroid by thyroid function tests, 6% were euthyroid, 3% had Hashimoto's thyroiditis, and 1% was hypothyroid. At the time of diagnosis of thyroid dysfunction, more than 90% of patients had a palpably diffuse or nodular goiter on examination.

A close temporal relationship between the onset of thyroid orbitopathy and the diagnosis of hyperthyroidism has been found in numerous studies. Approximately 40% to 60% of patients with hyperthyroidism have or will develop thyroid orbitopathy within 1 year after the diagnosis of hyperthyroidism [9]. The onset of thyroid orbitopathy may occur before a diagnosis of hyperthyroidism in 20% patients, at the same time as the diagnosis of hyperthyroidism in 40%, and after the diagnosis of hyperthyroidism in 40% of patients [3]. As a result, 20% of patients with thyroid orbitopathy are clinically euthyroid at the time of diagnosis, and 80% are clinically hyperthyroid. Euthyroid patients can develop clinical signs and symptoms of thyroid orbitopathy, although their disease course tends to be less severe [12].

Numerous studies have reported similar findings that orbitopathy typically presents within 1 year before or after the diagnosis of hyperthyroidism [9,13–15]. In 1996 Bartley et al [10] found that thyroid orbitopathy was diagnosed within 6 months before the diagnosis of thyroid dysfunction in 20% patients, was concurrent with the diagnosis of hyperthyroidism in 20%, developed in the 6 months after the diagnosis of hyperthyroidism in 22%, and developed more than 6 months after diagnosis of hyperthyroidism in another 35%.

For prognosis, Rootman [3] reported that approximately 36% of patients with thyroid orbitopathy remain the same or worsen clinically after 1 year. Risk factors or prognostic indicators of progressive and severe thyroid orbitopathy are

1. Male gender
2. Age greater than 50 years
3. Rapid onset of symptoms under 3 months
4. Cigarette smoking
5. Diabetes
6. Severe or uncontrolled hyperthyroidism
7. Presence of pretibial myxedema
8. High cholesterol levels
9. Peripheral vascular disease

These indicators should be explained in detail to all patients presenting with thyroid-related orbitopathy.

In patients with both thyroid orbitopathy and diabetes, the use of corticosteroids is limited because of the effect on glycemic control. Orbital irradiation is contraindicated because of its contribution to retinopathy. Recent onset of the orbitopathy in relation to the thyroid metabolic disorder may also portend a worse orbital process.

Smoking is an important risk factor for progressive and severe thyroid orbitopathy [16–19]. Patients with thyroid orbitopathy have greater than twice the incidence of smoking compared with the general population. This finding suggests there is an increased risk of orbitopathy in patients who smoke or are around those who smoke [18]. The severity of orbitopathy is also greater in smokers. In one recent study, patients who had restrictive myopathy and diplopia within $20°$ of primary position had a significantly higher incidence of cigarette smoking (90%) than patients without restrictive myopathy (63%). In addition, the incidence of compressive optic neuropathy was slightly higher in smokers [18].

In addition to an increased incidence and severity of thyroid orbitopathy, smoking decreases the effectiveness of medical treatment [19–21]. The association between the number of cigarettes smoked daily and the increased incidence of severe disease has been recognized previously [19]. In 2003, Eckstein [21] found that smoking affects the response of orbitopathy to treatment in a dose-dependent manner. The response to treatment, measured by proptosis, clinical activity score, and motility, was delayed and significantly poorer in smokers.

Smoking also increases the relapse rate of thyroid orbitopathy, particularly in males [22,23]. Although the precise mechanism underlying the association between cigarette smoking and thyroid orbitopathy is not clearly defined, patients should be strongly advised to refrain from smoking.

Because thyroid orbitopathy is part of an autoimmune process, patients may have concomitant systemic diseases. Myasthenia gravis is found in 1% of patients with thyroid dysfunction [11]. Other coexisting disorders that have been reported include rheumatoid arthritis, diabetes, ulcerative colitis, Crohn's disease, Paget's disease, pernicious anemia, vitiligo, pituitary adenoma, and breast or colon carcinoma. A complete systemic history and evaluation therefore is indicated in all patients with thyroid orbitopathy.

Diagnosis of thyroid orbitopathy

Evolution of classification systems

The most widely used classification system for thyroid orbitopathy was the NOSPECS classification, which was introduced by Werner and the American Thyroid Association in 1969 [24]. The NOSPECS system was based on the presence and severity of certain signs and symptoms: stare, lid lag, proptosis, tearing, photophobia, conjunctival injection or chemosis, eyelid fullness, lagophthalmos, diplopia, extraocular muscle involvement, corneal changes, and optic nerve involvement. The mnemonic, NOSPECS, stood for N-no signs or symptoms; O-only signs; S-soft tissue involvement; P-proptosis of 3 mm or more; E-extraocular muscle involvement and restriction; C-corneal involvement; and S-sight loss caused by optic nerve involvement.

The NOSPECS system was modified in 1977 to account for differences among different ethnic groups in the upper limits of normal proptosis (18 mm for whites, and 22 mm for blacks) [25,26].

In 1981, Sergott et al [27] argued that an assessment for disease activity needed to be included in the classification system, because patients with more active disease tend to respond differently to therapy than do patients with quiescent disease. A clinical disease activity index was devised that incorporated indicators of active, progressive orbitopathy:

1. Injection over the horizontal extraocular muscles
2. Pain with ocular motility
3. Resistance to globe retropulsion
4. Decreased visual acuity
5. Acquired dyschromatopsia on pseudoisochromatic color plate testing

Numerous other classification systems were similarly reported in an attempt to provide more reproducible and objective criteria for the characterization and prognostication of thyroid orbitopathy [28]. Limitations were found in all the proposed classification systems and modifications, however. Resistance to retropulsion and injection over extraocular muscle insertions were unreliable predictors for disease activity. Results of treatment studies showed that these systems yielded unclear prognostication [28–31].

In 1992, the major international thyroid societies agreed to abandon the NOSPECS classification because the system characterized disease activity poorly, did not represent a continuous progression of clinical disease, relied on subjective criteria, and had little to no prognostic value [28,32].

The distinction between the acute inflammatory stage and the indolent noninfiltrative stage remained important in determining patient management. In 1993 Kendler [9] presented six clinical indices of thyroid orbitopathy that were applied to patients grouped by age and gender: soft tissue inflammation, muscle impairment, visual acuity, Hertel measurement, intraocular pressure difference in upgaze, and corneal staining. Patients older than age 50 years more frequently had an acute or subacute onset of orbitopathy over less than 4 weeks, as well as asymmetric disease. In patients older than age 50 and in men, the severity of restricted motility, decreased visual acuity, soft tissue inflammation, and increased intraocular pressure on upgaze were also greater [9].

In 1995, Bartley [33] proposed a diagnostic algorithm for thyroid orbitopathy that was simple, clinical, and reproducible. The diagnosis of thyroid orbitopathy is made if eyelid retraction is present with abnormal thyroid function studies, with exophthalmos 20 mm or greater, with optic nerve dysfunction, or with extraocular muscle involvement. The findings may be unilateral or bilateral. If eyelid retraction is not present, the diagnosis is made if exophthalmos, optic nerve dysfunction, or extraocular muscle involvement is concurrent with abnormal thyroid function studies.

In 1997, Mourits [34] developed a clinical activity score that distinguished patients with active orbitopathy from those with fibrotic end-stage disease. This assessment of clinical activity explains why 35% of patients with thyroid orbitopathy do not respond to immunosuppressive management. The clinical activity score is based on four classic signs of inflammation:

pain (at rest or with eye movement), redness (eyelid or conjunctiva), swelling (eyelid, chemosis, caruncle, proptosis), and impaired function (motility, visual acuity). A point is given for each finding, yielding a score ranging from 0 to 10. The study found that the clinical activity score has a high predictive value for the outcome of immunosuppressive treatment in thyroid orbitopathy. Patients with a higher clinical activity score (more active orbital disease) tend to respond better to immunosuppressive treatment with oral prednisone or orbital irradiation. Disease activity is therefore a prime prognostic indicator of therapeutic outcome.

Rootman [3] also advocates characterizing thyroid orbitopathy by activity and severity. Mild disease, characterized by lid lag, eyelid retraction, lagophthalmos, and mild proptosis, is typically found in younger patients and may occasionally resolve with medical control of the thyroid dysfunction. Moderate active disease consists of increasing and persistent signs and symptoms, including intermittent myopathy that eventually stabilizes within 1 year. With increasing disease severity and activity, mass effects and cicatricial changes within the orbit manifest as progressive exophthalmos, restrictive myopathy, and an orbital apex syndrome with optic neuropathy.

Clinical evaluation

A comprehensive history and review of systems is warranted in all patients suspected of having thyroid orbitopathy. A review of systems should include any history of unplanned weight loss, increased appetite, heat or cold intolerance, difficulty sleeping, proximal muscle weakness of the limbs, and mood lability or anxiety. The thyroid gland should be palpated. Infiltrative pretibial myxedema and thyroid acropathy, characterized by clubbing and subcutaneous fibrosis of the fingers, may be seen occasionally [3,8]. All patients should be referred to an endocrinologist or internist, if not already involved, for further medical evaluation and management of the systemic disorder.

The orbital manifestations can be divided into soft tissue features, eyelid abnormalities, myopathy, and orbital apex compression.

Soft tissue features

External signs of inflammatory disease include chemosis, conjunctival hyperemia, eyelid and periorbital injection, and edema. The periorbital swelling may initially be intermittent, presenting upon awakening and improving throughout the day. Orbital fat prolapse with fullness of the eyelids may occur and may or may not be present with eyelid edema.

Patients may describe frequent tearing, ocular surface irritation, ocular fatigue with reading, and mild pain on eye movement. Severe pain is not typical; however, many patients complain of a constant retrobulbar aching or pressure. Increased ocular surface exposure results in complaints of burning, sandiness, grittiness, mucus discharge, tearing, photophobia, and blurred vision.

Any decrease in visual acuity requires an assessment for abnormalities of the tear film, corneal surface, and optic nerve. Slit-lamp examination may demonstrate conjunctival injection, particularly prominent over the extra-ocular muscle insertions onto the globe. Any combination of proptosis, upper and lower eyelid retraction, and lagophthalmos predisposes the corneal surface to dryness and exposure keratitis. Exposure keratitis may range from minimal superficial punctate staining of the inferior cornea to superior limbic keratoconjunctivitis [3,8,22] to severe keratitis and even corneal ulceration. Primary lacrimal gland dysfunction may be present in thyroid orbitopathy, and some patients may show evidence of altered protein composition of tears or altered rate of tear production [35].

Eyelid abnormalities

Eyelid retraction is the most common clinical sign of thyroid orbitopathy, present in approximately 75% patients at diagnosis and in 91% of patients at some point in the clinical course (Fig. 1). Other common findings, and their frequencies, are exophthalmos (62%), restrictive myopathy (43%), and optic neuropathy (6%). Only 5% of patients demonstrate the full spectrum of eyelid retraction, hyperthyroidism, exophthalmos, optic neuropathy, and restrictive myopathy [11].

It has been suggested that the upper eyelid retraction in thyroid orbitopathy is caused by sympathetic overaction of Müller's muscle, increased sensitivity to circulating catecholamines, or fibrosis and functional shortening of the levator palpebrae superioris muscle, Müller's muscle, and even conjunctiva. The upper eyelid retraction in thyroid orbitopathy has a characteristic temporal flare, with the retraction curving higher laterally than along the medial eyelid. Care should be taken to avoid a misdiagnosis of ptosis of the contralateral eyelid in instances of mild eyelid retraction (Fig. 2). Lower eyelid retraction may result from similar changes within the capsulopalpebral fascia and lower eyelid retractors. Concomitant proptosis tends to accentuate the appearance of both upper and lower eyelid retraction.

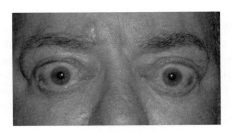

Fig. 1. Typical clinical presentation of severe thyroid orbitopathy, showing marked upper and lower eyelid retraction, axial proptosis, lagophthalmos, and conjunctival injection over the extraocular muscle insertions.

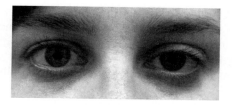

Fig. 2. Patient with mild retraction of the right upper eyelid. Mild retraction without superior scleral show may be misdiagnosed as ptosis of the contralateral eyelid.

Although eyelid retraction is most frequently associated with thyroid orbitopathy, other causes for eyelid retraction must be excluded, such as neurogenic causes, other myogenic causes, cirrhosis, congenital causes, or following trauma or surgery [36].

Because of eyelid retraction and proptosis, mean vertical palpebral fissure heights are greater in patients with thyroid orbitopathy (12 mm) than in normal patients (9 mm) [37]. Inferior scleral show is as common as superior scleral show. Anatomically, the inferior rectus muscle, which is the most frequently involved muscle in thyroid orbitopathy, has terminal fibrous attachments (called the capsulopalpebral fascia) that connect to the lower eyelid (Fig. 3). Because of this attachment, fibrotic contracture of the inferior rectus muscle or direct involvement of the capsulopalpebral fascia results in retraction of the lower eyelid.

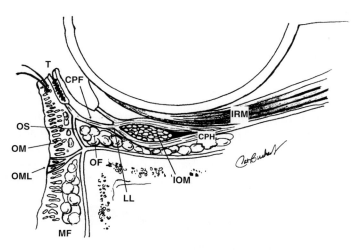

Fig. 3. Normal lower lid anatomy in cross-section. Fibrotic contracture of the inferior rectus muscle, the muscle most frequently involved in thyroid orbitopathy, may result in lower eyelid retraction because of terminal fibrous attachments called the capsulopalpebral fascia that connect to the lower eyelid. CPF, capsulopalpebral fascia; CPH, capsulopalpebral head; IOM, inferior oblique muscle; IRM, inferior rectus muscle; LL, Lockwood's ligament; MF, malar fat; OF, orbital fat; OM, orbicularis muscle; OML, orbitomalar ligament; OS, orbital septum; T, tarsus.

Levator function is normal or high in many patients with exophthalmos [38]. Other studies report that, as the eyelid retraction increases, maximum levator function may decrease [3]. In some instances, very low levator function may be found in patients with compressive optic neuropathy because of significant inflammatory infiltration and fibrosis around the levator muscle [38]. Upper eyelid crease height may be slightly higher in thyroid orbitopathy because of attenuation of the levator aponeurosis from frequent eyelid squeezing to relieve chronic ocular surface irritation and exposure [8]. Therefore, in patients with orbitopathy, a degree of ptosis may counterbalance or mask the eyelid retraction initially.

Other characteristic eyelid findings include lid lag and von Graefe's sign [39]. Lid lag is detected by asking the patient to fixate on a target high above the head and then maintain fixation as the target is slowly lowered. Lid lag is the static manifestation when the eyelid remains elevated and does not completely descend with downgaze (Fig. 4). Because the eyelid fails to move in conjunction with the eye, the superior sclera is temporarily visible as the patient looks down. von Graefe's sign is the slow, delayed downward movement of the upper eyelid on downgaze. The eyelid may sometimes display a staccato or saccadic movement [40]. Similarly, the lower eyelid may demonstrate lag on upgaze.

Incomplete and infrequent blinking (Stellwag's sign), spasmodic retraction of the upper eyelid during fixation in primary position resulting in a widened palpebral fissure (Dalrymple's sign), tremor of the gently closed lids (Rosenbach's sign), difficulty in everting the upper eyelid (Gifford's sign), and resistance to downward pull of the upper eyelid (Grove's sign) can also occur. With the patient in downgaze, Grove's sign is positive when the upper eyelashes are grasped and resistance to downward pulling of the eyelid is felt. Resistance indicates probable involvement of the levator muscle [41].

Myopathy

Inflammation and edema of the extraocular muscles, with subsequent deposition of glycosaminoglycans, collagen, and eventual fibrosis, correlate with the symptoms and signs of progressive myopathy. A common presenting symptom is binocular diplopia that is initially intermittent and gradually becomes chronic. The diplopia is first noticed in upgaze or

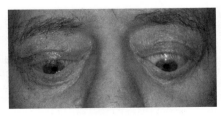

Fig. 4. Lid lag, or incomplete descent of the upper eyelid (*left eye*) may be seen in thyroid orbitopathy.

downgaze, because of the propensity of the disorder to affect the vertical rectus muscles, and may eventually progress to diplopia in primary gaze. Vision may blur with saccadic movements because of decreased peak saccadic velocity from increased muscle size [3]. With increasing severity of myopathy, a pulling or pressure sensation occurs, followed in some instances by pain with eye movement.

On examination, the most common motility abnormality is limitation of elevation caused by fibrosis of the inferior rectus muscle, which results in diplopia on upgaze. The medial rectus is second most frequently involved, followed by the superior rectus/levator complex, and then the lateral rectus muscle. Involvement of the lateral rectus muscle alone would be atypical for thyroid orbitopathy. Multiple muscles may be involved, and involvement of the two orbits may be asymmetric. Vertical or horizontal globe displacement occurs with progressive fibrosis of the muscles.

Thyroid orbitopathy is the most common cause of both unilateral and bilateral exophthalmos, defined as an exophthalmometry measurement of 2 mm or more above the normal limit. Mean exophthalmometer readings are significantly greater in thyroid orbitopathy (22 mm; SD, 3.5) than in normal patients without any orbital process (16 mm; SD, 2.5) [42]. Although in normal patients mean exophthalmometer readings are typically larger in males than females, no statistically significant differences were found in patients with orbitopathy when grouped by gender or age. Other studies reported similar exophthalmometer readings of 20 mm in thyroid orbitopathy [43]. Variations in the normal exophthalmometer measurements among different ethnic populations should always be taken into consideration: the upper normal limit is 20 mm in whites, 22 mm in African Americans, and 18 mm in Asians [26,44,45].

The proptosis in thyroid orbitopathy is usually bilateral but may be asymmetric, giving the clinical impression of unilateral proptosis. The proptosis is axial in direction; displacement of the globe in any other direction suggests another diagnosis. Unilateral proptosis is common and may occur in 13% of patients, more often in men than in women [9]. Because the globe is displaced anteriorly, the proptosis is partially limited by the orbital septum and the posterior attachment of the extraocular muscles at the apex. When the pressure within the retrobulbar tissues exceeds the forces counteracting proptosis, acute subluxation of the globe anterior to the eyelids may occur.

Mean exophthalmometer readings do not necessarily correlate with incidence of optic neuropathy [42]. In some cases, prominent exophthalmos may prevent optic nerve compression by auto-decompressing the orbital tissues anteriorly.

Progressive restrictive myopathy also manifests as an increase in intraocular pressure during upgaze caused by restriction of the inferior rectus muscle. An elevation in intraocular pressure during upgaze of more than 4 mm Hg is considered abnormal [3]. Others consider an increase of

6 mm Hg or more in upgaze to be abnormal [8]. Increases in intraocular pressure during upgaze may be found in up to 60% of patients and tend to be greater in men (7.8 mm Hg) than in women (5.8 mm Hg) [9,46].

Ocular hypertension, or elevated intraocular pressure in primary position, may also be found in patients with thyroid orbitopathy. Although the precise mechanism of development is unknown, the hypertension has been attributed to increased intraorbital pressure associated with proptosis, increased episcleral venous pressure secondary to orbital congestion, increased mucopolysaccharide deposition in the trabecular meshwork, a direct thyrotoxic effect, or a predisposed genetic association between thyroid disease and glaucoma [46–49].

One study [47] found that the mean intraocular pressure in eyes with proptosis of 19 mm or more was 20 mm Hg, whereas the pressure in eyes with proptosis less than 19 mm was 17 mm Hg. The difference was statistically significant, suggesting that proptosis may contribute to ocular hypertension. Cockerham et al [50] found that 24% of patients with thyroid orbitopathy had intraocular pressures greater than 22 mm Hg. Although all these patients had enlarged extraocular muscles on CT scans, enlarged muscles, limited motility, proptosis, or diplopia was not found to be predictive of progression to glaucoma. Only the duration of orbitopathy was correlated significantly with progression to glaucoma, occurring in 2% of patients at 12 years after the diagnosis of thyroid orbitopathy. Therefore, patients with chronic thyroid orbitopathy may require frequent follow-up for assessment of optic nerve damage.

Orbital apex compression

The clinical examination should include testing for visual acuity, color vision, motility, examination for an afferent pupillary defect, and fundoscopy to detect optic disc swelling or pallor. The optic nerve head appearance may be normal in 47% of patients with optic neuropathy [51].

Optic neuropathy is the most common cause of blindness in thyroid orbitopathy, with a prevalence of 5% to 8% in patients with thyroid orbitopathy [3,51]. Its onset is insidious and may be masked by other symptoms. Patients are usually male, older than 50 years of age, have a later onset of thyroid disease, and often have diabetes (16%) [9,51,52]. Optic neuropathy is usually bilateral, but up to one third of cases may be unilateral [9,52].

Most cases of optic neuropathy are caused by compression of the optic nerve by the enlarged extraocular muscles at the orbital apex, referred to as type II orbitopathy (Fig. 5A). Although patients usually have proptosis, optic neuropathy can occur without significant proptosis in patients whose tight orbital septum limits anterior globe displacement despite increased retrobulbar pressure. Rarely, optic neuropathy can occur without significant muscle enlargement. In this small subgroup, the optic neuropathy may be associated with stretching of the optic nerve caused by increased orbital

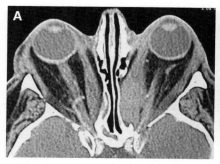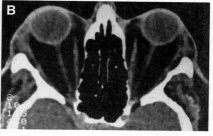

Fig. 5. (*A*) Axial CT scan of a patient with type II orbitopathy. Enlarged extraocular muscles may result in crowding of the optic nerve at the orbital apex. The tendinous muscle insertions near the globe are not involved. Significant proptosis, with the globes completely anterior to the zygoma, medial bowing of the lamina papyracea caused by pressure of the enlarged orbital tissues, and bony remodeling without erosion are also seen. (*B*) Axial CT scan of a patient with type I orbitopathy. Significant fat volume expansion, rather than muscle enlargement, causes increased orbital volume and severe proptosis. The lacrimal glands are also enlarged.

volume or compression of the nerve by increased orbital fat rather than muscle (type I orbitopathy; Fig. 5B) [3,53].

The clinical parameters most highly correlated with extraocular muscle volume and thus with risk for optic neuropathy are measurements of ocular motility. The greater the severity of restrictive myopathy, reflecting fibrotic, less compliant muscles, the greater the suspicion should be for compressive optic neuropathy [3,53,54]. Greater increases in intraocular pressure on upgaze of 9 mm Hg or more may also reflect apical compression [3]. Proptosis is less helpful or consistent in assessing the risk of optic neuropathy [42,54].

Optic neuropathy can occur in a significant number of patients (53%) with visual acuities of 20/40 or better. Visual field defects are present in 66%, and an afferent pupillary defect is seen in 35%. A swollen or pale optic disc is found in only 53% [51]. Color vision testing using the Farnsworth-Munsell 100-hue test is a sensitive indicator of optic nerve dysfunction. Pseudoisochromatic Ishihara plates, in contrast, rarely identify an acquired color defect unless optic neuropathy is severe, making Ishihara plates a suboptimal screening test for optic nerve involvement. The pattern-reversal visual evoked potential test is another sensitive test for detecting early optic neuropathy and may be useful in following patients after treatment [51].

Diagnostic tools

In patients with suspected thyroid orbitopathy, radioimmunoassay tests can be used to detect thyroid dysfunction. Hyperthyroidism may be detected by measuring increased serum free thyroxine and serum free triiodothyronine or a low TSH response to thyroid-releasing hormone stimulation. A more sensitive test known as TSH-IRMA (immunoradiometric assay) may reliably distinguish normal from hyperthyroid states and often is used in conjunction with free thyroxine measurements [55,56].

Positive tests for various thyroid antibodies help support the diagnosis of autoimmune thyroid disorder. In Graves' disease, antithyroglobulin antibodies are present in approximately 30% of patients, and antimicrosomal antibodies are found in 60%. Thyrotropin receptor antibodies are present in up to 95% of patients with untreated Graves' hyperthyroidism and in approximately 50% of patients with euthyroid Graves' disease [57].

A baseline visual field should be performed in all patients suspected of having optic nerve involvement, because serial visual fields are useful in following patients for progression of compressive optic neuropathy. They are also helpful in assessing a patient's response to medical therapy. Most frequently, a paracentral scotoma, enlarged blind spot, or inferior altitudinal defect occurs with compressive optic neuropathy. Other visual field defects may occur, including a nerve fiber bundle defect, vertical step, cecocentral scotoma, or generalized constriction [51].

Imaging

Orbital imaging for thyroid orbitopathy permits identification of enlarged extraocular muscles within the orbit, whether in unilateral, bilateral, or asymmetric disease. Many patients with clinical unilateral exophthalmos have thickening of the extraocular muscles in both orbits, with less involvement and enlargement in the subclinical orbit. This bilateral muscle thickening helps distinguish thyroid orbitopathy from other diseases that may cause muscle enlargement, such as idiopathic orbital inflammation, orbital myositis, arteriovenous fistulas, and metastatic carcinoma.

Ultrasonography may detect early thyroid disease in patients without clinical orbital findings or abnormal thyroid levels. One study showed that A-scan ultrasonography demonstrated enlarged extraocular muscles in patients with unilateral proptosis who were found to have thyroid dysfunction on subsequent laboratory tests [58]. Enlargement of the extraocular muscles may also be visualized with B-scan ultrasound techniques [59]. Ultrasonography of the extraocular muscles may also demonstrate a lower internal reflectivity in active disease than in inactive disease [60]. Assessment of extraocular muscle involvement at the orbital apex is less reliable using ultrasound than by CT scan.

Routine CT scanning is not necessary in all patients with a typical clinical and laboratory presentation of thyroid orbitopathy. A CT scan of the orbit is necessary if optic neuropathy is suspected to evaluate the orbital apex status. It is also indicated in patients with atypical motility disturbances or nonaxial proptosis to rule out other causes and before performing orbital decompression. Orbital CT may detect subclinical enlargement of the extraocular muscles on the contralateral side in 50% to 90% of patients [7].

The most characteristic CT findings in thyroid orbitopathy are ovoid enlargement of the extraocular muscles that spares the tendinous muscle insertions and axial globe proptosis. The inferior rectus muscle is most commonly enlarged, followed in frequency by the medial, superior, and lateral rectus muscles. The radiologic involvement of the extraocular muscles correlates to the restrictive myopathy found on clinical examination. Feldon and Weiner [61,62] found that the degree of extraocular muscle enlargement, determined by volumetric analysis of orbital CT scans, correlated with the degree of clinical orbitopathy. A linear relationship between worsening orbitopathy and both horizontal and total extraocular muscle volumes was found. Medial bowing of the lamina papyracea caused by pressure of the enlarged orbital tissues, bone remodeling without erosion, lacrimal gland enlargement, and normal orbital fat radiodensity can also be seen (Fig. 5) [4,7].

Orbital apex crowding is a sensitive indicator for the presence of optic neuropathy and is best assessed with coronal CT scans (Fig. 6). Enlargement of the extraocular muscles at the orbital apex with crowding of the optic nerve and a dilated superior ophthalmic vein may be clearly visualized [51]. Thyroid orbitopathy caused by fat expansion (type I) can also be distinguished from extraocular muscle enlargement (type II).

Because MRI is more expensive than CT imaging, CT scans are more commonly performed to evaluate the orbital involvement. MRI has been reported to be useful in distinguishing between active and inactive disease, however. Acute inflammation present within extraocular muscles results in a higher water content that demonstrates longer T2 times. Therefore, T1- and T2-weighted images may differentiate the active edematous disease stage from the inactive fibrotic muscle stage [63]. This information could help determine which patients have acute inflammatory disease that would respond better to radiation therapy and which have chronic fibrosis that tends to be refractory to radiation therapy [64].

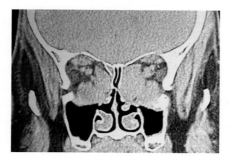

Fig. 6. Coronal CT scan of the orbital apex in a patient with compressive optic neuropathy. The posterior portions of the extraocular muscles are markedly enlarged, resulting in crowding of the optic nerve. The lateral rectus muscle is the least involved muscle.

Differential diagnosis

On clinical examination, the complete differential for eyelid retraction or proptosis should be considered if there is no prior history of thyroid disorder [36]. The motility disturbances should be distinguished from disturbances arising from other causes, such as a superior oblique palsy, trauma, or myasthenia gravis.

When acute orbital inflammation is present, the differential diagnosis includes idiopathic orbital inflammation (orbital pseudotumor), myositis, orbital cellulitis, or scleritis. Imaging can aid in determining the likely cause. Myositis is more often unilateral, involving a single muscle, with characteristic muscle tendon involvement on ultrasonography or CT. Ultrasonography may be more helpful than CT in detecting tendon involvement. The tendon enlargement in myositis is not a consistent finding, however. Rapid onset of symptoms and significant pain on extraocular movement is also more typical in idiopathic orbital inflammation and myositis. In contrast to thyroid orbitopathy, on CT scanning idiopathic orbital inflammation demonstrates involvement of the muscles and also the orbital fat, perineural connective tissues, Tenon's space, and the sclera, which may be seen as a circumferential "ring" sign outlining the globe. A medial subperiosteal abscess and adjacent sinus disease may indicate orbital cellulitis.

The most common cause of extraocular muscle enlargement on CT is thyroid disease, followed by idiopathic orbital inflammation and myositis. Unlike thyroid orbitopathy, idiopathic orbital inflammation most commonly involves the medial rectus (57%), followed by the lateral rectus (36%) [65]. Other causes of muscle enlargement include primary or local tumor invasion (lymphoma, rhabdomyosarcoma, meningioma) (26%), metastatic tumor (20%), vascular anomalies (cavernous hemangioma, carotid-cavernous fistula), and infection (orbital cellulitis, cysticercosis). Primary and metastatic tumors usually involve a single muscle and produce a nodular lesion with discrete borders. Adjacent bony erosion or remodeling may be present. An enlarged superior ophthalmic vein and uniform, moderate enlargement of the rectus muscles may indicate venous congestion from a carotid-cavernous fistula or from an insidious low-flow dural sinus fistula.

Medical management of thyroid orbitopathy

Principles and indications for treatment

The decision of whether, when, and how to treat thyroid orbitopathy and its manifestations depends on the careful diagnosis of the findings related to thyroid orbitopathy and on assessment of the stage of orbitopathy. As detailed in the previous section, the first assessment must be whether the disease is immunologically active or inactive. Patients with inactive disease may be amenable to observation or elective surgical correction of functional or cosmetic defects. Active disease may be further differentiated into moderate versus severe disease. Patients with moderate disease may be amenable to observation, conservative medical treatment, or elective surgery, whereas those who progress toward more severe disease may require intensive medical management and possibly urgent surgical intervention [3]. At every stage of treatment, protection of the optic nerve is paramount. All other thyroid orbitopathy–related changes are correctable, but vision loss from compressive optic neuropathy is nearly always permanent.

Of the three disease categories—inactive, moderately active, and severely active—most patients fall into the moderately active category. In most patients with moderately active disease, disease resolves spontaneously, with either observation or conservative, supportive medical treatment [66]. In a study by Bartley et al [67], 74% of patients in an incidence-cohort study required only supportive treatment or observation alone.

It is critical to distinguish between activity and severity of thyroid orbitopathy, because both are relevant to treatment decisions. Whereas the periorbital signs of activity indicate the degree of an ongoing, antigen–antibody response with activation of lymphocytes and fibroblasts in the orbit, severity is gauged by the consequences of the activity. Examples include eyelid retraction, proptosis, ocular surface disease, expansion of orbital fat, extraocular muscle thickening and restriction, strabismus, diplopia, and compressive optic neuropathy.

When a patient first presents to the clinician's office, it can be a challenge to identify the stage of disease activity and severity during a single examination. As discussed previously, external signs, such as periorbital edema and erythema, can be a valuable gauge of inflammatory activity within the orbit. Patients with substantial activity therefore can often be triaged to a treatment regimen without the need for a follow-up visit to assess progression [3]. Patients with severe proptosis and optic neuropathy without marked inflammatory signs can present a dilemma. On one hand, they could have nonprogressive manifestations of old, burned-out disease [66]; on the other hand, there is a small subset of patients whose substantial orbital inflammation and consequent optic nerve compression are masked by an externally quiet-appearing periorbita. Neigel et al [51] showed that most patients with optic neuropathy had quiet to mildly inflamed periorbita, and that there was no difference in the incidence of periorbital inflammatory signs in those with and without optic neuropathy.

Treatment of thyroid disease

The treatment of thyroid orbitopathy requires close coordination with an endocrinologist, because achievement of a euthyroid state helps control orbitopathy. It is thought that permanent euthyroidism or hypothyroidism (necessitating supplementation) results in a decrease of thyroid-autoreactive lymphocytes and thus in thyroid orbit antigenic cross-reactivity [68].

Currently, three options exist for the control of hyperthyroidism: thyroid suppression, thyroidectomy, and thyroid ablation with radioactive iodine. Thyroid suppression with drugs such as propylthiouracil and surgical thyroidectomy are associated with lower rates of worsening of activity than is radioablation. Tallstedt and Lundell [69] showed that orbitopathy worsened in 33% of patients treated with radioablation, compared with 10% of those treated with thyroid suppressants and 16% of those treated with thyroidectomy. In a meta-analysis, Marcocci et al [68] showed that 17% of patients treated with radioactive iodine had worsening of orbitopathy, but this percentage dropped to zero with concomitant use of oral glucocorticoids. Bartalena et al [70] also demonstrated prevention of radioiodine-induced orbital inflammation with concomitant steroids. In some studies, thyroidectomy was shown not to cause any worsening of thyroid orbitopathy [68,71]. Many endocrinologists feel that radioactive iodine offers the best long-term control of hyperthyroidism [3] and is therefore worth the controllable risk of worsening of orbital disease activity. In their clinical practice, the authors limit concomitant steroids to patients with either mild-to-moderate orbital inflammatory activity or impending crowding of the orbital apex. In either subset of patients, and especially the latter, increased activation is highly undesirable.

Medical treatment of mild thyroid orbitopathy

As discussed previously, most patients with thyroid orbitopathy have sufficiently mild disease to require only supportive measures until the orbital disease inactivates spontaneously. Although it is a useful diagnostic criterion for the physician, periorbital edema can range from a cosmetic nuisance to disfiguring for the patient. Nighttime head elevation and cool compresses often suffice for temporary reduction of mild edema, particularly before important business or social engagements. Although the use of diuretics has been debated in the past [72], it is not part of the authors' current clinical practice. Patients with severe periorbital edema are usually triaged to receive systemic steroids or radiation, which helps reduce the edema because it reduces the inflammatory activity.

Ocular surface irritation is an issue for many thyroid orbitopathy patients, manifesting as an annoying irritation and sometimes frightening patients because of blurred vision and photophobia. Complaints of blurring that do not match Snellen visual acuity are a hallmark of punctuate epithelial keratopathy and often are accompanied by foreign-body sensation or mild grittiness. A topical lubricating regimen often suffices [66]; the authors advocate methylcellulose tears four times daily and optional lubricating ointment at bedtime. Eyelid lag and lagophthalmos must be ruled out; if they are present, bedtime lubricating ointment and possibly eyelid taping or a corneal moisture chamber are recommended. Topical steroids may be added if there is a substantial component of ocular surface inflammation, as discussed later.

As discussed earlier, smoking is a significant risk factor for the development and progression of thyroid orbitopathy. Smoking cessation plays a significant role in the reduction of symptoms and signs of orbital inflammatory activity. In the authors' practice, the patient's subjective reports of improvement often exceed the physical findings of improvement, helping to reinforce patient adherence to a smokefree lifestyle.

The treatment of eyelid retraction and strabismus, although mostly surgical, has begun to include medical modalities such as botulinum toxin [73–77]. The surgical approaches to these problems are discussed later. Indications for treatment are inactive to mildly active orbital inflammation and stable eyelid, strabismus, and orbital measurements lasting for 6 months or more. Treatment of eyelid retraction may be considered in patients with more active disease if corneal decompensation is occurring. Depending on the degree of disfigurement and ocular surface irritation, correction of eyelid retraction may be functional or cosmetic. In a 2001 pilot study, Träisk and Tallstedt [76] demonstrated improvement in eight of nine patients, with variable responses to the same dose and unpredictable duration of effect. Uddin and Davies [77] reported a variable but satisfactory response to transconjunctival injection of botulinum toxin A in 10 of 11 patients. Duration of effect varied from 1 to 40 months; three patients suffered transient diplopia. Morganstern et al [74] showed variable reduction in marginal reflex distance in 17 of 18 patients with active orbital inflammation. In summation, transconjunctival or transcutaneous treatment of upper eyelid retraction with botulinum toxin A seems to offer variable but often acceptable improvement in patients who do not want or who are not candidates for surgery.

The association between thyroid orbitopathy and glaucoma is controversial. Glaucoma may be misdiagnosed if the intraocular pressure is not measured in 5° downgaze [3], which minimizes pressure of the extraocular muscles on the globe. Supporting this precaution are the findings of Kikkawa et al [78] that treatment of restrictive myopathy with botulinum toxin A causes a reduction in intraocular pressure. Karadimas et al [79] showed no association between glaucoma and circulating TSH or free triiodothyronine levels. Finally, intraocular pressure is often found to decline in patients undergoing orbital decompression [3]. In the authors' clinical practice, the few patients who have abnormally high intraocular pressures in 5° downgaze are referred to glaucoma subspecialists for evaluation.

Medical treatment of moderate to severe thyroid orbitopathy

Well-established treatments for moderately to severely active thyroid orbitopathy include corticosteroids, external beam radiation, and, more recently, immunosuppressants. Several newer modalities, including plasma-pheresis, somatostatin analogues and intravenous, are unproven, demon-strated in one study only, or have yet to achieve mainstream use.

Glucocorticoids have been used in the treatment of thyroid orbitopathy for more than 40 years [66]. Their efficacy has been demonstrated against many features specific to thyroid orbitopathy, including suppression of B and T lymphocytes, cytokine inhibition [80], and reduction of chemotactic recruitment of other leukocytes. Smith et al [81,82] demonstrated in vitro reduction in glycosaminoglycan synthesis by cultured orbital fibroblasts using glucocorticoids.

Oral corticosteroids have long been a mainstay in the treatment of both active orbital inflammation and acute optic neuropathy. Treatment usually begins at doses of 60 to 100 mg/day of prednisone [66]; long, slow tapers over several months are usually necessary [3,66]. Kazim et al [83] demonstrated an improvement in orbital pain, diplopia, and proptosis in one third of patients treated with prednisone. There was a similar improvement in signs related to acute optic neuropathy—visual acuity, color vision and afferent pupillary defect—in 50% of patients treated with prednisone. Wiersinga et al [84] noted that 66% of patients treated with an oral prednisone taper beginning at 60 mg/day had some reduction in the NOSPECS score, an outcome comparable in their study to that of orbital irradiation. Limitations of oral corticosteroids include the side effects associated with their long-term use, including weight gain, acne, hirsutism, weakness, insomnia, personality changes, osteoporosis, secondary infections, glucose intolerance, and full-blown Cushing's syndrome [3].

In recent years, pulsed intravenous (IV) corticosteroids have become an increasingly popular treatment for moderate to severe orbital inflammation and is the treatment most commonly used used by one of the authors (JGR). The regimen includes 1 g methylprednisolone delivered intravenously over 1 hour, three times in 1 week (typically Monday/Wednesday/Friday) [3]. No oral steroid taper follows the IV pulse. Improvement in inflammatory signs and symptoms is typically seen in 4 to 6 weeks [3], but one author (JGR) has seen early improvement as soon as 1 to 2 weeks. Side effects are typically much less frequent and severe than with long-term treatment with oral steroids [3].

Several studies have characterized the efficacy of pulsed IV cortico-steroids, although none has included a prospective, randomized comparison with oral steroids or orbital irradiation. In a meta-analysis, Bartalena et al [66] describe a nearly 80% initial response to IV corticosteroids, compared with 60% for oral corticosteroids. Ohtsuka et al [85] showed a statistically significant reduction in extraocular muscle hypertrophy 1 and 6 months following pulsed IV steroids, but their steroid pulse was followed by a 3-month oral steroid taper. The same group demonstrated the same reduction in muscle hypertrophy following pulsed IV steroids with and without orbital irradiation following the steroid pulse [86]. In the treatment of dysthyroid optic neuropathy, pulsed IV methylprednisolone caused a marked short-term improvement in visual acuity in five of five patients [87].

Attempts have been made to assess the predictability of response to pulsed IV steroids. An uncontrolled study demonstrated that orbital scintigraphy may predict response to pulsed IV methylprednisolone [88]. Another study demonstrated an association between IV steroid response and high serum TSH-receptor antibody levels [89].

In an attempt to minimize systemic side effects from corticosteroids, Marcocci et al [90] prospectively compared oral prednisone therapy with orbital irradiation combined with retrobulbar methylprednisolone. Sixty percent of patients in the oral prednisone group showed improvement, but only 25% in the retrobulbar group showed improvement. Other uncontrolled studies have shown similar results [66].

Orbital irradiation has been shown to provide improvement in signs and symptoms of acute orbital inflammation, although it has been surrounded with increased controversy lately. It has been in use for more than 6 decades and, before the advent of pulsed IV corticosteroids, represented a mainstay in the treatment of orbital inflammation caused by thyroid orbitopathy. The mechanism for action of orbital radiotherapy involves both the suppression of lymphocytes, which are highly radiosensitive, and alteration of the helper/suppressor T-lymphocyte ratio [66].

In several studies, orbital irradiation has been shown to improve periorbital edema, erythema, and pain, especially when treatment is initiated early in the disease process, when the inflammatory activity is presumably more acute. Beckendorf et al [91] showed that 76% of patients treated had partial or complete response with these symptoms, but little improvement was seen in proptosis or ocular motility disorders unless they were treated very early in their disease course. Patients treated in the first 7 months of the disease course had better results than those treated later. Likewise, Lloyd and Leone [92] demonstrated improved response in patients treated early in the course of disease, with initial improvement noted at 4 to 6 weeks after initiation of treatment. Their study and a study by Rush et al [93] demonstrated improvement in early compressive optic neuropathy with orbital irradiation, highlighting irradiation, as well as for orbital decompression surgery, as a potential treatment for early compressive optic neuropathy.

There is controversy concerning the treatment of ocular motility disorders with radiation. Although Beckendorf et al [91] demonstrated occasional improvement in ocular motility after irradiation, and only early in the disease process, Mourits et al [94] showed more encouraging results. In a randomized, placebo-controlled (sham-irradiation), prospective trial, 60% of irradiated patients had improvement in diplopia, compared with 31% in the control group at 24-week follow-up. Nonetheless, 75% of the irradiated patients still eventually underwent strabismus surgery.

Echographic measurements have also shown a decrease in extraocular muscle size following external beam radiation that is stable beyond 12 months [95].

Some recent studies have argued that orbital irradiation has little efficacy. In a retrospective review of 90 patients, van Ruyven et al [96] showed that there was no change in proptosis, a subclinical change in ocular motility, no change in visual acuity, and a reduction of periorbital soft tissue signs that could not be differentiated from the normal disease course. In a prospective, randomized, placebo-controlled clinical trial of orbital radiotherapy, Gorman et al [97] showed no improvement at 3- or 6-month intervals in proptosis, muscle or fat volume, range of extraocular movements, area of diplopia fields, or vertical palpebral fissure width. At 1 year there was still no difference between irradiated orbits and the sham-irradiated orbits in the same patients and no correlation between lack of response and clinical activity score [98]. Nonetheless, those who favor radiotherapy for active thyroid orbitopathy argue that the Gorman study did not focus on patients early in the disease course who had more active orbital inflammation.

As with any treatment, external beam radiation has its risks. The lifetime risk for fatal malignancies (0.3% as a population average [99]) may discourage some clinicians from offering this treatment to younger patients. There have been reports of radiation retinopathy, but these reports were associated with errors in dosage calculations and radiotherapy technique [100]. In the same study cohort in which his colleagues argued that radiotherapy offered no benefit for thyroid orbitopathy [97,98], Robertson et al [101] demonstrated de novo appearance of retinal microvascular abnormalities in five eyes in three patients. Of the three patients, one already had microvascular abnormalities in the contralateral eye before radiotherapy.

Immunosuppressants may be useful in patients who do not respond to other modalities or who cannot tolerate steroids. Azathioprine, methotrexate, cyclophosphamide, and cyclosporine can all be used, but hematologic monitoring is necessary [3]. Some orbital surgeons may feel comfortable administering these medications themselves; others, including the authors, prefer to enlist the help of a rheumatologist who has experience administering immunosuppressants safely.

Surgical management of thyroid orbitopathy

Most patients with thyroid orbitopathy have mild symptoms and require only local supportive or medical measures to control eye manifestations. A minority of patients with severe disease (3%–5%) may need aggressive treatments that require a multidisciplinary approach.

Two important developments in the surgical management of thyroid-related orbitopathy have occurred in the last few decades. The first development, a philosophy currently followed by most treating physicians, is that decompression surgery should be done when patients are first medically stabilized. Although there are indications for acute surgical intervention, most of the acute phase of the disease is managed with a medical approach [102]. Medical management of the disease allows the spontaneous regression of inflammation and proptosis, thus avoiding tissue manipulation in the setting of inflammation. It also may reduce the surgical risk of hemorrhage and postoperative edema, making the surgical results more predictable.

The second development has been the ability to visualize the orbital contents with CT and MRI. Before the development of CT scanning, there was little understanding of the expansion of the orbital contents. CT and MRI scanning have expanded the understanding of the role of ocular muscles, orbital fat, soft tissue, bone thickness, and their relationships to each other in the orbit. These factors and related pathology can assist the surgeon by making outcomes more predictable.

A staged approach to surgical rehabilitation is accomplished by expanding the orbit, then addressing any strabismus, and finally retracting excessive skin and soft tissue with eyelid surgery [3].

Orbital decompression

Orbital decompression as a treatment for thyroid orbitopathy has traditionally been indicated for patients with exposure keratitis, compressive optic neuropathy, and severe orbital inflammation with pain [102]. In recent years, an increasing number of patients with disfiguring proptosis are being surgically treated for aesthetic reasons.

Dollinger [103] described the first orbital decompression in 1911. Since then, many different techniques and approaches have been developed, including one-, two-, and three-wall decompressions with orbital fat removal Each technique results in a more-or-less successful reduction and improvement of proptosis.

Major disadvantages of decompression include the risk of postoperative muscle imbalance and diplopia. Potential complications of orbital decompression include blindness, bleeding, diplopia, periorbital numbness, sinusitis, and lid or globe malposition. There is evidence for decreased incidence of diplopia with balanced decompression of both the medial and lateral walls [104,105].

Common approaches to the orbit for decompression surgery, including transantral, coronal, transcaruncular, inferior fornix, the lateral canthal, upper eyelid and, more recently, the endonasal endoscopic approach, have been well described in the literature [106–115]. The different approaches are not reviewed in detail here. Most orbital surgeons have a repertoire that includes a subset of these procedures and must be able to familiarize themselves adequately with the relevant anatomy and risks. In addition, these procedures often are customized further to suit the individual needs and expectations of the patient.

Often the complex nature of the disease process requires repeated visits and documentation of stability over time before nonurgent surgery. Both medical and surgical management of compressive optic neuropathy may be required. If medical treatment is ineffective, orbital decompression may be performed as the definitive treatment of compressive optic neuropathy [51].

The traditional approach to decompression of the optic nerve is by decompressing the medial wall and floor of the orbit. In addition, lateral decompression can be taken to the posterior diploic space at the apex, a technique favored by one of the authors (JGR). Because this technique carries a high likelihood of a cerebrospinal fluid (CSF) leak, surgeons attempting this approach should be comfortable managing intraoperative CSF leaks.

The medial decompression must be taken posteriorly to the orbital apex. Medial wall removal should not extend above the frontoethmoidal suture to prevent serious bleeding from the anterior and posterior ethmoidal arteries and any potential CSF leaks. After bony orbital decompression, the periorbita is opened, allowing the orbital contents to prolapse through the surgical osteotomy.

Goldberg et al [116] described the inferomedial orbital strut and the importance of its preservation. It was further characterized radiographically by Kim et al [117] and lies between the ethmoid and maxillary bones. If the strut is removed during surgery, there may be an inferomedial shift in globe position, causing diplopia.

Orbital fat decompression without bony removal has been described for thyroid orbitopathy without apical compression. This procedure can either be done alone or in combination with bony decompression [115,118,119].

Strabismus surgery

Diplopia, which may be very disabling, is typically caused by fibrosis of the extraocular muscles resulting from the disease itself. In addition, it may result from displacement of the eyes after orbital decompression. Patients need to be stabilized for at least 6 months before consideration for strabismus surgery [120,121].

The goal for strabismus surgery is to achieve single, binocular vision in primary gaze and, ideally, in downgaze for reading. Patients should understand that the expectation of single, binocular vision in all positions of gaze may not be reasonable and that multiple strabismus surgeries and prisms may be required. In addition, because these procedures may be unpredictable, adjustable sutures are often placed to help the surgeon determine the appropriate position postoperatively. These issues must be discussed with patients and family before surgery.

Because of the restrictive myopathy related to thyroid orbitopathy, recession, rather than resection, is the predominant procedure. When feasible, adjustable-suture surgery is recommended, because these procedures can be less predictable than strabismus surgery on nonrestricted muscles. Forced ductions should be checked before and after surgery. Freeing of all adhesions and connections between the lower lid retractors and the inferior rectus muscle is helpful in reducing restriction. It is advised not to operate simultaneously on more than two muscles per eye, to prevent ocular ischemic syndrome. Generally, with multiple muscle involvement, one can correct about 2.5 to 3.0 diopters of deviation per millimeter of recession. With single muscle involvement, on the other hand, approximately 3 to 5 diopters can be achieved with 1 mm of recession [3].

Surgery of the inferior rectus deserves special mention. Inferior rectus recession may decrease upper lid retraction but often results in lower lid retraction despite dissection of the lower lid retractors. Because the inferior rectus has subsidiary actions (eg, excyclotorsion, adduction), inferior rectus recessions may lead to a component of intorsion and A-patterns.

As mentioned previously, under medical management of thyroid orbitopathy, botulinum toxin may be of benefit in some patients with thyroid orbitopathy who have small-angle diplopia of less than 6 months' duration. In addition, the use of botulinum toxin has been recently reported for treatment of upper eyelid retraction [74].

Lid-lengthening surgeries

Surgery to reduce retraction of the upper and lower eyelids is the most common surgery that thyroid orbitopathy patients undergo. It can improve both the patient's appearance and the ocular surface exposure symptoms. Eyelid surgery should take place after strabismus surgery, which follows orbital decompression, if needed [66]. Surgeons performing eyelid recession should be familiar with the anatomy of the muscles of the upper and lower eyelids because the relevant anatomy can be more difficult to characterize surgically than in normal individuals [66].

Upper lid retraction may be treated by either an internal (transconjunctival) approach to Müller's muscle or as an external approach (lid crease incision) to the levator muscle. A combination of the two approaches may be required [122]. One of the authors (CAB) prefers the internal approach; another (JGR) uses the internal approach for less than 3 mm of retraction and the external approach to treat 3 mm or more of retraction. Both techniques are usually performed under local anesthesia or very light IV sedation, so the patient can sit up repeatedly for evaluation of the eyelid height, symmetry, and contour.

For the internal approach, the eyelid is everted over a Desmarres retractor. A light cutting cautery or a radiofrequency handpiece is used to incise the conjunctiva at the superior edge of the tarsus and to disinsert Müllers muscle from the superior border of tarsus. The muscle is dissected from the underlying levator muscle using either the incisional handpiece or blunt dissection, and the incision is carried laterally for the upper length of the upper tarsal border.

The external approach begins with an upper eyelid crease incision and sharp dissection through the orbicularis and layers of the orbital septum using the incisional handpiece. The attachments between the central fat pad and the levator muscle, much stronger than those typically encountered in a routine blepharoptosis repair, are lysed. Often, bands of cicatrix on the surface of the levator can be palpated by strumming them with the tip of the incisional handpiece before activating it. The bands of cicatrix are individually lysed with the handpiece. Particular attention is given to the lateral horn of the levator to decrease the temporal flare of the eyelid margin typical in patients with thyroid-related eyelid retraction. For marked retraction, the levator muscle can be disinserted from the tarsus entirely and recessed by attaching it to the tarsus on hangback sutures, essentially performing the opposite of an external levator repair for blepharoptosis.

Lower eyelid retraction has traditionally been treated with placement of spacer grafts. Ear cartilage, hard palate, human acellular dermis, polytetrafluoroethylene, and porous polyethylene spacers have been described and are commonly used [123–127]. Hard palate grafting has been shown to have less postoperative contraction than acellular dermis [128]; the main disadvantage to this otherwise successful technique is potential donor site complications [129].

Horizontal tightening procedures, such as lateral canthopexy and lateral tarsal strip, increase scleral show in patients with proptosis and are not recommended. In the horizontally tight eyelid, lateral canthal advancement is a useful adjunct to enhance the effect of retractor recession and reduction of temporal flare.

Blepharoplasty

Blepharoplasty is the last phase of restorative surgery in thyroid orbitopathy and typically is performed to debulk excess anterior orbital fat for cosmesis. Lower lid blepharoplasty can be performed with a transconjunctival approach, unless there is a marked excess of lower eyelid skin. Upper lid blepharoplasty is performed transcutaneously with conservative skin excision. It is important to remember that excess skin excision may cause lagophthalmos. In addition, dacryopexy may be required if lacrimal gland prolapse is present.

References

[1] Felberg N, Sergott R, Savino P, et al. Lymphocyte subpopulations in Graves' ophthalmopathy. Arch Ophthalmol 1985(103): p. 656–9.

[2] Morris J, Hay I, Nelson R, et al. Clinical utility of thyrotropin-receptor antibody assays: comparison of radioreceptor and bioassay methods. Mayo Clin Proc 1988;63:707.

[3] Rootman J, Dolman P. Thyroid orbitopathy. In: Rootman J, editor. Diseases of the orbit: a multidisciplinary approach. Philadelphia: Lippincott Williams & Wilkins; 2003. p. 169–212.

[4] Trokel S, Jakobiec F. Correlation of CT scanning and pathologic features of ophthalmic Graves' disease. Ophthalmology 1981;88:553–64.

[5] Campbell R. Immunology of Graves' ophthalmopathy: retrobulbar histology and histochemistry. Acta Endocrinol (Copenh) 1989;121(Suppl 2):9.

[6] Kemp E, Rootman J. Lipid deposition within the extra-ocular muscles of a patient with dysthyroid ophthalmopathy. Orbit 1989;8:45–8.

[7] Rothfus W, Curtin H. Extraocular muscle enlargement: a CT review. Radiology 1984;151: 677–81.

[8] Tucker S, Tucker N, Linberg J. Thyroid orbitopathy. In: Tasman W, Jaeger E, editors. Duane's clinical ophthalmology. Philadelphia: Williams & Wilkins; 2005. Chapter 36.

[9] Kendler D, Lippa J, Rootman J. The initial clinical characteristics of Graves' orbitopathy vary with age and sex. Arch Ophthalmol 1993;111:197–201.

[10] Bartley G, Fatourechi V, Kadrmas E, et al. Chronology of Graves' ophthalmopathy in an incidence cohort. Am J Ophthalmol 1996;121:426–34.

[11] Bartley G, Fatourechi V, Kadrmas E, et al. Clinical features of Graves' ophthalmopathy in an incidence cohort. Am J Ophthalmol 1996;121:284–90.

[12] Prummel M, Wiersinga W, Mourits M, et al. Effect of abnormal thyroid function on the severity of Graves' ophthalmopathy. Arch Intern Med 1990;150:1098–101.

[13] Burch H, Wartofsky L. Graves' ophthalmopathy: current concepts regarding pathogenesis and management. Endocr Rev 1993;14:747–93.

[14] Gorman C. Temporal relationship between onset of Graves' ophthalmopathy and diagnosis of thyroid toxicosis. Mayo Clin Proc 1983;58:515–9.

[15] Garrity J, Fatourechi V, Bergstralh E, et al. Results of transantral orbital decompression in 428 patients with severe Graves' ophthalmopathy. Am J Ophthalmol 1993;116: 533–47.

[16] Haag E, Asplund K. Is endocrine ophthalmopathy related to smoking? Br J Med 1987;295: 634–5.

[17] Bartalena L, Martino E, Marcocci C. More on smoking habits and Graves' ophthalmopathy. J Endocrinol Invest 1989;12:733–7.

[18] Nunery W, Martin R, Hienz G, et al. The association of cigarette smoking with clinical subtypes of ophthalmic Graves' disease. Ophthal Plast Reconstr Surg 1993;9: 77–82.

[19] Mann K. Risk of smoking in thyroid-associated orbitopathy. Exp Clin Endocrinol Diabetes 1999;107:S164–7.

[20] Wiersinga W, Bartalena L. Epidemiology and prevention of Graves' ophthalmopathy. Thyroid 2002;12:855–60.

[21] Eckstein A, Quadbeck B, Mueller G, et al. Impact of smoking on the response to treatment of thyroid associated ophthalmopathy. Br J Ophthalmol 2003;87:773–6.

[22] Chavis P. Thyroid and the eye. Curr Opin Ophthalmol 2002;13:352–6.

[23] Kimball L, Kulinskaya E, Brown B, et al. Does smoking increase relapse rates in Graves' disease? J Endocrinol Invest 2002;25:152–7.

[24] Werner S. Classification of the eye changes of Graves' disease. J Clin Endocrinol Metab 1969;29:982–4.

[25] Werner S. Modification of the classification of the eye changes of Graves' disease. Am J Ophthalmol 1977;83:725–7.

[26] Werner S. Modification of the classification of the eye changes of Graves' disease: recommendations of the Ad Hoc Committee of the American Thyroid Association. J Clin Endocrinol Metab 1977;44:203–4.

[27] Sergott R, Felberg N, Savino P, et al. Graves' ophthalmopathy—immunologic parameters related to corticosteroid therapy. Invest Ophthalmol 1981;20:173–82.

[28] Bartley G. Evolution of classification systems for Graves' ophthalmopathy. Ophthal Plast Reconstr Surg 1995;11:229–37.

[29] Wiersinga W, Prummel M, Mourits M, et al. Classification of the eye changes of Graves' disease. Thyroid 1991;1:357–60.

[30] Gorman C. Clever is not enough: NOSPECS is form in search of function. Thyroid 1991;1: 353–5.

[31] Gorman C. The measurement of change in Graves' ophthalmopathy. Thyroid 1998;8: 539–43.

[32] Frueh B. Why the NOSPECS classification of Graves' eye disease should be abandoned, with suggestions for the characterization of this disease. Thyroid 1992;2:85–8.

[33] Bartley G, Gorman C. Diagnosis criteria for Graves' ophthalmopathy. Am J Ophthalmol 1995;119:792–5.

[34] Mourits M, Prummel M, Wiersinga W, et al. Clinical activity score as a guide in the Management of Patients with Graves' ophthalmopathy. Clin Endocrinol (Oxf) 1997;47: 9–14.

[35] Khalil H, deKeizer R, Kijlstra A. Analysis of tear proteins in Graves' ophthalmopathy by high performance liquid chromatography. Am J Ophthalmol 1988;106:186–90.

[36] Bartley G. The differential diagnosis and classification of eyelid retraction. Ophthalmology 1996;103:168–76.

[37] Frueh B, Musch D, Garber F. Lid retraction and levator aponeurosis defects in Graves' eye disease. Ophthalmic Surg 1986;17(4):216–20.

[38] Frueh B, Garber F, Musch D. The effect of Graves' eye disease on levator muscle function. Ophthalmic Surg 1986;17(3):142–5.

[39] Harvey J, Anderson R. Lid lag and lagophthalmos: a clarification of terminology. Ophthalmic Surg 1981;12(5):338–40.

[40] von Graefe A. Über Basedow'sche Krankheit. Deutsche Klinik 1864;16:158–9.

[41] Grove A. Surgery of the orbit. In: Spaeth G, editor. Ophthalmic surgery: principles and practice. Philadelphia: W.B. Saunders; 1982. p. 439–42.

[42] Frueh B, Musch D, Garber F. Exophthalmometer readings in patients with Graves' eye disease. Ophthalmic Surg 1986;17(1):37–40.

[43] Day R. Ocular manifestations of thyroid disease: current concepts. Trans Am Ophthalmol Soc 1959;57:572–601.

[44] Amino N, Yuasa T, Yabu Y, et al. Exophthalmos in autoimmune thyroid disease. J Clin Endocrinol Metab 1980;51:1232–4.

[45] Migliori M, Gladstone G. Determination of the normal range of exophthalmometric values for black and white adults. Am J Ophthalmol 1984;98:438–42.

[46] He J, Wu Z, Yan J, et al. Clinical analysis of 106 cases with elevated intraocular pressure in thyroid-associated ophthalmopathy. Yan Ke Xue Bao [Eye Science] 2004;20:10–4.

[47] Ohtsuka K. Intraocular pressure and proptosis in 95 patients with Graves Ophthalmopathy. Am J Ophthalmol 1997;124:570–2.

[48] Kalmann R, Mourits M. Prevalence and management of elevated intraocular pressure in patients with Graves' orbitopathy. Br J Ophthalmol 1998;82:754–7.

[49] Danesh-Meyer H, Savino P, Deramo V, et al. Intraocular pressure changes after treatment for Graves' orbitopathy. Ophthalmology 2001;108:145–50.

[50] Cockerham K, Pal C, Jani B, et al. The prevalence and implications of ocular hypertension and glaucoma in thyroid-associated orbitopathy. Ophthalmology 1997;104:914–7.

[51] Neigel J, Rootman J, Belkin R, et al. Dysthyroid optic neuropathy: the crowded orbital apex syndrome. Ophthalmology 1988;95:1515–21.

[52] Trobe J. Optic nerve involvement in dysthyroidism. Ophthalmology 1981;88:488–92.

[53] Anderson R, Tweeten J, Patrinely J, et al. Dysthyroid optic neuropathy without evidence of extraocular muscle involvement. Ophthalmic Surg 1989;20:568–74.

[54] Feldon S, Muramatsu S, Weiner J. Clinical classification of Graves' ophthalmology, identification of risk factors for optic neuropathy. Arch Ophthalmol 1984;102: 1469–72.

[55] Spencer C. Clinical utility and cost-effectiveness of sensitive thyrotropin assays in ambulatory and hospitalized patients. Mayo Clin Proc 1988;63:1214–22.

[56] Toft A. Use of sensitive immunoradiometric assay for thyrotropin in clinical practice. Mayo Clin Proc 1988;63:1035–42.

[57] Gorman C. Thyroid function testing: a new era. Mayo Clin Proc 1988;63:1026.

[58] Shammos H, Minckler D, Ogden C. Ultrasound in early thyroid orbitopathy. Arch Ophthalmol 1980;98:277–9.

[59] Werner S, Coleman D, Franzen L. Ultrasonic evidence of a consistent orbital involvement in Graves' disease. N Engl J Med 1974;290:1447–50.

[60] Polizzi A, Camoriano G, Panarello S, et al. Relationship between extra-ocular muscle echobiometry and tonometry in Graves' disease. Ital J Ophthalmol 1989;3:187.

[61] Feldon S, Weiner J. Clinical significance of extraocular muscle volumes in Graves' ophthalmopathy: a quantitative computed tomography study. Arch Ophthalmol 1982;100: 1266–9.

[62] Feldon S, Lee C, Muramatsu S, et al. Quantitative computed tomography of Graves' ophthalmopathy: extraocular muscle and orbital fat in development of optic neuropathy. Arch Ophthalmol 1985;103:213–5.

[63] Nugent R, Belkin R, Neigel J, et al. Graves' orbitopathy: correlation of computed tomography and clinical findings. Radiology 1990;177:675–82.

[64] Just M, Kahaly G, Higher H, et al. Graves' ophthalmopathy: role of MR imaging in radiation therapy. Radiology 1991;179:187–90.

[65] Patrinely J, Osborn A, Anderson R, et al. Computed tomographic features of nonthyroid extraocular muscle enlargement. Ophthalmology 1989;96:1038–47.

[66] Bartalena L, Pinchera A, Marcocci C. Management of Graves' ophthalmopathy: reality and perspectives. Endocr Rev 2000;21(2):168–99.

[67] Bartley G, Fatourechi V, Kadrmas E, et al. The treatment of graves' orbitopathy in an incidence cohort. Am J Ophthalmol 1996;121:200–6.

[68] Marcocci C, Bartalena L, Tanda M, et al. Graves' ophthalmopathy and I-131 therapy. Q J Nucl Med 1999;43(4):307–12.

[69] Tallstedt L, Lundell G. Radioiodine treatment, ablation, and ophthalmopathy: a balanced perspective. Thyroid 1997;7(2):241–5.

[70] Bartalena L, Marcocci C, Bogazzi F, et al. Use of corticosteroids to prevent progression of Graves' ophthalmopathy after radioiodine therapy for hyperthyroidism. N Engl J Med 1989;321(20):1349–52.

[71] Marcocci C, Bruno-Bossio G, Manetti L, et al. The course of Graves' ophthalmopathy is not infuenced by near total thyroidectomy: a case-control study. Clin Endocrinol (Oxf) 1999;51:503–8.

[72] Char D. Thyroid eye disease. Br J Ophthalmol 1996;80:922–6.

[73] Mills M, Coats D, Donahue S, et al. Strabismus surgery for adults: a report by the American Academy of Ophthalmology. Ophthalmology 2004;111:1255–62.

[74] Morganstern K, Evanchan J, Foster J, et al. Botulinum toxin type A for dysthyroid upper eyelid retraction. Ophthal Plast Reconstr Surg 2004;20(3):181–5.

[75] Shih M, Liao S, Lu H. A single transcutaneous injection with Botox for dysthyroid lid retraction. Eye 2004;18:466–9.

[76] Traisk F, Tallstedt L. Thyroid associated ophthalmopathy: botulinum toxin A in the treatment of upper eyelid retraction–a pilot study. Acta Ophthalmol Scand 2001;79: 585–8.

[77] Uddin J, Davies P. Treatment of upper eyelid retraction associated with thyroid eye disease with subconjunctival botulinum toxin injection. Ophthalmology 2002;109: 1183–7.

[78] Kikkawa D, Cruz R, Christian W, et al. Botulinum A toxin injection for restrictive myopathy of thyroid-related orbitopathy: effects on intraocular pressure. Am J Ophthalmol 2003;135:427–31.

[79] Karadimas P, Bouzas E, Topouzis F, et al. Hypothyroidism and glaucoma: a study of 100 hypothyroid patients. Am J Ophthalmol 2001;131:126–8.

[80] Bartalena L, Marcocci C, Bogazzi F, et al. Glucocorticoid therapy of Graves' ophthalmopathy. Exp Clin Endocrinol 1991;97:320–8.

[81] Smith T. Dexamethasone regulation of glycosaminoglycan synthesis in cultured human fibroblasts: similar effects of glucocorticoid and thyroid hormone therapy. J Clin Invest 1984;64:2157–63.

[82] Smith T, Bahn R, Gorman C. Hormonal regulation of hyaluronate synthesis in cultured fibroblasts; evidence for differences between retroocular and dermal fibroblasts. J Clin Endocrinol Metab 1989;69:1019–23.

[83] Kazim M, Trokel S, Moore S. Treatment of acute Graves orbitopathy. Ophthalmology 1991;98:1443–8.

[84] Wiersinga W, Smit T, Schuster-Uittenhoeve A, et al. Therapeutic outcome of prednisone medication and of orbital irradiation in patients with Graves' ophthalmopathy. Ophthalmologica 1988;197:75–84.

[85] Ohtsuka K, Sato A, Kawaguchi S, et al. Effect of high-dose intravenous steroid pulse therapy followed by 3-month oral steroid therapy for Graves' ophthalmopathy. Jpn J Ophthalmol 2002;46:563–7.

[86] Ohtsuka K, Sato A, Kawaguchi S, et al. Effect of steroid pulse therapy with and without orbital radiotherapy on Graves' ophthalmopathy. Am J Ophthalmol 2003;135:285–90.

[87] Guy J, Fagien S, Donovan J, et al. Methylprednisolone pulse therapy in severe dysthyroid optic neuropathy. Ophthalmology 1989;96:1048–53.

[88] Colao A, Lastoria S, Ferone D, et al. Orbital scintigraphy with (111-In-diethylenetriamine pentaacetic acid-D-Phe-1)-octreotide predicts the clinical response to corticosteroid therapy in patients with Graves' ophthalmopathy. J Clin Endocrinol Metab 1998;83(11):3790–4.

[89] Mori S, Yoshikawa N, Horimoto M, et al. Thyroid stimulating antibody in sera of Graves' ophthalmopathy patients as a possible marker for predicting efficacy of methylprednisolone pulse therapy. Endocr J 1995;42:442–8.

[90] Marcocci C, Bartalena L, Panicucci M, et al. Orbital cobalt irradiation combined with retrobulbar or systemic corticosteroids for Graves' ophthalmopathy: a comparative study. Clin Endocrinol (Oxf) 1987;27:33–42.

[91] Beckendorf V, Maalouf T, George J, et al. Place of radiotherapy in the treatment of Graves' orbitopathy. Int J Radiat Oncol Biol Phys 1999;43(4):805–15.

[92] Lloyd W, Leone C. Supervoltage. Orbital radiotherapy in 36 cases of Graves' disease. Am J Ophthalmol 1992;113:374–80.

[93] Rush S, Winterkorn J, Zak R. Objective evaluation of improvement in optic neuropathy following radiation therapy for thyroid eye disease. Int J Radiat Oncol Biol Phys 2000;47(1):191–4.

[94] Mourits M, van Kempen-Hartveld M, Garcia M, et al. Radiotherapy for Graves' orbitopathy: randomised placebo-controlled study. Lancet 2000;355:1505–9.

[95] Erickson B, Harris G, Lewandowski M, et al. Echographic monitoring of response of extraocular muscles to irradiation in Graves' ophthalmopathy. Int J Radiat Oncol Biol Phys 1995;31(3):651–60.

[96] van Ruyven R, van den Bosch W, Mulder P, et al. The effect of retrobulbar irradiation on exophthalmos, ductions and soft tissue signs in Graves' ophthalmopathy: a retrospective analysis of 90 cases. Eye 2000;14:761–4.

[97] Gorman C, Garrity J, Fatourechi V, et al. Prospective A. Randomized, double-blind, placebo-controlled study of orbital radiotherapy for Graves' ophthalmopathy. Ophthalmology 2001;108:1523–34.

[98] Gorman C. Radiotherapy for Graves' ophthalmopathy: results at one year. Thyroid 2002; 12(3):251–5.

[99] Broerse J, Snijders-Keilholz A, Jansen J, et al. Assessment of a carcinogenic risk for treatment of Graves' ophthalmopathy in dependence on age and irradiation geometry. Radiother Oncol 1999;53:205–8.

[100] Kinyoun J, Kalina R, Brower S, et al. Radiation retinopathy after orbital irradiation for Graves' ophthalmopathy. Arch Ophthalmol 1984;102:1473–6.

[101] Robertson D, Buettner H, Gorman C, et al. Retinal microvascular abnormalities in patients treated with external beam radiation for Graves ophthalmopathy. Arch Ophthalmol 2003; 121:652–7.

[102] Bartalena L, Marcocci C, Pinchera A. Treating severe Graves' ophthalmopathy. Baillieres Clin Endocrinol Metab 1997;11:521–36.

[103] Dollinger J. Die Druckentlastung der Augenhohle durch Entfernung der auberen Orbitaland bei hochgradigem Exophthalmus (Morbus Basedowii) und konsekutiver Hornhauterkrankung. Dtsch Med Wochenschr 1911;37:1888–90.

[104] Goldberg R, Perry J, Hortaleza V, et al. Strabismus after balanced medial plus lateral wall versus lateral wall only orbital decompression for dysthyroid orbitopathy. Ophthal Plast Reconstr Surg 2000;16(4):271–7.

[105] Unal M, Ieri F, Konuk O, et al. Balanced orbital decompression combined with fat removal in Graves ophthalmopathy: do we really need to remove the third wall? Ophthal Plast Reconstr Surg 2003;19(2):112–8.

[106] Cruz A, Leme V. Orbital decompression: a comparison between trans fornix/trans-caruncular inferomedial and coronal inferomedial plus lateral approaches. Ophthal Plast Reconstr Surg 2003;19(6):440–5.

[107] Stewart W, Levin P, Toth B. Orbital surgery: the technique of coronal scalp flap approach to the lateral orbitotomy. Arch Ophthalmol 1988;106(12):1724–6.

[108] Walsh T, Ogura J. Transantral orbital decompression for malignant exophthalmos. Laryngoscope 1957;67:545–68.

[109] Leone C, Piest K, Newman R. Medial and lateral wall decompression for thyroid ophthalmopathy. Am J Ophthalmol 1989;108:160–6.

[110] Shorr N, Baylis H, Goldberg R, et al. Transcaruncular approach to the medial orbit and orbital apex. Ophthalmology 2000;107:1459–63.

[111] Shore J. The fornix approach to the inferior orbit. Adv Ophthal Plast Surg 1987;6: 377–85.

[112] McCord C. Orbital decompression for Graves' disease: exposure through lateral canthal and inferior fornix incision. Ophthalmology 1981;88:533–40.

[113] Graham S, Brown C, Carter K, et al. Medial and lateral orbital wall surgery for balanced decompression in thyroid eye disease. Laryngoscope 2003;113(7):1206–9.

[114] Stiglmayer N, Mladina R, Tomic M, et al. Endonasal endoscopic orbital decompression in patients with Graves' ophthalmopathy. Croat Med J 2004;45(3):318–22.

[115] Ettl A. Die Orbitadekompression bei endokriner Orbitopathie: Indikationen, Techniken, Ergebnisse und Komplikationen. Klin Monatsbl Augenheilkd 2004;221(11):922–6.

[116] Goldberg R, Shorr N, Cohen M. The medial orbital strut in the prevention of postdecompression dystopia in dysthyroid ophthalmopathy. Ophthal Plast Reconstr Surg 1992;8(1):32–4.

[117] Kim J, Goldberg R, Shorr N. The inferomedial orbital strut: an anatomic and radiographic study. Ophthal Plast Reconstr Surg 2002;18(5):355–64.

[118] Adenis J, Robert P, Lasudry J, et al. Treatment of proptosis with fat removal orbital decompression in Graves' ophthalmopathy. Eur J Ophthalmol 1998;8(4):246–52.

[119] Robert P, Camezind P, Adenis J. Techniques de decompression graisseuse. J Fr Ophtalmol 1004:27(7):845–50.

[120] Maillette de Buy Wenniger-Prick L, van Mourik-Noordenbos A, Koornneef L. Squint surgery in patients with Graves' ophthalmopathy. Doc Ophthalmol 1986;61:219–21.

[121] Mourits M, Koornneef L, van Mourik-Noordenbos A, et al. Extraocular muscle surgery for Graves' ophthalmopathy: does prior treatment influence surgical outcome? Br J Ophthalmol 1990;74(8):481–3.

[122] Fichter N, Schittkowski M, Guthoff R. Die Behandlung der Oberlidretraktion bei endokriner Orbitopathie durch die Rucklagerung des Levatorkomplexes. Klin Monatsbl Augenheilkd 2004;221(11):933–40.

[123] Feldman K, Putterman A, Farber M. Surgical treatment of thyroid-related lower eyelid retraction: a modified approach. Ophthal Plast Reconstr Surg 1992;8(4):278–86.

[124] Cohen M, Shorr N. Eyelid reconstruction with hard palate mucosa grafts. Ophthal Plast Reconstr Surg 1992;8(3):183–95.

[125] Karesh J, Fabrega M, Rodrigues M, et al. Polytetrafluoroethylene as an interpositional graft material for the correction of lower eyelid retraction. Ophthalmology 1989;96(4): 419–23.

[126] Tan J, Olver J, Wright M, et al. The use of porous polyethylene (Medpor) lower eyelid spacers in lid heightening and stabilisation. Br J Ophthalmol 2004;88(9):1197–200.

[127] Brock W, Bearden W, Tann T, et al. Autogenous dermis skin grafts in lower eyelid reconstruction. Ophthal Plast Reconstr Surg 2003;19(5):394–7.

[128] Sullivan S, Dailey R. Graft contraction: a comparison of acellular dermis versus hard palate mucosa in lower eyelid surgery. Ophthal Plast Reconstr Surg 2003;19(1):14–24.

[129] Wearne M, Sandy C, Rose G, et al. Autogenous hard palate mucosa: the ideal lower eyelid spacer? Br J Ophthalmol 2001;85(10):1183–7.

ELSEVIER
SAUNDERS

Otolaryngol Clin N Am
38 (2005) 1075–1098

OTOLARYNGOLOGIC
CLINICS
OF NORTH AMERICA

Surgical Management of Essential Blepharospasm

Bhupendra C.K. Patel, MD, FRCS, FRC Ophth

*Division of Facial Plastic Reconstructive and Cosmetic Surgery, John Moran Eye Center,
University of Utah, 50 North Medical Drive, Salt Lake City, UT 84132, USA*

There are few conditions seen by the facial plastic surgeon as disabling as blepharospasm. The anguish and frustration felt by patients suffering from this disease are profound. Although many conditions treated by the facial plastic surgeon are amenable to surgical intervention, blepharospasm is unique in that the majority of patients will not go on to need surgical treatment. To that end, it is important to understand the natural course of the disease and the overall response of patients to medical treatments. Thus one can identify the best candidates for surgical intervention.

Blepharospasm is a progressive involuntary contraction of the entire orbicularis oculi muscles (pretarsal, preseptal, and periorbital) and the procerus, depressor supercilii, and corrugator muscles (Fig. 1). The onset is usually spontaneous with the spasms being bilateral, intermittent, or persistent.

Isolated spasm involving the orbicularis oculi, procerus, depressor supercilii, and corrugator muscles is termed essential blepharospasm. As many as 80% of patients exhibit dystonic movements of other facial, oral, mandibular, or cervical muscles and many patients with essential blepharospasm go on to develop such associated spasms. Appropriate medical and surgical treatment of blepharospasm requires a clear understanding of the clinical features and differential diagnosis of the condition [1–26].

Clinical features

The mean age of onset of benign essential blepharospasm is 56 years. Blepharospasm is seen in 1 in 10,000 patients seeking medical attention;

Supported in part by an unrestricted grant from Research to Prevent Blindness, Inc., New York, to the Department of Ophthalmology, University of Utah.

E-mail address: bhupendra.patel@hsc.utah.edu

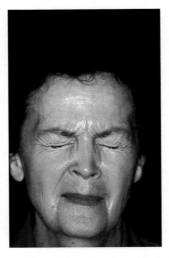

Fig. 1. Essential blepharospasm. Contractions involve orbicularis, procerus, and corrugator muscles. Lower face is uninvolved.

women outnumber men by 3:1. The onset is heralded by variable episodes of increased blinking lasting seconds to minutes. The increased blinking may initially be unilateral or predominantly unilateral and progress to bilateral involvement over time. If the spasm remains unilateral, the patient has hemifacial spasm, although unilateral blepharospasm secondary to a thalamomesencephalic lesion has been described.

The increased blinking gradually progresses to involuntary spasms of eyelid closure causing functional blindness in an estimated 12% of patients. A fluctuating course characterized by remissions and exacerbations is usual. The rate of progression of the disease is extremely variable. It is impossible to predict which patients with orbicularis spasm will progress.

In 1910 Henry Meige, a French neurologist described a condition characterized by blepharospasm and facial, mandibular, oral, lingual, and laryngeal spasms and called it "spasm facial median." Although Meige has been credited with the first description of blepharospasm, Talkow in 1870 described a patient with similar findings, as did Horatio C. Wood in presentations at the University of Pennsylvania in the 1870s. The combination of lower facial movements accompanying eyelid spasms is also referred to as cranial-cervical dystonia or Meige's syndrome (Fig. 2). In individuals with lower facial involvement, several areas may spasm simultaneously.

One of the first documentations of blepharospasm is thought to be in a painting by the Flemish artist Brueghel, who in the sixteenth century painted a woman with apparent blepharospasm with facial and neck involvement. The term "Brueghel's syndrome" is used when extensive mandibular involvement is a major component of the disease. As many as 50% of patients with both blepharospasm and oromandibular involvement also

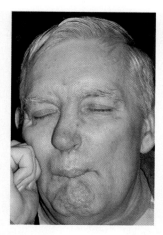

Fig. 2. Meige's syndrome: blepharospasm with lower face involvement. Note pursing of lips.

develop a variety of other dystonias including torticollis, antecollis, trunk spasms, and dystonic posturing of limbs. Multiple other muscle groups may be involved, including those of the respiratory tract, palate, pharynx, neck, abdomen, and trunk. The intensity of the spasms may be variable, and only careful examination may reveal involvement of some groups. All these features may also be seen in Meige's syndrome. Thus blepharospasm, Meige's, and Brueghel's syndrome seem to be a spectrum of facial dystonias, and strict classifications in individual patients can be difficult.

Bright sunlight, stress, fatigue, driving, reading, and many other factors may precipitate blepharospasm. Sleep, relaxation, walking, and talking may improve the spasms. Some patients learn to avoid situations that aggravate the condition; others develop techniques using other muscles innervated by the facial nerve or acts of mental concentration to decrease the frequency and intensity of the spasms. These tricks include humming, singing, whistling, yawning, coughing, mouth opening, nose pinching, chewing gum, eating, talking continuously, rubbing the eyelids or covering one eye, and solving puzzles or problems. A common method of relieving a prolonged episode of spasms is applying pressure on particular parts of the face (Fig. 3).

The protractors (the corrugator, procerus, depressor supercilii, and the orbicularis oculi muscles) are responsible for eyelid closure; the retractors (the levator, Mueller's, and frontalis muscles) open the upper eyelids. The constant contraction of these opposing forces, along with attempts to manually prize the lids open, leads to a number of periocular problems in blepharospasm patients. Stretching of the skin with loosening of its attachment to orbicularis oculi leads to dermatochalasis. Eyebrow ptosis results from weakened fascial support with the brows lying below the superior orbital rims (also known as Charcot's eyebrow sign of blepharospasm). Blepharoptosis occurs secondary to attenuation and disinsertion of

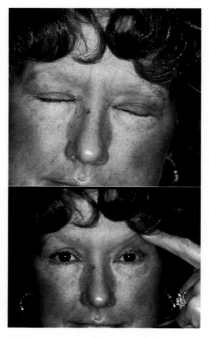

Fig. 3. Some patients with blepharospasm find trigger zones that help relieve an attack of blepharospasm. This woman with essential blepharospasm found pressure on the left forehead helped relieve her blepharospasm.

the levator aponeurosis. The droopy skin, brows, and eyelids can block the patient's superior visual field even when the eyelids are not in spasm, further compounding the patient's functional problems. Stretching of the medial and lateral canthal tendons also occurs secondary to the spasms in orbicularis oculi muscles and may lead to ectropion or entropion of the lower lids as well as phimosis of the lid fissures (Fig. 4).

In advanced stages, patients develop severe eyelid spasms that render them functionally blind, socially reclusive, and unable to work or care for themselves. Some patients have difficulty opening their lids (apraxia of lid opening), further compounding their problems. Involvement of lower facial muscles and other muscle groups may lead to trouble eating with resulting poor nutrition and weight loss. Involuntary vocalizations (such as grunting, frequent throat clearing, or respiratory noises), dysphagia, and respiratory difficulties may also develop.

Differential diagnosis

A thorough ophthalmic and neurologic examination is essential to establish a diagnosis of benign essential blepharospasm. Reflex irritation of

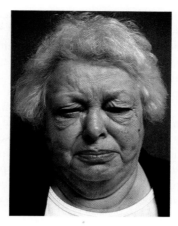

Fig. 4. Long-standing blepharospasm will exacerbate normal aging changes leading to more pronounced brow ptosis, dermatochalasis, lower eyelid laxity, and phimosis of eyelid fissures.

the eyes is the commonest cause of blepharospasm; it may be caused by corneal irritation from keratitis sicca, spastic entropion, eyelash abnormalities, or blepharitis. Patients with ocular pain and photophobia secondary to anterior uveitis or posterior subcapsular cataracts may also demonstrate reflex blepharospasm. Symptoms of dryness of eyes, grittiness, irritation, or photophobia may be seen in more than 50% of patients presenting with blepharospasm, as can demonstrable ocular surface or eyelid pathology.

Hemifacial spasm usually begins with fasciculation of the periocular orbicularis and surrounding muscles and gradually spreads to involve the lower facial muscles innervated by the facial nerve. The spasms are involuntary, aggravated by stress, and usually persist during sleep. There is often underlying facial weakness in hemifacial spasm, whereas normal or increased facial strength is present in blepharospasm.

Blepharospasm is occasionally associated with Parkinson's disease or progressive supranuclear palsy. These patients also have difficulty in opening the eyelids even when they are not in spasm (apraxia of lid opening).

Dopamine stimulators and nasal decongestants containing antihistamines and sympathomimetics have been reported to cause blepharospasm. Meige's syndrome may occur in patients receiving long-term neuroleptic treatment, and this observation supports the role of dopaminergic mechanisms in the origin of Meige's syndrome. Other causes of secondary Meige's syndrome include neurodegenerative disorders and chronic administration of levodopa.

Orbicularis myokymia is characterized by localized fascicular contractions within the orbicularis muscle and is usually unilateral. Temporary orbicularis myokymia is common after physical exertion, caffeine consumption, emotional stress, or fatigue. It is rarely seen with brain stem lesions such as glioma, multiple sclerosis, and Guillain-Barré syndrome.

Habitual spasms or facial tics of variable frequency can resemble blepharospasm.

In hysterical blepharospasm, the spasms are under volitional control and are not improved by rest or worsened by fatigue. This condition is usually seen in younger patients.

Apraxia of eyelid opening is a nonparalytic motor abnormality characterized by difficulty in initiating lid elevation and may occur with or without blepharospasm. Patients with apraxia have a characteristic high-arched brow caused by the contracting frontalis muscle. Some patients with apraxia of eyelid opening do not demonstrate the classic high-arched brow, however (Fig. 5). Many patients with blepharospasm have underlying apraxia of eyelid opening. The author and colleagues have found that as many as 50% of patients with blepharospasm show evidence of apraxia of eyelid opening.

Therapy

Many blepharospasm sufferers have tried numerous modes of therapy, including biofeedback, acupuncture, hypnosis, faith healing, herbal therapies, and relaxation therapy, with limited relief.

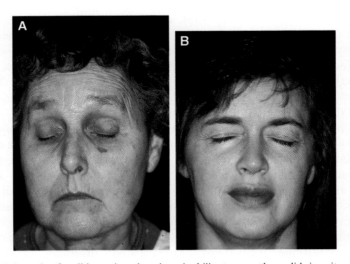

Fig. 5. (*A*) Apraxia of eyelid opening: there is an inability to open the eyelids in spite of marked contraction of frontalis muscle with associated elevation of brows. (*B*) Not all patients with apraxia of eyelid opening demonstrate marked overaction of the frontalis muscle and arched brow. Some patients have difficulty initiating elevation of the upper eyelids and also show mild overt spasm of the orbicularis oculi. Some of these patients may have overaction of the pretarsal orbicularis oculi muscle. This subset of patients is often helped with pretarsal injections of botulinum toxin.

Pharmacotherapy

Several drugs have been reported to ameliorate specific types of blepharospasm, although their efficacy seems to be limited and temporary in most cases. The list includes antipsychotics, affective disorder agents, antianxiety agents, stimulants, sedatives, parasympathomimetics, antimuscarinics, catecholamine synthesis inhibitors, alphamethyl P-tyrosine, antihistamines, and anticonvulsants.

Anti-Parkinsonian drugs have been tried because of an association with Parkinson's disease. Muscle relaxants (baclofen, orphenadrine, diazepam) have been helpful to some extent in the occasional patient. The author and colleagues have found orphenadrine useful for lower facial and neck spasms that continue after myectomy or botulinum toxin injections.

Chemical myectomy

Various attempts have been made to achieve a chemical denervation or myectomy of the orbicularis muscle. In animals, local injection of doxorubicin has the ability to cause atrophy of the orbicularis oculi muscle fibers with sparing of the surrounding tissues. It has been tried with mixed success as a form of chemical myectomy in blepharospasm patients. Research into chemical myectomy continues, but currently few surgeons use this modality for the treatment of blepharospasm.

Botulinum-A toxin

The pioneering work by Scott and co-workers on the use of botulinum toxin for selective weakening of extraocular muscles has led to its establishment as a form of treatment for a diverse range of conditions. Botulinum-A toxin is the best temporary treatment available for the orbicularis spasms seen in blepharospasm and hemifacial spasm. Botulinum-A toxin interferes with acetylcholine release from nerve terminals, resulting in temporary paralysis of the injected muscles. As many as 86% of all blepharospasm patients can be appropriately managed with the use of botulinum toxin alone.

Surgical treatment

Functionally impaired patients with blepharospasm who have not tolerated or responded well to medication or botulinum-A toxin are candidates for surgical intervention.

The aim of surgery is

- To correct or improve the functional and, by inference, the cosmetic changes associated with blepharospasm (brow ptosis, dermatochalasis, ptosis, lash ptosis, canthal dystopia, ectropion, and others)

- To reduce the severity of spasms
- To decrease the dosage of botulinum toxin and increase the interval between treatments
- To improve apraxia of eyelid opening

Patients with marked ptosis, brow ptosis, dermatochalasis, temporal hooding, and lash ptosis may respond to botulinum toxin reasonably well and still be disabled by the underlying changes that are exacerbated in these patients. Such disabling changes can be ascertained by asking the patient to squeeze the eyelids a few days after injection of botulinum toxin; the effects of the botulinum toxin can be gauged by observing the force of the periorbital and eyelid muscles. In such patients, surgical improvement of the underlying changes alone may give the patient relief. When such surgery to improve the structural changes is undertaken, myectomy is usually performed at the same time to improve the response to botulinum toxin.

True failures of botulinum toxin will have significant squeezing of the eyelids and periorbital muscles after the injections. The author and colleagues have found that many so-called failures have the secondary changes described previously or have apraxia of eyelid opening.

Surgical options

Although it is recognized that the source of blepharospasm probably resides in the midbrain, little progress has been made in identifying factors responsible for this disabling condition. Surgical therapeutic efforts have therefore tried to address the nerve carrying the impulses resulting in the overaction of the muscles (facial nerve) or manipulation of the muscles involved (various forms of myectomy).

Peripheral facial neurectomy

Before the myectomy procedure was available, peripheral facial neurectomy was considered the only effective surgical procedure for blepharospasm. Peripheral facial neurectomy involved alcohol injections to produce chemical necrosis of the nerve, surgical sectioning of the nerve, percutaneous thermolysis of the nerve, or, in the surgical technique that was used most frequently, selective peripheral facial nerve avulsion.

Many patients and physicians, however, were dissatisfied with the high recurrence rate and untoward side effects following selective resection of the facial nerve. These side effects included paralytic ectropion, epiphora, lagophthalmos, exacerbation of upper lid dermatochalasis, lip paresis, drooping of the mouth, collection of saliva in the parotid gland necessitating aspiration, and loss of facial expression. Many patients undergoing facial nerve avulsion require secondary procedures to correct eyelid malpositions and lagophthalmos. Grandas et al found a recurrence of symptoms in 22 of 27 patients within a year of bilateral facial nerve avulsions. McCord and associates compared the results of facial nerve avulsion (Reynold's procedure) and myectomy for blepharospasm in two groups of 22 patients each and found that secondary procedures were required 4.5 times more frequently after neurectomy. The patients' subjective response to the surgical results plus their acceptance of the procedure was also higher with myectomy. Researchers at the Mayo clinic in Rochester, Minnesota, and at Moorfields Eye Hospital in England have also concluded that myectomy is superior to neurectomy in treating blepharospasm. Frueh and colleagues found that 82% of blepharospasm patients had satisfactory relief of symptoms after upper and, if necessary, lower myectomy and concluded that myectomy should be the preferred technique. They also found that patients with essential blepharospasm are just as likely to respond adequately to surgery as patients with associated lower facial muscle involvement (Meige's syndrome). Facial neurectomy aggravates all the preexisting anatomic, functional, and cosmetic eyelid deformities in patients with blepharospasm (brow ptosis, dermatochalasis, lateral canthal tendon laxity, and blepharoptosis). Thus most surgeons have abandoned neurectomy in favor of myectomy. Differential section of the seventh nerve should not be completely discarded, however. Surgeons with a meticulous approach to surgical dissection, careful follow-up, and careful attention to selective neurectomy claim a high level of satisfaction with this approach (Robert Small, personal communication, 2002). Also, a recent review by Fante and Frueh showed that although 85% of patients with blepharospasm could be controlled with botulinum toxin injections alone, and 97% of patients were helped by botulinum toxin with protractor myectomy, an additional 2% of patients could be helped with the addition of one or two differential sections of the facial nerve. Therefore, as an adjunct in refractive cases, differential sectioning of the facial nerve may still be a reasonable option.

Myectomy

Myectomy refers to resection of the protractor muscles; it may include some or all of these muscles and also may include some nasal muscles (Fig. 6). The first description of a limited resection of the orbicularis oculi muscle to treat blepharospasm appeared in 1925. Other isolated reports followed. In 1951, Fox reported a case of postencephalitic blepharospasm caused by Parkinson's disease. He treated it with resection of the orbicularis of both upper and lower lids, leaving the pretarsal fibers intact. Five years after the surgery, the patient had some return of the blepharospasm but was independent and employed. Fox noted that this technique was not as effective in the treatment of essential blepharospasm. He later recommended resection of both the upper and lower orbicularis oculi muscle, sparing the pretarsal fibers, and he used a frontalis sling at the same time to allow opening of the lids. This technique had limited success, possibly because of the pretarsal muscle sparing.

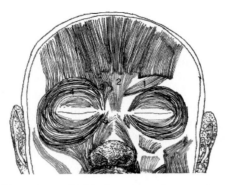

Fig. 6. Muscles treated in patients with blepharospasm. 1, corrugator; 2, procerus muscle; 3, depressor supercilii; 4, orbicularis oculi; 5, levator labii superioris and nasalis.

Limited resection of orbicularis oculi from the upper and lower lids was performed by enthusiasts in the following three decades. In 1981, Gillum and Anderson modified the Fox procedure with the complete removal of the orbicularis oculi, corrugator, superciliaris, and procerus muscles as well as the orbicularis muscle in the extended temporal raphe region. Some surgeons refer to this technique as a neuromyectomy, because the peripheral facial nerve branches that traverse the muscle are also removed.

The original description by Gillum and Anderson advocated upper and lower myectomy with a suprabrow incision. This procedure led to considerable morbidity with lymphedema and unpredictable positions of upper and lower eyelids. Patients were patched with a firm dressing for 3 to 4 days. Subsequently, Gillum and Anderson advocated performing surgery on one side at a time separated by 2 to 3 weeks. This approach still led to numerous problems, and the results were not entirely predictable or symmetrical. Complications included complete loss of sensation in the distribution of the supraorbital and supratrochlear nerves, loss of brow hairs, and unacceptable brow scars. More recently, only upper myectomy was advocated to prevent the variable and sometimes significant degree of lymphedema that patients developed. Lower myectomy was proposed for patients who continued to have significant lower eyelid and midfacial squeezing after upper myectomy and was delayed by several months.

Although some very reasonable functional and cosmetic results were obtained, some patients were concerned by the appearance of suprabrow scars and by variable lid scars, depressions, lagophthalmos, and a skeletonized look (Fig. 7).

Transfer of excised muscle as free grafts into the areas of muscle resection to prevent postoperative depressions has shown good results. Problems with the suprabrow incisions and sacrifice of the supraorbital and supratrochlear nerves and vessels remain when the full myectomy approach is used, however. The author and colleagues have applied advances in endoscopic

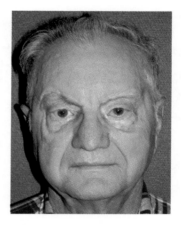

Fig. 7. A patient who presented for management of effects of a previous full myectomy through a suprabrow incision. He had had a lower myectomy several years previously. The patient has marked brow scars, lower lid retraction, lagophthalmos, corneal exposure keratopathy, chronic chemosis, and depressions over the areas of myectomy.

surgery to perform a full myectomy with acceptable aesthetic and functional results.

Full upper myectomy: endoscopic and upper eyelid approach

In patients with the full constellation of signs associated with severe blepharospasm and secondary periorbital changes, the author and colleagues advocate upper myectomy as the initial procedure. They have developed a myectomy that reduces many of the problems seen with the original full myectomy using suprabrow incisions.

The extent of brow ptosis is assessed with the patient sitting up in the usual way. The corrugator and procerus muscles, which may overact significantly in patients with blepharospasm, are assessed, and any depressions in the glabellar area are marked. The forehead is marked as in a standard endoscopic brow lift, with marking of the temporal arcuate line, the corrugator and procerus muscles, the supraorbital notches, and the zygomatic arch and lateral orbital rim. Unlike a standard endoscopic brow lift, in this approach the dissection is extended to below the zygomatic arch, and the release of the superior orbital rim periosteum is extended down to the lateral orbital rim (Fig. 8). This technique allows appropriate elevation of the tail of the brow, which needs to be more aggressive than in a standard brow lift. The excessive contracture of the orbicularis oculi muscle also causes deep temporal rhytids in the crow's feet.

The author and colleagues use two paracentral and two temporal incisions in the brow lift and corrugator and procerus myectomy. The dissection planes are as in a standard endoscopic brow lift: subperiosteal in

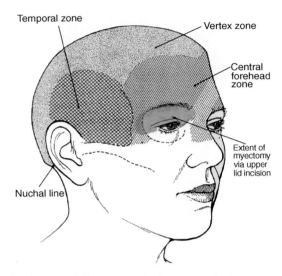

Fig. 8. The central and temporal dissections differ from a standard endoscopic brow lift in that the dissection is carried centrally much further down the nasal bone, and the temporal dissection extends lower down the lateral orbital rim and onto the zygomatic arch. This technique allows correction of the nasal "champion pucker" often seen in patients with blepharospasm and also allows correction of the marked temporal brow and eyelid changes seen.

the zone between the two arcuate lines and deep to the superficial temporal fascia in lateral to the arcuate lines. Endoscopic front-biting forceps, scissors, and cautery are used to avulse and weaken the procerus and corrugator muscles. The supraorbital neurovascular bundles are preserved in the endoscopic dissection. The periosteum is released from one lateral orbital rim to the other across the forehead. Over the supraorbital and supratrochlear neurovascular bundles, a spreading motion is used to separate the periosteum without injuring the neurovascular structures. The author and colleagues have found that dissecting the periosteum off the nasal bridge, with the dissection carried all the way down the nasal bone, gives a much better improvement in the marked horizontal nasal rhytids (the "champion pucker") often seen in patients with blepharospasm (Fig. 9).

Once the dissection is medial to the supraorbital neurovascular bundle, the insertion of the corrugator, depressor supercilii, and the procerus muscle may be weakened by using long Mayo scissors in a crosshatch manner. Some of the supratrochlear nerves may be sacrificed in this maneuver. The author and colleagues have not found long-term anesthesia to be a problem using this technique. The corrugator, depressor supercilii, and procerus muscles are weakened aggressively using any modality with which the surgeon is comfortable. Local excision, avulsion, cauterization, and laser all work well. The author and colleagues insert soft tissue (temporalis fascia or

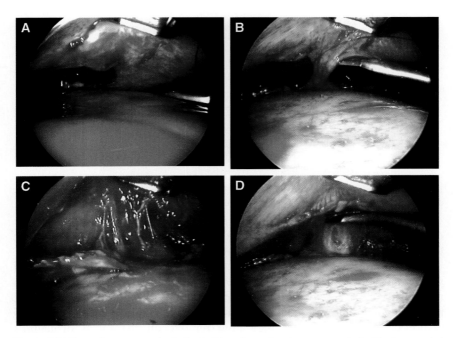

Fig. 9. (*A*) The periosteum can be incised with a sharp elevator or separated with sharp-ended scissors. In patients with blepharospasm, this dissection and release are performed aggressively. (*B*) A rotational motion of the endoscopic elevator tears the periosteum without injuring the surrounding nerves and vessels. (*C*) The supraorbital neurovascular bundle can be safely separated from the surrounding corrugator muscle, which is then weakened with avulsion, cauterization, or a combination of the two. (*D*) Dissection of the procerus muscle and skin off the nasal bridge all the way down the nasal bone allows correction of horizontal rhytids as well as nasal skin ptosis.

orbicularis oculi muscle) into the glabellar region to prevent a depression and to prevent the glabellar area from scarring down to the periosteum (Fig. 10).

Excess upper eyelid skin is marked before surgery, but care is taken to avoid being overly aggressive with this resection, because the brow elevation and the corrugator and procerus muscle weakening is more aggressive than with a cosmetic brow lift. Before the brow is fixated, the upper eyelid incisions are made, and the upper eyelid tissue is resected. The author and colleagues remove skin and orbicularis muscle within the confines of the marked excess in the upper eyelids. Thereafter, skin hooks are placed at the upper border of the incision. A Paufique forceps and a Stevens scissors are used to develop a dissection plane between skin and muscle. Skin necrosis and injury are avoided if the small subcutaneous vessels are not cauterized and the assistant properly manipulates the skin hooks to allow observation of both the surgical plane and the scissors' blades through the thin overlying skin. Visualization of all dissection planes through the incision is further enhanced with a fiberoptic headlight. Particular care is taken to resect as much of the orbital

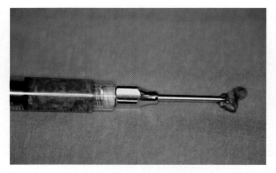

Fig. 10. Temporalis fascia, resected muscle, and fat are used with a 12-gauge needle to fill in any depressions that may form during myectomy surgery.

orbicularis oculi as possible, especially in the superomedial quadrant where there is overlap of the corrugator, depressor supercilii, and procerus muscles.

The author and colleagues used to leave a small (2–3 mm) strip of pretarsal orbicularis muscle around the margin of the eyelid to help maintain voluntary closure. They have noted, however, that it is almost impossible to remove too much orbicularis oculi muscle in patients with severe blepharospasm, and they now remove all the tarsal orbicularis possible through the lid crease incision. The dissection is carried almost to the lid margin but stops short of the hair roots.

The forehead is then elevated and fixated. The author and colleagues use bone tunnels and a 2-0 Surgidek suture to give a permanent elevation without the use of screws that have to be removed. Any method of fixation that the surgeon prefers may be used, including buried screws, absorbable screws, and the Endotine forehead fixation device (Coapt Systems Inc., Palo Alto, CA). The temporal brow lift is performed aggressively and with a proper release of the periosteum down the lateral orbital rim. Patients with blepharospasm have marked droop of the tail of the brow with secondary crow's feet and lateral tissue redundancy. Therefore the dissection in this temporal region and over the lateral orbital rim must be aggressive.

Patients with severe ptosis have a levator advancement, although in most patients it is necessary only to reapproximate the levator to the tarsus. The eyelid crease incision facilitates removal of the eyelid margin orbicularis and aponeurotic fixation and helps form a good crease. It also avoids wrinkling of the pretarsal skin and improves eyelash position.

Before closure, bleeding points and vessels in spasm are meticulously cauterized with a bipolar unit to prevent hematoma formation. When done endoscopically and with adequate hemostasis, suction drains are rarely necessary. A firm forehead turban dressing is applied, and ice is used on the eyelids. Three to 4 days of systemic steroids also seems to decrease swelling. Hematomas should be treated with suture removal, expression of the clots, and cauterization of residual bleeding points. Patients are instructed to use artificial tears and nightly ointment for several weeks to prevent exposure keratopathy secondary to lagophthalmos. Complete healing occurs between 3 months and 1 year after surgery (Figs. 11, 12).

Alternative full upper myectomy

The author and colleagues are not proponents of the alternative full upper myectomy, but it has been described in the literature and warrants discussion. In patients without a significant degree of brow ptosis, the upper myectomy may be performed using an upper eyelid skin crease incision; with a medial upper eyelid crease incision, the corrugator superciliaris and the procerus muscles may be removed (Fig. 13). The efficiency of this approach may be limited in patients with prominent glabellar regions, because the approach using incisions in the upper eyelid skin crease may be difficult. Also, weakening of the muscles is achieved blindly when using this approach; therefore the surgeon may find it difficult to weaken the muscles effectively. Although this approach may give a moderate lift to the medial brow, substantial brow ptosis cannot be addressed. The author and colleagues have not been impressed with the longevity of the internal brow lift in cosmetic patients or in patients with blepharospasm. Similarly, sculpting the temporal brow fat may improve brow position moderately, but the results are not impressive. The author and colleagues have observed that most patients have deflation of facial fat, including the brow fat pad, necessitating repositioning, not removal, of the fat.

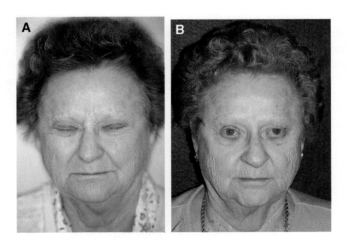

Fig. 11. (*A*) Patient with marked blepharospasm, brow ptosis, dermatochalasis, and ptosis. (*B*) Three years after an endoscopic myectomy and upper myectomy with tissue-transfer technique: note absence of depressions and scars, good position of the upper lid, absence of chemosis. Lower myectomy was not done. Patient still receives botulinum toxin but needs a smaller and less frequent dose. This patient still gets apraxia of eyelid opening, which is generally not helped by the myectomy technique.

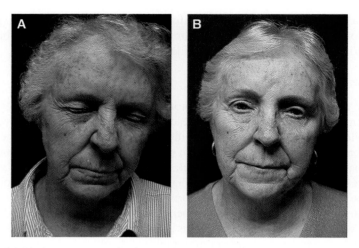

Fig. 12. (*A*) Blepharospasm, ptosis, dermatochalasis, and apraxia of eyelid opening. (*B*) Two years after endoscopic myectomy with brow lift, upper myectomy, and levator advancement. Patient still has apraxia of eyelid opening and needs botulinum toxin.

Limited upper myectomy

Indications

Many patients with good response to botulinum-A toxin have secondary functional and cosmetic soft tissue changes of brow ptosis, upper dermatochalasis, ptosis, and lash ptosis. In the absence of a marked brow ptosis, the author and colleagues undertake what they term a "limited myectomy." This procedure is ideally suited to patients with a good or decreasing response to botulinum-A toxin who desire correction of dermatochalasis and ptosis and are willing to continue receiving botulinum-A toxin injections after surgery. Many of the younger patients with blepharospasm who get an insufficient response to botulinum toxin do well with the limited myectomy.

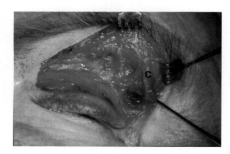

Fig. 13. The corrugator muscle (C) may be approached through the incision in the upper eyelid skin crease and weakened. In the author and colleague's experience, the efficiency of this approach is less than ideal.

Technique

The preseptal and orbital orbicularis are excised through a skin crease approach together with a blepharoplasty to correct dermatochalasis and levator aponeurosis repair to correct ptosis (Fig. 14). The myectomy includes excision of the lateral raphe. The author and colleagues have found that extending the excision of the orbicularis oculi to the lateral raphe to include the muscle above and below the lateral canthal angle gives some degree of weakening of the lower orbicularis oculi. This approach does not generally require support of the lateral lower eyelid with a lateral canthoplasty and does not lead to a lower eyelid ectropion.

A partial weakening of the procerus and corrugator muscles may be achieved by dissecting medially from the medial extent of the upper eyelid incision onto the nasal bridge and in the glabellar area. Adequate lighting and retraction are necessary. Even so, this dissection can be extremely bloody and, in the author's experience, does not achieve complete weakening of the

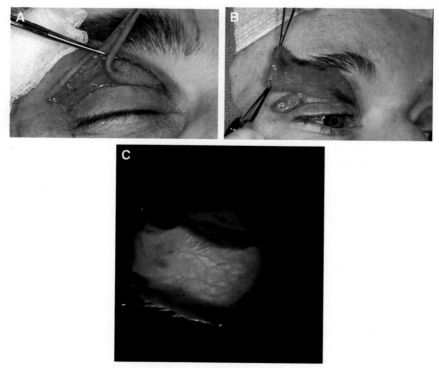

Fig. 14. (*A–C*) The skin is separated from the orbicularis oculi muscle by a meticulous dissection. Separation of the muscle from the overlying skin is aided by the use of transillumination to protect the skin and the dermal vessels. The orbicularis oculi muscle is removed in one or more pieces. The best way to separate the muscle from the overlying skin is to use a combined blunt separation and cutting motion.

corrugator and procerus muscles. There is also a significant risk of injury to branches of the supraorbital and supratrochlear nerves and vessels. The author and colleagues generally attempt to achieve whatever weakness is possible. In men with prominent supraorbital rims and glabellar regions, access through these incisions is difficult.

The author and colleagues have noted that the amount of botulinum-A toxin required is usually reduced after a limited myectomy. The patient must not expect to be completely free from botulinum-A toxin, however, and some patients eventually require a full myectomy, especially if the procerus and corrugator muscle components become more substantial. The limited myectomy requires only slightly more healing time than a standard cosmetic or reconstructive eyelid operation. When appropriate patients are chosen for a limited myectomy, the functional and cosmetic outcome is gratifying (Fig. 15).

Lower myectomy

A lower blepharoplasty incision is used for a lower myectomy. When aggressive pretarsal, septal, and orbital orbicularis oculi muscle resections were performed, complications of lower lid retraction, ectropion, and lagophthalmos were common, particularly because almost all patients undergoing lower myectomy also had had upper myectomies. Therefore the author and colleagues now resect the preseptal orbicularis and the orbital orbicularis (Fig. 16) and weaken the levator labii superioris, which is responsible for the rabbit sign seen in blepharospasm (Fig. 17). This

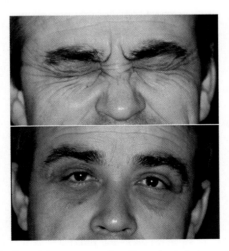

Fig. 15. This patient had partial response to botulinum toxin but was incapacitated by severe blepharospasms as soon as the effect of the toxin started to wear off, as early as 4 weeks after injections. He responded well to a limited myectomy; subsequent botulinum toxin injections gave him longer relief.

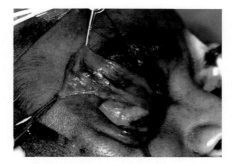

Fig. 16. Excision of the preseptal and orbital lower eyelid orbicularis oculi muscle.

squeezing of the levator labii superioris can be a source of considerable discomfort to the patient and is frequently missed when injecting botulinum toxin. Hemostasis is best achieved if a plane is developed between the orbicularis and skin. An en bloc excision is performed down to the inferior orbital rim using a technique similar to that described for upper myectomy. The skin is elevated gently with skin hooks, and the muscle is excised with the help of retroillumination. The orbital septum is left intact. The author and colleagues never remove orbital fat during upper or lower myectomies. A tarsal tuck procedure is performed to tighten the lateral canthus and lower lid and to help avoid or correct ectropion, entropion, or phimosis. With good surgical technique and proper hemostasis, a drain is rarely required after lower myectomy, and the dressings may be removed in a day or two.

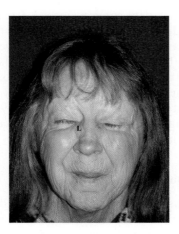

Fig. 17. Overaction of the levator labii superioris and, to some degree, the nasalis muscles produces the "rabbit sign" in some patients with blepharospasm; this condition can cause considerable disability.

Results

The healing process after full myectomy may take several months. In most cases, patients are able to keep their eyes open immediately after the operation. Considerable swelling, lymphedema, and ecchymosis—varying greatly from patient to patient—may be present early in the postoperative period. The number of patients requiring lower myectomy after upper myectomy is variable. Studies have shown that between 20% and 35% of patients later require a lower myectomy.

In the author and colleagues' experience, myectomy has improved visual disability in more than 90% of cases of blepharospasm. As is true with all forms of therapy, results are best in isolated blepharospasm. In Meige's and Brueghel's syndromes, myectomy provides a great deal of relief visually, but the patient is often disabled by persistent lower facial spasms.

In most cases of blepharospasm, secondary functional and cosmetic improvement in brow ptosis, blepharoptosis, dermatochalasis, canthal tendon laxity, and lower eyelid deformities is achieved after complete postoperative healing. Although, when healing is complete, there is frequently a cosmetic improvement over the preoperative appearance, myectomy should not be considered or indicated as a cosmetic procedure. Even when tissue-transfer techniques, as discussed previously, are used, the outcome of myectomy procedures do not meet cosmetic requirements in most patients.

Use of botulinum toxin after myectomy

Statistics concerning the number of patients who are completely free of the need for botulinum toxin are difficult to come by. Anecdotal remarks claiming complete cure of most patients, with no further use of botulinum toxin, should be regarded with caution. Indeed, Chapman et al found that all of their patients undergoing myectomy after 1990 (when botulinum toxin became commercially available) needed postoperative botulinum toxin. The author and colleagues have found that most patients need a lower dose of botulinum toxin, and the interval between treatments is usually longer after myectomy. When results are assessed over years rather than months, however, it is apparent that some patients, especially those with apraxia of eyelid opening, continue to be disabled by the disease. Most continue to need botulinum toxin in varying doses.

Apraxia of eyelid opening

Many cases of blepharospasm have apraxia of eyelid opening as well, and this condition is more difficult to manage. Some patients have a combination of marked blepharospasm as well as apraxia of eyelid opening. In others, the apraxia is the predominant feature. Even when the eyelid spasms have been appropriately treated with botulinum toxin or with myectomy, the apraxia of eyelid opening persists. Patients close their eyelids and use their brows and other facial muscles in an attempt to elevate their eyelids. Whereas in patients with true ptosis with very poor levator function, brow elevation succeeds in elevating the upper eyelids to some extent, the effort in patients with apraxia is less successful. Patient frequently have trigger points, usually somewhere on the face, that they use to initiate opening of the eyelids. When patients are able to open their eyes, the lids remain open with effort, only to descend without warning and to the obvious consternation of the patient.

Many patients with apraxia of eyelid opening have a levator-disinsertion type of ptosis. The use of myectomy and levator advancement is helpful in patients with apraxia of eyelid opening. The myectomy weakens the antagonist to the levator muscle, and the levator advancement puts the lid to its maximal mechanical advantage.

The use of frontalis slings is sometimes indicated in patients with apraxia of eyelid opening. The author and colleagues generally reserve these measures for patients who have already had a myectomy and levator advancement. Also, many patients with apraxia of eyelid opening do not use their brows efficiently, so the use of a sling is not particularly useful. Close observation of the patient, sometimes over an extended period, is necessary before appropriate surgical decisions can be made. The author and colleagues have found that, with appropriate use of myectomy, levator advancement, and postoperative use of botulinum toxin in the pretarsal residual orbicularis, most patients with apraxia of eyelid opening can be helped. A very small number of patients are candidates for a frontalis sling.

Complications

All patients experience ecchymosis of the periorbital region. Skin necrosis has been described in the literature, but the author and colleagues have not encountered that problem. Postoperative hematomas should be drained immediately to avoid necrosis of overlying tissues, secondary infection, and optic nerve damage. Supraorbital nerve damage was much more common when suprabrow incisions were used. After an endoscopic approach, hypoesthesia or anesthesia may be noted postoperatively for a number of weeks but usually resolves within a few months. Patients often describe itching and pins-and-needles sensations for a number of months after surgery.

Exposure keratitis may be an early problem, but no permanent visual loss has occurred in the author and colleagues' patients. Artificial tears and ocular lubricants are used in the early postoperative period. Less common complications include chronic lymphedema, which may last up to a year. This problem was more frequent when simultaneous upper and lower myectomies were performed. Chronic lymphedema in the lower lids increases the risk of retraction or ectropion. Partial loss of brow hairs was often seen with the direct brow incisions but is rare with the endoscopic approach. Blepharoptosis secondary to inadvertent levator aponeurotic disinsertions can occur. Ectropion and lower eyelid retraction are potential complications of lower eyelid surgery, but the frequency of these conditions has been greatly reduced by the simultaneous use of the tarsal tuck procedure and sparing of the lower eyelid pretarsal orbicularis oculi. Although regeneration of the nerves and recurrence of blepharospasm are common after facial neurectomies, muscles do not regenerate after myectomy. Patients often experience residual eyelid twitching and some degree of blepharospasm, necessitating the continued use of botulinum toxin at a lower dose and less frequently than previously. Postoperative lower facial spasms, which are not corrected with these procedures, may respond to orphenadrine citrate or other antispasmodics.

Cosmetic concerns should not be overlooked in these patients. Even the most effective complete myectomy leaves some scarring, and this scarring sometimes becomes more obvious with the passage of time because of secondary involutional changes that occur. The brow scars, even with meticulous closure with wound eversion, are never ideal; therefore, the endoscopic approach is eminently preferable. Use of the resected tissues to augment the depressions that otherwise form with aggressive myectomy is a useful addition to this procedure. The rate of long-term recurrence of blepharospasm after such muscle transfer remains to be determined, however.

Only a small number of patients have required touch-up operations to remove muscle that was missed at the initial surgery. In the author and colleagues' experience, low doses of botulinum-A toxin are usually required in these patients. After myectomy, patients often experience more discomfort during injections. The author and colleagues frequently apply topical anesthetic cream 45 minutes before injecting these patients. Most patients with Meige's syndrome who did not have lower eyelid myectomy initially have required this operation later to relieve the continual spasms involving the lower eyelid or require botulinum toxin injections in the lower eyelids. Some patients with Meige's syndrome and most patients with essential blepharospasm are functionally rehabilitated without the lower eyelid portion of the operation.

Because blepharospasm disorders are progressive, lower facial involvement may worsen after myectomy or any other therapy. Most patients, however, have obtained good, permanent improvement in their visual disabilities caused by blepharospasm, Meige's syndrome, or hemifacial spasm, and some have even obtained considerable relief from lower facial and neck spasms after myectomy.

Summary

At present there is no cure for blepharospasm and related dystonias. Systemic medications help some patients. Debilitating blepharospasm continues in most cases, however, rendering many of these patients functionally blind. Botulinum-A toxin is the best temporary therapy and is successful in keeping 86% of patients reasonably well controlled. For the remaining patients, myectomy is currently the best long-term therapy. In patients who do not respond appropriately to botulinum toxin or myectomy (2% of all blepharospasm patients), a selective neurectomy has been found to be helpful.

An inherent disadvantage of all available treatments is that they address end organs and not the source of this disease. It is hoped that the future will bring a better understanding of the etiology and pathophysiology of blepharospasm and the other facial dystonias, so that management can be directed toward the cause and prevention of the disease rather than treatment of the side effects of these debilitating diseases.

References

[1] Jankovic J. Clinical features, differential diagnosis and pathogenesis of blepharospasm and cranio-cervical dystonia. In: Bosniak SG, Smith BC, editors. Advances in ophthalmic plastic and reconstructive surgery–blepharospasm. New York: Pergamon Press; 1985. p. 67–93.

[2] Marsden CD. Blepharspasm: oromandibular dystonia syndrome (Brueghel's syndrome). A variant of adult-onset torsion dystonia. J Neurol Neurosurg Psychiatry 1976;39:1204–9.

[3] Meige H. Les convulsion de la face une form clinique de convulsion faciale, bilaterale et mediane. Rev Neurol 1970;10:437–43.

[4] Talkow J. Klonische Krampfe der Angelinder: Neurotomie der supraorbitalnerven. Klin Montasbl Augenheilkd 1870;8:129–45.

[5] Tolosa ES. Clinical features of Meige's disease (idiopathic orofacial dystonia). Arch Neurol 1981;38:147–51.

[6] Bird AC, McDonald WI. Essential blepharospasm. Trans Ophthalmol Soc U K 1975;95: 250–3.

[7] Lepore FE. So-called apraxias of lid movement. Adv Neurol 1988;49:85–90.

[8] Tolosa E, Marti MJ. Blepharospasm-oromandibular dystonia syndrome (Meige's syndrome): clinical aspects. Adv Neurol 1988;49:73–84.

[9] Elston JS. A new variant of blepharospasm. J Neurol Neurosurg Psychiatry 1992;55(5): 369–71.

[10] Baker L, Wirtschafter JD. Experimental doxorubicin myopathy. A permanent treatment for eyelid spasms? Arch Ophthalmol 1987;105:1265–8.

[11] McLoon LK, Bauer G, Wirtschafter J. Quantification of muscle loss in the doxorubicin-treated orbicularis oculi of the monkey. Effect of local injection of doxorubicin into the eyelid. Invest Ophthalmol Vis Sci 1991;32(5):1667–73.

[12] Patel BCK, Anderson RL. Blepharospasm. ophthalmic practice 1993;11:293–302, 312.

[13] Gillum WN, Anderson RL. Blepharospasm surgery: anatomic approach. Arch Ophthalmol 1981;99:1056–62.

[14] Jones TW, Waller RR, Samples JR. Myectomy for essential blepharospasm. Mayo Clin Proc 1985;60:663–6.

[15] McCord CD, Coles WH, Shore JW, et al. Treatment of essential blepharospasm. I. Comparision of facial nerve avulsion and eyebrow-eyelid muscle stripping procedure. Arch Ophthalmol 1984;102:266–8.

[16] Bates AK, Halliday BL, Bailey CS, et al. Surgical management of essential blepharospasm. Br J Ophthalmol 1991;75:487–90.

[17] Frueh BR, Callahan A, Dortzbach RK, et al. The effects of differential section of the VII nerve on patients with intractable blepharospasm. Trans Am Acad Ophthalmol 1976;81: 595–602.

[18] Grandas F, Elston J, Quinn N, et al. Blepharospasm: a review of 264 patients. J Neurol Neurosurg Psychiatry 1988;51(6):767–72.

[19] Frueh BR, Musch DC, Bersan TA. Effects of eyelid protractor excision for the treatment of benign essential blepharospasm. Am J Ophthalmol 1992;113(6):681–6.

[20] Patel BCK. Endoscopic brow lifts: pearls and nuances. Review of Ophthalmology 1998; 5(12):70–3.

[21] Yen MT, Anderson RL. Orbicularis oculi muscle graft augmentation after protractor myectomy in blepharospasm. Ophthal Plast Reconstr Surg 2003;19(4):287–96.

[22] Fante RG, Frueh BR. Differential section of the seventh nerve as a tertiary procedure for the treatment of benign essential blepharospasm. Ophthal Plast Reconstr Surg 2001;17:276–80.

[23] Chapman KL, Bartley GB, Waller RR, et al. Follow-up of patients with essential blepharospasm who underwent eyelid protractor myectomy at the Mayo Clinic from 1980 through 1995. Ophthal Plast Reconstr Surg 1999;15:106–10.

[24] Frueh BR, Musch DC, Bersane TA. Effects of eyelid protractor excision for the treatment of benign essential blepharospasm. Am J Ophthalmol 1992;113:681–6.

[25] Gurdjian ES, Williams HW. The surgical treatment of intractable cases of blepharospasm. JAMA 1928;91:2053–6.

[26] Frazier CH. The surgical treatment of blepharospasm. Ann Surg 1931;93:1121–8.

ELSEVIER
SAUNDERS

Otolaryngol Clin N Am
38 (2005) 1099–1107

OTOLARYNGOLOGIC
CLINICS
OF NORTH AMERICA

Endoscopic Lacrimal Surgery

Eric B. Baylin, MD[a,b,]*,
Geoffrey J. Gladstone, MD, FAACS[a,b,c,d]

[a]*Department of Ophthalmology, William Beaumont Hospital, 3535 West Thirteen Mile Road,
Royal Oak, MI 48073, USA*
[b]*Consultants in Ophthalmic and Facial Plastic Surgery, PC, 29201 Telegraph #305,
Southfield, MI 48034, USA*
[c]*Department of Ophthalmology, Michigan State University School of Medicine,
A217 Clinical Center, East Lansing, MI 48824, USA*
[d]*Departments of Ophthalmology and Otolaryngology, Wayne State University School of
Medicine, 4717 St. Antoine Boulevard, Detroit, MI 48201, USA*

Preoperative evaluation

Modern endoscopic lacrimal surgery provides excellent views and access to lacrimal structures, affording successful resolution of epiphora for many patients. The approach to a tearing patient, however, begins with awareness of the multitude of possible causes. Although lacrimal drainage system obstructions incite selected cases of epiphora, other causes may be seen with the same or greater frequency. Causes of tearing can occur in isolation or in concert, and a careful history and clinical evaluation of these factors should focus treatment appropriately.

Any ocular irritant can cause reflex tearing. Dry eyes are one of the most common causes, which may be as simple as aqueous insufficiency. Poor tear quality resulting from abnormal mucus or oil components of tears can cause subnormal aqueous adherence or rapid evaporation, however. Slit-lamp examination with and without fluorescein staining reveals the extent of corneal surface decompensation. Measurements of basal tear secretion and tear breakup time provide semiquantitative data as well.

Malposition of the eyelids can also contribute to epiphora. A retracted or ectropic eyelid increases ocular exposure and tear evaporation. Ectropion often leads to punctual eversion with significant epiphora. An entropic eyelid with or without trichiasis mechanically irritates the eye, resulting in reflex tears. Take note of the eyelid margin for signs of meibomian gland

* Corresponding author.
E-mail address: lebaylin@comcast.net (E.B. Baylin).

0030-6665/05/$ - see front matter © 2005 Elsevier Inc. All rights reserved.
doi:10.1016/j.otc.2005.05.004

inspissation, inflammation, and scarring. Always examine the conjunctival cul-de-sac for signs of inflammatory or infectious conditions and the presence of symblepharon.

Tear drainage does not merely depend passively on gravity. A well-described lacrimal pump mechanism relies on eyelid structural integrity. Horizontal eyelid laxity, seen with involutional eyelid changes or with facial nerve paresis, impairs pump function. Facial nerve palsy can also lead to incomplete blink excursion and lagophthalmos, which are potential causes of reflex tearing. A clue to less obvious or partially healed facial paralysis is the absence of medial movement of the lower eyelid punctum during a blink phase.

Once this survey is complete, attention can be turned to the lacrimal apparatus. For ease of understanding, the lacrimal system can be anatomically separated into upper and lower divisions. The upper division begins at the punctum and continues through the canaliculi until reaching the lacrimal sac. The lacrimal sac and nasolacrimal duct comprise the lower or distal portion. Beginning proximally, the punctum, by virtue of stenosis or eversion, can cause epiphora. These issues are simply addressed by puncto-plasty or eyelid repositioning, respectively. Endoscopic lacrimal surgery treats obstructions distal to the punctum.

Some external clues can guide diagnosis. For instance, if there are signs of dacryocystitis, such as mucocele, discharge, or tenderness over the lacrimal sac, the lower system is partially or completely obstructed. Remember that swelling above the medial canthal tendon is most consistent with lacrimal sac tumor and should prompt imaging before surgery. Discharge or debris in the tear lake usually indicates blockage in the lower system; upper system blockage usually results in passage of mucoid debris into the nose.

A dye disappearance test is sometimes used to demonstrate lacrimal outflow capacities. In short, a fluorescein drop is placed in both eyes, with the expectation that clearance of the dye occurs in approximately 5 minutes from a normal eye. An abnormal result is nonlocalizing, indicating pump failure or outflow obstruction at any point within the apparatus. The mainstay of diagnosis is probing and irrigation of the lacrimal system. Probing with a Bowman probe or 23-gauge irrigating cannula detects canalicular stenosis or blockage. Inability to pass a probe and palpate the lacrimal bone indicates canalicular blockage, whereas difficult passage indicates narrowing. A stenotic canaliculus may be amenable to silastic tubing intubation before consideration of more invasive surgery. Attempts can sometimes be made to repair a localized canalicular obstruction, as done for traumatic canalicular lacerations. To test the lower system, the lower canaliculus is irrigated with saline or water. The patient should taste water in the back of the throat with minimal force on the syringe. The upper punctum is observed for reflux, which is abnormal in any amount. A distinction is made between partial and complete obstruction, but even partial obstructions can cause clinically significant tearing.

Nasal endoscopy is critical in preoperative evaluation for two important reasons. The first is to evaluate the relation of the septum to the lateral nasal wall. Deviation of the nasal septum can preclude endoscopic surgery if crowding is severe. Moreover, when a Jones tube is placed, successful surgery relies on adequate space for the distal end of the tube to drain tears. If necessary, a septoplasty should be performed at least 1 month before endoscopic conjunctivodacryocystorhinostomy (CDCR) to allow for optimal medialization of the septum. Intranasal tumors are the second reason warranting preoperative nasal endoscopy. Benign and malignant tumors can cause outflow obstruction, and knowledge of their presence is essential to guide the most rational treatment course.

Indications and advantages of endoscopic lacrimal surgery

When a diagnosis of lacrimal system obstruction is made, treatment is surgical. Dacryocystorhinostomy (DCR) bypasses a nasolacrimal duct blockage when the upper division of the system is intact. More proximal obstruction requires bypass of the canalicular system with CDCR. Selection of the appropriate operation is obvious when careful preoperative evaluation has occurred. Despite this, a subtle abnormality in the canalicular system sometimes requires CDCR as a secondary procedure once DCR has failed. An infrequent indication for CDCR is idiopathic hypersecretion, a diagnosis of exclusion. Shirmer testing reveals higher than normal basal tear secretion, and a comprehensive search for other causes should be exhausted.

DCR and CDCR can be approached externally or intranasally. An endoscopic approach to lacrimal surgery has advantages that are common to both procedures. Avoiding a skin excision eliminates scarring and accidental severing of the angular vessel. Therefore, there is less ecchymosis and edema. Once a surgeon has surmounted the steep learning curve of endoscopic surgery, both procedures can increase the efficiency of surgery by eliminating steps of the external approach. Visualization is enhanced for both procedures. An adequate ostium can be ensured, and access to the lacrimal fossa is facilitated for inspection and potential biopsy.

The endoscopic approach offers benefits specific to the CDCR procedure as well. Disruption of the medial canthal tissues with an external incision imposes a healing response and edema that can alter tissue position with time. Eliminating tissue manipulation with an endonasal approach may secure the proximal placement of the Jones tube. If the desired 45° downward angle of the tube is altered, gravity-driven drainage of tears can be impaired. An additional benefit of endoscopic CDCR is the excellent intraoperative visualization of the distal tube position. A short tube risks overgrowth of lateral nasal wall mucosa, whereas a long tube can abut the nasal septum. Either situation is best addressed at the time of surgery before the tube heals into position. Another important relation appreciated endoscopically is that of the distal end of the tube to the middle turbinate. Even after infracture of the middle turbinate, a partial turbinectomy may be necessary for a successful postoperative course.

Surgical techniques

Endoscopic dacryocystorhinostomy

The patient is asked to clear the nasal passage approximately 30 minutes before surgery. Two sprays of a nasal decongestant, 0.05% oxymetazoline, are administered to the nasal cavity on the surgical side. After 5 minutes, administration of nasal decongestant is repeated. The patient is then brought into the operating room and sedated. Although most patients tolerate the procedure under monitored intravenous sedation, some patients require general anesthesia. Under sedation, an 18-in length of 0.5-in gauze soaked in a 4% cocaine solution is packed in the area of the middle turbinate for 5 minutes. After removal of the gauze, local anesthesia using a 50:50 mixture of 2% lidocaine with 1:100,000 epinephrine with 0.75% bupivacaine with 1:200,000 epinephrine is injected into the submucosa of the anterior middle turbinate, uncinate process, and lateral nasal wall. The injection is given under direct visualization with the endoscope, and blanching of the mucosa is noted. With the endoscope, another strip of cocaine-soaked gauze is replaced between the lateral nasal wall and middle turbinate for at least 5 more minutes. This further shrinks the mucosa and provides more working area during surgery. Hemostasis is the most important factor in maintaining an excellent view during endoscopic lacrimal surgery. To avoid frustration and unnecessary surgical challenges, it is imperative to follow a strict regimen like that detailed here. After the second nasal packing is placed, time is available to drape the patient, scrub, and set up the video monitor. A sterile field is not required.

The nasal packing is removed, and the endoscope is placed within the nose. Occasionally, the middle turbinate is infractured with the blunt end of a periosteal elevator to enable an unobstructed view of the uncinate process and avoid blocking of the ostium. This maneuver is performed gently to avoid potential cerebrospinal fluid (CSF) leaks, because the middle turbinate attaches directly to the cribriform plate superiorly. Now, the sharp end of the periosteal elevator is used to incise the mucosa at the anterior border of the uncinate process. This demarcates the posterior border of the osteotomy. In preparation for the osteotomy, the mucosa overlying the lacrimal fossa is cauterized with a guarded monopolar cautery. The boundaries for cautery extend 10 mm anterior to the uncinate process and 10 mm inferior to the root of the middle turbinate. Care is taken to avoid cautery of the middle turbinate, which causes scarring and potential lateralization of the turbinate. Once cauterized, the mucosa is removed with

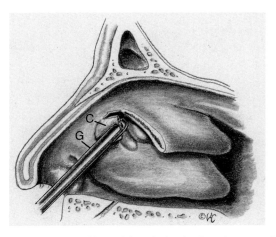

Fig. 1. DCR bone removal. Bone (C) overlying the lacrimal sac is removed with a Kerrison rongeur (G). (*Courtesy of* Frank A. Nesi, MD; with permission.)

the sharp edge of a periosteal elevator in a downward motion exposing the underlying bone. Blakesley forceps are used to clear any mucosal fragment still in the way. Clearing the mucosa reduces bleeding during bone removal.

Bone removal begins at the posterior edge of the exposed bone using a medium-sized 90° Kerrison rongeur (Fig. 1). This site corresponds to the site of the previous incision over the uncinate process. Several bites with the rongeur anteriorly and superiorly expose the underlying lacrimal sac. After punctal dilation, a size 0 Bowman probe is passed through the upper canalicular system and tents the posterior wall of the lacrimal sac (Fig. 2). The tented sac is then incised vertically with a sickle blade (Fig. 3). Enlargement of the sac opening is performed with the same blade or by gently tearing the mucosa with Blakesley forceps. Silastic tubing is passed through the canaliculi, the ostium, and the nose. Under mild tension, tubes are tied in a square knot (Fig. 4). A 3-mm section of a Robinson catheter may be tied over this knot to facilitate repositioning in the event of tube prolapse. No dressing or medication is required after surgery.

Endoscopic conjunctivodacryocystorhinostomy

The surgical procedure for endoscopic CDCR entails the steps of endoscopic DCR, starting with patient preparation for removal of bone overlying the lacrimal sac. Opening of the posterior sac wall is not necessary. Once the osteotomy is created, a tract for the Jones tube is formed with a 12-gauge angiocatheter. A bend is placed in the angiocatheter before placement to assist anterior placement of the tube. In a 45° infero-medial direction, the angiocatheter is advanced through the middle of the caruncle. Excision of the caruncle is not recommended, because this

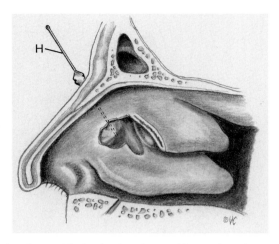

Fig. 2. DCR tenting the sac. The lacrimal sac is tented internally with a Bowman probe (H). (*Courtesy of* Frank A. Nesi, MD; with permission.)

promotes internal migration of the Jones tube. Endoscopic visualization is used as the needle passes through the lacrimal fossa and into the nasal cavity. Adjustments of position are made at this time. The needle is retracted, leaving the plastic catheter in place. A 9-in 14-gauge guidewire is passed through the catheter and held securely, and the catheter is then removed. A 4-mm × 19-mm Gladstone-Putterman modified Jones tube is then passed over the wire. This tube was designed with an internal flange 4 mm distal to the external flange. The added flange functions like an

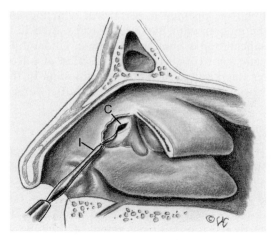

Fig. 3. DCR sac incision. An incision is made in the lacrimal sac (C) with a sickle blade (I). (*Courtesy of* Frank A. Nesi, MD; with permission.)

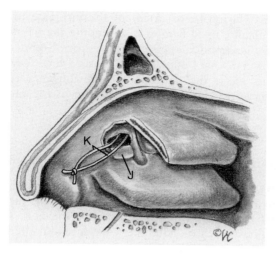

Fig. 4. DCR tube in place. The final appearance of the ostium is shown, with silastic tubing (K) in place and a mucosal flap (J) below the tubing. (*Courtesy of* Frank A. Nesi, MD; with permission.)

arrowhead to secure the tube against internal and external migration or ejection with forceful nose blowing, sneezing, or coughing. The modified tube inserts in a similar fashion as the original design except that a palpable click is felt when the internal flange traverses the medial canthal tissues. Both thumbnails are used on the external flange to lock the tube into position effectively. Ideally, the distal end of the tube is situated midway between the lateral wall and septum. In the event that the tube length is not appropriate, a longer or shorter tube may be inserted with the guidewire in place. Tube exchange is performed carefully to avoid shattering the glass tube. If forceps do not deliver the tube easily, a 2-0 silk suture may be wrapped around the proximal end to aid in gentle extraction. Once the proper tube is inserted, the guidewire is removed. To encourage the tube to heal without internal migration, a 6-0, double-armed, silk suture is double wrapped around the external flange. Both needles are passed through the medial canthus and tied over skin with a sterile rubber band bolster. The bolster is removed 1 week after surgery. No dressing or medications are needed after surgery.

Special surgical considerations

Occasionally, the distal end of the Jones tube may be too proximal to the middle turbinate. This situation risks tube occlusion and external migration. Intraoperative partial middle turbinectomy evades these complications. The procedure is straightforward. Local anesthetic is injected into the substance of the turbinate. The posterior extent of the turbinate to be removed is crushed with a small curved hemostat. Bounding the offending portion of the turbinate, the hemostat is applied to the superior border, attempting to join the compressed areas. Following the crushed lines, curved endoscopic turbinate scissors incise the portion of turbinate. Persistent connections often require gentle twisting with Blakesley forceps for amputation of the piece.

Postoperative care and management of complications

Postoperative care for endoscopic DCR is rather simple. The main precaution is to avoid eye rubbing, which can extract the tube. If the silastic tubing prolapses, the patient can try to blow the nose forcefully while occluding the opposite nostril. After a few unsuccessful attempts, the tubing can be temporarily taped to the nose or cheek to avoid ocular irritation. In a cooperative patient, the tube can be repositioned easily. Minor prolapse is sometimes amenable to external feeding of the tube back into the nose. When this is attempted with more significant prolapse, the tubing often curls into the lacrimal sac and later recoils. In this instance, the tube should be pulled back into the nasal cavity using bayonet forceps. An endoscope aids in tube localization, but the Robinson catheter is often visible with only a speculum. Before entering the nose, a nasal decongestant can be used to shrink the mucosa and to help with minor bleeding. In addition, an inhaled mucosal anesthetic can be used for comfort. Ideally, the tube should be left in place for at least 3 months. At this time, the tube is cut at the canthus and the patient forcefully expels the tubing. Occasionally, the tube needs to be manually retrieved. Retesting of the lacrimal system is now performed with irrigation.

Postoperative care and complications of endoscopic CDCR can be more involved. Patient satisfaction remains a vital indication of surgical success or failure. Objective evaluation of surgical outcome involves classification of tube drainage. A grading system is used by observing drainage of administered drops of water to the medial canthal area. Class I drainage is defined as spontaneous disappearance of water. Class II drainage implies that water travels down the tube with exaggerated nasal inspiration. Class I and II drainage is usually consistent with a positive subjective patient response. When the tube can be irrigated with a syringe, class III drainage is present, whereas class IV drainage indicates tube obstruction. Epiphora is not improved in either of these two scenarios.

Poor postoperative drainage results from misplacement or displacement of the tube. Tears cannot enter a tube that is displaced anteriorly. The course of action is to reposition the Jones tube more posteriorly. The tube must be removed, usually by wrapping a 2-0 silk suture around the external flange to minimize tube breakage. Contraction of medial canthal tissues around the tube can necessitate the use of Westcott scissors to release the tube. The 12-gauge angiocatheter re-enters the caruncular tissues posteriorly in relation to previous placement. Jones tube insertion follows as previously described.

Similarly, in cases of posterior placement, the tube is repositioned more anteriorly. Exaggerated posterior positioning of the Jones tube causes ocular irritation and risks conjunctival blockage of the proximal tube opening.

Internal migration of the tube also causes obstruction of the proximal end, and possibly the distal end, of the Jones tube. When caruncular tissues are needlessly excised, inward displacement is more likely. Removing these tubes can be challenging. Sometimes, a soft instrument is used intranasally to coax the tube outward. Westcott scissors are used to release contracted medial canthal tissues overlying the external flange. Once the tube is exposed, 2-0 silk suture can aid in extraction. Dissection should be purposeful to cause minimal disruption of the medial canthal tissues. In the event of extensive tissue manipulation, subsequent replacement of the tube should await adequate healing. This reduces the probability of repeated internal migration.

External displacement of the tube precludes tear entry and may cause eyelid irritation. Occasionally, manual pressure can relock the Jones tube in position. Intranasal examination may reveal a treatable cause of this migration. Possibilities include contact with the nasal septum, which requires placement of a shorter tube. As mentioned previously, a partial turbinectomy is necessary if the middle turbinate pushes on the distal end of the tube.

Sometimes, even a perfectly placed Jones tube can be blocked by redundant conjunctiva. Simple chemosis may resolve with a depo-steroid injection, but excess tissue resection can also be curative. Topical or depo-steroid may be used to quiet irritation of the medial canthal tissues.

ELSEVIER
SAUNDERS

Otolaryngol Clin N Am
38 (2005) 1109–1117

OTOLARYNGOLOGIC
CLINICS
OF NORTH AMERICA

Facial Lifting with "APTOS" Threads: Featherlift

M.A. Sulamanidze, MD[a], T.G. Paikidze, MD[a],
G.M. Sulamanidze, MD[a], Janet M. Neigel, MD[b],*

[a]TOTALCharm, Clinic of Plastic and Aesthetic Surgery, Moscow, Russia
[b]Private Practice, 101 Old Short Hills Road, Suite 204, West Orange, NJ 07052, USA

As the human face ages, it is known to be characterized by uneven focal ptosis of the soft tissues of the frontal, infraorbital, zygomatic, buccal, mental, and submental areas. The fat tissue in the zygomatic area is closely connected to the skin and the arch of the zygomatic bone by the solid intersection of the superficial musculoaponeurotic system (SMAS) and is rarely sagging [1]. The subcutaneous fat of the adjacent areas (infraorbital, buccal, malar, and partially mandibular) is suspended from under the soft tissues of the zygomatic areas (Fig. 1). Therefore, the skin of a young person is smooth and even. Gradually, under the effect of different causes (eg, age, degree of development of subcutaneous fat, structural pattern of the subcutaneous fat with its relation to the SMAS, along with mimic and masticatory muscles), gravitational sagging occurs in the areas where the connections are weak or the influence is more intensive (Fig. 2). Therefore, lachrymal grooves appear, the nasolabial fold deepens, and wrinkling starts to be more evident [2].

In addition, much importance in the causation of involutional alterations in the suborbicular areas is attached by some researchers [3] to the gradual sliding down of such formations as the suborbicular ocular fat (SOOF).

In the lower portions of the face, the neurovascular bundle that originates from the mental orifice of the lower jaw prevents sagging of the subcutaneous fat. In addition to the neurovascular bundle, a more or less solid adhesion of soft tissues along the lower edge of the jaw line prevents the sagging. The so-called "overhanging" of tissues appears along with wrinkles [4]. The surgical intervention of uplifting and excision of excessive skin is the radical solution to correcting these deformities.

* Corresponding author.
E-mail address: jmn@eyelid.com (J.M. Neigel).

SULAMANIDZE et al

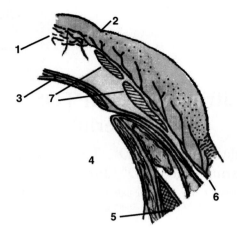

Fig. 1. Diagram of a horizontal dissection through the subzygomatic and buccal areas. 1, Circular muscle of mouth; 2, nasolabial pleat; 3, buccal muscle; 4, oral cavity; 5, masseter; 6, SMAS; 7, large and small jugal muscles.

In 1974, craniofacial and then plastic surgeons began to implement surgery of uplifting soft tissues under the SMAS. The surgeons put forward a postulate on the role of aging effects and the facial skeleton. The bravest of them changed over to supraperiosteal as well as subperiosteal SMAS uplifting. Such operations were even possible with the help of endoscopic equipment [5–7]. Beginning at approximately the same time, rejuvenating the face and neck was attempted through different methods. Various types

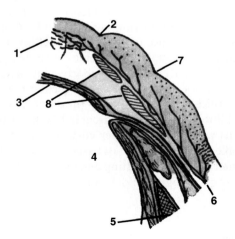

Fig. 2. Same diagram, with involutional alterations. 1, Circular muscle of mouth; 2, nasolabial pleat; 3, buccal muscle; 4, oral cavity; 5, masseter; 6, SMAS; 7, tear trough; 8, large and small jugal muscles.

of skin peeling and contour injection plasty of soft tissues with a variety of gels, along with skin reinforcement with special 20-karat golden threads, were performed [8,9]. Usually, the number of different methods described to solve a single problem suggests that few have borne the test of time, failing to win consensus.

Surgical intervention on a much grander scale has been characterized by a lengthy rehabilitation period fraught with possible complications and the expectation that the efficiency and natural appearance as well as the long-term results would not be comparable with the severity of the intervention performed [10].

If one fills in those wrinkles and folds with any implant, for example, hyaluronic acid gel, this can result in puffiness with unnatural contours, and the center of gravity of the face would be visually shifted downward. Using chemical peels makes it possible to obtain skin reduction, most notably of the superficial layers, but not tightening of the underlying flabby tissues. This does not attain uplift or a new contour to the face.

There is no doubt that one must retain these tissues in their old place before one can give the aging face a more juvenile appearance. The aim of the present study consists of improving the cosmetic outcome of surgical treatment of patients suffering from facial ptosis, using a new specially designed suturing material, simplifying the surgical technique, and decreasing the severity and duration of the postoperative period.

Material and methods

In our practice, we use a new technique of uplifting through suturing of flabby soft tissues of the aging face with special suturing material and stable fixation in a new esthetically advantageous position.

This technique is performed with the help of a new suturing material that we devised and called "APTOS" (RF patent 2139734, International Priority PST/RU 99/00263, dated July 29, 1999). The APTOS thread can be made of a metal, polymeric, or biologic material that is biocompatible with the human body. During the manufacturing process, the smooth thread (eg, made of polypropylene) is constructed with dents, cogs, or barbs, thus creating slant edges with sharp ends (Fig. 3). These cogs enable the thread to travel one way with the soft tissues. After the thread is inserted under the

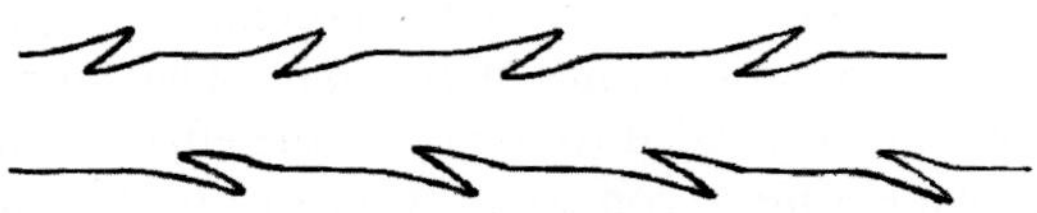

Fig. 3. Diagram of the longitudinal section of the APTOS thread with unilaterally directed cogs.

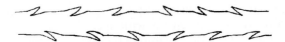

Fig. 4. Diagram of the longitudinal section of the APTOS thread with bilateral (converging) direction of the cogs.

skin, the cogs prevent the thread from moving in the opposite direction. This creates a uniform and symmetric gathering of the soft tissues, which uplifts them and provides a new volumetric contour.

To fix the uplifted tissues in the required position, the thread is provided with variously directed (convergent) cogs that provide support and fixation of the newly created contour inside the tissues (Fig. 4). The thread is inserted into the subcutaneous fat with the help of a guide, which is a long injection needle.

Surgical technique

In most cases, local anesthesia is used; 1% lidocaine solution is administered intradermally in the area of the entry and exit of the guide and along the area of the guide passage located in the fat (average consumption of 0.5–0.7 mL for one thread). The guiding needle is used to punch the skin along the previously marked contour before the area of desired lift at the required depth and is brought out at the place needed beyond the area of desired lift. Then, through one of the needle's orifices, the thread with converging cogs is inserted to give the soft tissues an upward lift. After the needle is removed, the remaining thread fixates the desired position of the tissues. If necessary, the ends of the threads are additionally pulled up. In doing so, each cog engages and supports a particular portion of the soft tissue. The threads smoothly shift and group the whole area of the soft tissues, which lie within the zone of the threads' action. After this, the thread ends are cut and allowed to retract under the skin.

To uplift separate portions of ptosed tissues, we have developed a special marking (Fig. 5). For example, lifting the buccozygomatic areas requires three threads to be passed under the skin from both sides: one long (8.5 cm) and two short (5 cm) threads, with the long one passed sufficiently deep within the fat tissue. After being stretched, this creates an uplift of the flabby buccal tissues and a round contour of the skin. The short thread passed parallel to the long one is needed to maintain the effect created by the long thread and to provide a more convex contour of the skin in this area. The second short thread passed subcutaneously along a steep arch from the zygomatic area toward the cheek makes it possible to replace the overhanging

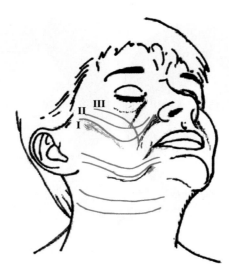

Fig. 5. Diagram of marking soft tissues of the face and neck in lifting with the APTOS thread.

above the nasolabial fold not only upward but laterally toward the cheekbones, thereby giving a smoother appearance and decreasing the lachrymal groove (tear trough).

To lift mental overhanging, we implant two long threads on each side parallel to the skin, not touching it from the inside, at a depth of 1 to 2 mm in the subcutaneous fat. Two APTOS threads (8.5 mm long) are passed in the submental area, improving the contour of the soft tissue of the subzygomatic areas.

Depending on the patient and individual peculiarities, other variants of implanting the threads are possible. The routine procedure is easy and quick to perform and is accompanied by minimal injury to the tissues, with little swelling and bruising experienced. The outcome is seen immediately, with a minimal short-term postoperative period (if any) and minimal postoperative restrictions (no abrupt chewing or facial expression and no facials, microdermabrasion, or massage for 2–3 weeks).

Since 1999, we have used the described technique on more than 250 patients; however, the present article deals with analyzing the outcomes of only 157 patients aged 22 to 77 years old (average age = 49 years). Most of these patients were women (94.4%). Of these patients, 130 underwent the placement of APTOS threads as the only procedure. The other 27 patients had additional procedures performed, such as peeling, liposuction and undercutting wrinkles with the wire scalpel.

The indications for correction of the contours of the face and neck with the APTOS threads were ptosis of tissues of the face and neck, a flabby and flat face, and poorly manifested esthetic contours.

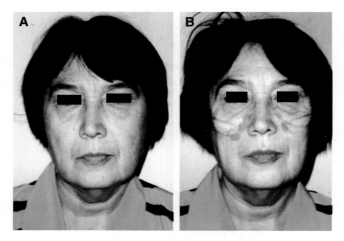

Fig. 6. Before (*A*) and immediately after (*B*) uplifting of the buccozygomatic areas.

Results and discussion

For the most part, this method was used to remove ptosis of the buccozygomatic areas (62%), which is related to the fact that it is these involutional alterations that the patients mainly worry about. In addition, the effect of the operation in these areas is visible immediately after the intervention and is especially expressive as well as long lasting (Fig. 6).

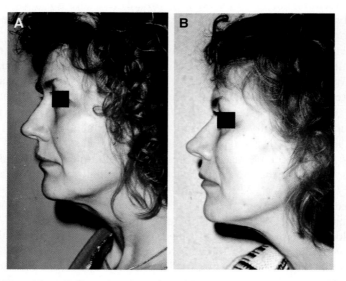

Fig. 7. Before (*A*) and 2 weeks after (*B*) uplifting of the buccozygomatic areas plus blepharoplasty.

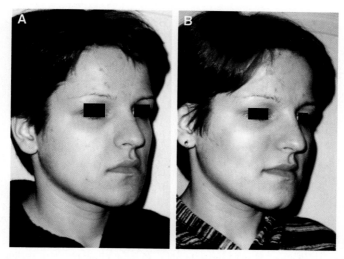

Fig. 8. Before (*A*) and 4 months after (*B*) uplifting of the buccozygomatic areas.

The immediate postoperative period up to 14 days was uneventful in most of the patients (Fig. 7). Only in 4 cases (2.5%) did we observe thread disruption attributable to unilateral weakening of edges and threads emerging to the cutaneous surface, thus requiring their removal and performance of a secondary implantation. We did not consider the cases of hypercorrection (9.5%), linear hemorrhage along the passage of the thread (9.5%), or skin indraft at the entrance and exit sites (14.6%) as

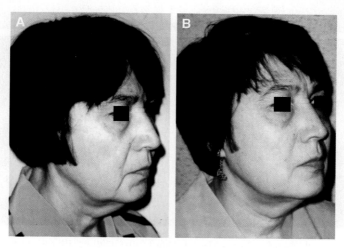

Fig. 9. Before (*A*) and 6 months after (*B*) lifting of the whole face.

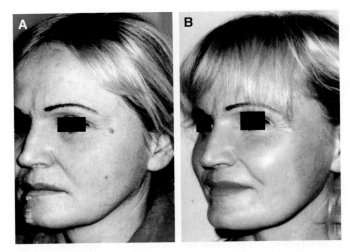

Fig. 10. Before (*A*) and 12 months after (*B*) facial lifting plus skin peeling.

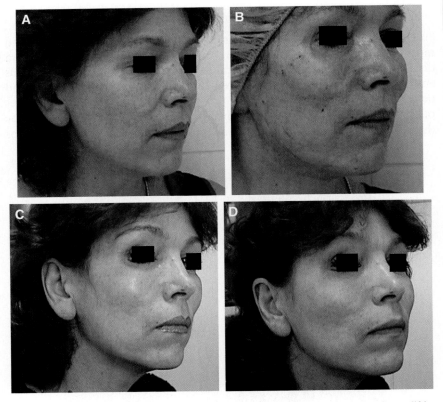

Fig. 11. Evolution of the face before (*A*), immediately after uplifting (*B*), 2 weeks after uplifting (*C*), and 1.5 months after uplifting (*D*).

complications, because all of these were easily corrected spontaneously or manually. No other complications or allergic reactions were noted.

Initially, we invited the patients to return during the postoperative period to follow up the duration of the effect achieved; however, later on, we were convinced that in most cases, the patients were satisfied with the obtained outcomes, and they only returned to continue other treatment. Additionally, the surgeons involved were quite satisfied with the short- and long-term outcomes, because the latter were good as well as permanent (follow-up from 2 months to 2.5 years after surgery; Figs. 8–11); therefore, we chose not to look for the evaluation criteria of the operations performed. Mention should only be made that at various points, 12 cases (8.9%) required unilateral or bilateral implantation of additional threads.

Summary

The use of the APTOS threads for lifting the tissues of the face and neck is a simple, conservative, cost-saving, and time-sparing procedure that leaves no visible traces of intervention on the skin. At the same time, the proposed technique proved efficient for correction of the jaw line and for lifting the flabby ptosed tissues in involutional facial alterations. Our experience proves that the described method can be an alternative technique to the classic methods of lifting and contour plasty of the jaw line with various implants.

References

[1] Mitz V, Peironye M. The superficial musculo-aponeurotic system in the parotid and cheek area. Plast Reconstr Surg 1976;58:80.

[2] Owsley JQ. Lifting the malar fat pad correction of prominent nasolabial folds. Plast Reconstr Surg 1993;91:463–74.

[3] Freeman MS. Transconjunctival sub-orbicularis oculi fat (SOOF) pad lift blepharoplasty. Arch Facial Plast Surg 2000;2.

[4] Sulamanidze MA, et al. Flabby, ageing face. A new approach. Presented at the World Congress on Aesthetic and Restorative Surgery. Mumbai February 2001.

[5] De la Plaza R, Arroyo JM. A new technique for the treatment of palpebral bags. Plast Reconstr Surg 1988;81:677–85.

[6] Hamra ST. The zygorbicular dissection in composite rhitidectomy: an ideal midface plane. Plast Reconstr Surg 1998;102(5):1646–57.

[7] Kazinnikova OG, Adamian AA. Age-specific changes in facial and cervical tissues, a review. Ann Plast Reconstr Aesth Surg 2000;1:52–61.

[8] Adamyan AA, et al. Clinical aspects of facial skin reinforcement with special (gold) surgical filaments. Ann Plast Reconstr Aesth Surg 1998;3:18–22.

[9] Sulamanidze MA, Sulamanidze GM, Paikidze TG. Wire scalpel for surgical correction of soft tissue contour defects by subcutaneous dissection. Dermatol Surg 2000;26(2):146–51.

[10] Skoog T. Plastic surgery. New methods and refinements. Stockholm: Almquist & Wiksell International; 1974. p. 301–3.

OTOLARYNGOLOGIC
CLINICS
OF NORTH AMERICA

Otolaryngol Clin N Am
38 (2005) 1119–1129

ELSEVIER
SAUNDERS

Cosmetic Uses of Injectable Phosphatidylcholine on the Face

Doris Maria Hexsel, MD[a],*, Marcio Serra, MD[b],
Taciana de Oliveira Dal'Forno, MD[c],
Debora Zechmeister do Prado, PHARM[d]

[a]*Cosmetic Dermatology Department, Brazilian Society of Dermatology, Brazil*
[b]*Sexually Transmitted Diseases Department, Brazilian Health Ministry,
Rio de Janeiro, RJ, Brazil*
[c]*Federal University of Rio Grande do Sul, Porto Alegre, RS, Brazil*
[d]*Doris Hexsel Dermatologic Clinic, Porto Alegre, RS, Brazil*

Intravenous phosphatidylcholine was initially used in cardiology for the treatment of lipid atheromas, hypercholesterolemia, fat embolism, and fatty deposits or plaque adhering to arterial walls [1–5]. It was also used for the treatment of mental disturbances and hepatic and cardiac conditions induced by medication, alcohol, pollution, virus, and toxins [6–9].

The first report of the cosmetic use of phosphatidylcholine was in Italy, where Maggiori [10] presented his work with phosphatidylcholine in the treatment of xanthelasmas.

In Brazil, the cosmetic use of phosphatidylcholine began on an off-label basis at the end of the 1990s. This article is a retrospective study using a sample of patients who were treated before phosphatidylcholine was prohibited in Brazil in January 2003.

The objective of this article is to report the authors' clinical experience in the use of phosphatidylcholine for the treatment of localized fatty areas of the face, which is a frequent complaint from some patients and is usually treated by liposuction, a more invasive procedure.

Anatomic aspects of facial fat

The facial outline is determined by the subcutaneous cellular tissue together with the facial musculature and the prominence of the parotid

---

* Corresponding author. Plinio Brasil Milano 476, Porte Alegre, RS 90520-000, Brazil.
E-mail address: dohexsel@zaz.com.br (D.M. Hexsel).

0030-6665/05/$ - see front matter © 2005 Elsevier Inc. All rights reserved.
doi:10.1016/j.otc.2005.05.002

glands [11]. A layer of fat covers the muscles and is distributed over the face in compartments of different shapes and volumes, such as Bichat's fatty pads in the malar region, which are responsible for the shape of the cheeks.

Adipose tissue has metabolic, thermal protective, and mechanical functions in addition to the esthetic effect of molding the body [12]. With aging, a redistribution of fat occurs and the deposits of fat become reduced in size; at the same time, there is a reduction in the function, size, and number of adipocytes as well as a reduction of preadipocyte differentiation, probably caused by alterations in important transcription factors, such as CCAAT/enhancer binding protein (C/EBP) and peroxisome proliferator activated receptor (PPAR) [13,14]. This also implies a change in the shape of the face, which acquires a more rounded form, similar to that of infancy, and the appearance of wrinkles and facial furrows. The redistribution of adipose tissue may also occur as an adverse effect of some chronic diseases, such as HIV/AIDS infection and Crohn's disease, for example.

In HIV infection, partial lipodystrophy occurs with the loss of peripheral fat in the face and limbs. One mechanism that causes this is the acceleration of apoptosis of adipose cells attributable to the mitochondrial toxicity caused by some antiretroviral drugs, mainly the nucleoside reverse transcriptase inhibitors (NRTIs). This process completely modifies the facial outline, with the loss of Bichat's fat pads as well as perioral, periocular, and other fat deposits and the resultant formation of large cavities in the face. These give the appearance of advanced age or terminal illness. At the same time, an accumulation of fat around the center of the body, such as the trunk and neck, may occur. In the face, the fat accumulation is seen with greater frequency in the parotid, lateral maxillary, and submandibular regions (Fig. 1), mainly in patients using protease inhibitors, although the mechanisms are as yet not well understood [15,16].

Available treatments of localized facial fat

Almost 20 years after its first application, liposuction is currently a procedure commonly used in the cervicofacial region [17]. Neck and facial liposuction requires smaller cannulas [18]. Smaller and shorter cannulas connected to a syringe or special machines creating negative pressure should be used for the jowl area to avoid oversuctioning [18].

The ideal conditions for the use of liposuction are the existence of sufficient elasticity of the skin, little excess skin, and sufficient subcutaneous adipose tissue to be suctioned. [17] Liposuction not only allows the flattening of contours but correction of sagging teguments, resulting in some skin retraction [17,19]. Submental liposuction is an adjunctive surgical procedure that allows relatively predictable soft tissue recontouring of the cervicofacial region [20].

A number of variations on the surgical techniques for face and neck liposuction have been described, including soft tissue shaver [21],

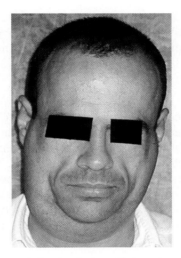

Fig. 1. Patient with fat accumulation in the parotid, lateral maxillary, and submandibular regions.

ultrasound-assisted lipectomy [22–24], intraoral transmental suction lipectomy [25], five-incision method combining machine-assisted and syringe aspiration [26], and submental suction-assisted lipectomy [27]. This latter technique has traditionally been reserved for younger patients or for older patients who are not face lift candidates. Thus, in general, for older patients, suction-assisted lipectomy is typically used as an adjunct for face and neck lifts [27].

The combination of well-tried and newly described liposuction techniques with techniques of facial or neck [28] lifting and augmentation [29] may offer enhancement of achievable results [30]. Liposuction may also be used in combination with laser resurfacing to improve the results, often with no increase in recovery time [31,32].

Injectable phosphatidylcholine

Phosphatidylcholine, for commercial ends, is mainly extracted from lecithins from vegetable species, such as soy, sunflower, and mustard. Lecithin from eggs is also a source of phosphatidylcholine [33].

In the composition of phosphatidylcholine extracted from soy, fatty acids like palmitic and stearic acids make up 19% to 24% of the total content. Monounsaturated fatty acids represent 9% to 11%, linoleic acid represents 56% to 60%, and alpha-linoleic acid represents 6% to 9%. Choline represents approximately 15% of the composition of phosphatidylcholine [33–35].

Chemically, phosphatidylcholine is also known as 1,2-diacyl-:ussn:ue-glycero-3-phosphocholine, PtdCho, and lecithin [34]. The phosphatidylcholine molecule consists of a head group (phosphorylcholine), a middle piece (glycerol), and two tails (the fatty acids, which vary). The phosphatidylcholine molecules present in the tissues of organisms may vary depending on the radical of the fatty acid linked to the molecule [34].

Action mechanism

The most widely recognized action mechanisms for phosphatidylcholine are those of an emulsifier and tensoactivator [36]. Rotunda and colleagues [36] affirm that phosphatidylcholine behaves as a detergent in the subcutaneous level, causing nonspecific lysis of fat cell membranes. These authors injected phosphatidylcholine and other detergents used in laboratories into pieces of pig skin. The viability and lysis of the cell membranes from the pig skin were evaluated after injection with these substances, and it was found that there was a significant loss of viability, membrane lysis, and breakdown of the architecture of the muscles and fats in the areas injected [36].

Components of the injectable solution

Injectable phosphatidylcholine is composed of the following chemical components:

- Phosphatidylcholine, USP 96%: as individually prepared and commercial injectable products, 5% phosphatidylcholine (5 g in each 100 mL of solution or 50 mg/mL) is used according to the monograph of the medicine registered with the United States Pharmacopoeia (USP) [34].
- Sodium deoxycholate or monoethanolamine deoxycholate: an active component that favors solubility of phosphatidylcholine and reduces its viscosity
- Benzyl alcohol: used as a preservative in injectable products
- Distilled water for reverse osmosis: the traditional vehicle for injectable preparations

Conservation and storage

Conservation and storage of the injectable 5% phosphatidylcholine preparation should be according to the manufacturer's recommendations and the specific legislation for injectable products. Phosphatidylcholine should be contained in brown glass vials because it suffers degradation when exposed to light. The manufacturer recommends that it should be kept under refrigeration (4°C–9°C), although there is no reference to this medicine being sensitive to temperature.

Materials and methods

From January 2001 to December 2002, 20 patients were given applications of phosphatidylcholine for the treatment of localized fat on the face. Of these 20 patients, 17 were female and 3 were male. Their age varied from 37 to 72 years for the women and from 32 to 47 years for the men. The mean age of the patients in the sample was 53.4 years. Three patients were HIV-positive.

The technique used for facial and neck treatment was subcutaneous infiltration with undiluted phosphatidylcholine (250 mg/5 mL), using a 0,5 × 13 G needle directly into the area of localized fat. Those areas with small fat deposits were infiltrated at only one central point, whereas in larger areas, the injections were at equidistant points of approximately 1 cm. At each application site, 0.2 mL was injected, totaling 0.2 to 5.0 mL (10–250 mg) per session. There were one to five sessions, with intervals of 3 to 4 weeks, according to the necessities of each patient, based on the initial medical evaluation and according to the results obtained from subsequent applications. The treated areas were the jaw line in 14 patients, the submental/chin region in 8 patients, the malar area in 3 patients, and the preauricular area in 2 patients.

The patients were asked to report any side effects that occurred during treatment. Digital photographs were taken before initiating treatment and at the end of the treatment course.

A follow-up questionnaire was administered by telephone up to 3 years after the last treatment. The satisfaction level of the patients with the treatment was evaluated as satisfied or unsatisfied. In those patients who responded that they were satisfied, the degree of reduction of localized fat was evaluated as discreet, moderate, or marked. Patients were also asked whether the reduction of localized fat was persistent up to 3 years after application.

Results

All the treated patients had pain, itching, and erythema on the first and second days after the injections. The edema remained visible for a maximum of 10 days after the treatment. Bruising was also observed at the treated sites and regressed spontaneously in the days immediately after treatment. No systemic side effect was reported by these patients. Although these side effects disappeared in a short time, they may cause more discomfort in facial areas than in body areas, where they can be hidden by clothing.

Of the sample of 20 patients, 18 (90% of the sample) reported a reduction in the deposits of localized fat on the face after phosphatidylcholine treatment. Of these 18 patients, 9 (50%) reported a marked reduction, 6 (33.3%) reported a moderate reduction, and 3 (16.6%) reported a discreet reduction. The 2 patients who did not report any improvement only had one application session.

In the group that reported improvement, 16 patients (80% of the sample) reported that the improvement persisted up to 3 years after the treatment

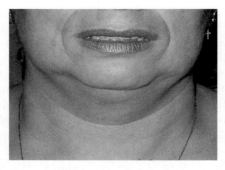

Fig. 2. Patient with fat accumulation before treatment with injections of phosphatidylcholine.

sessions. The three HIV-positive patients reported marked and persistent improvements.

Discussion

The youthful face is characterized by its rounded aspect and the presence of adequate volumes of bone, teeth, fat, and collagen. The reabsorption of these volumes and the redistribution of the fat in some deposit areas of the lower face lead to an aged appearance. Treatment of the aging process has led to a demand for specific treatments, such as fillers, lasers, botulinum toxin, and other methods (eg, those that can remove localized accumulations of excess fat). With liposuction, there is a potential risk when dealing with small volumes of fat in the face.

The demand for ever less-invasive techniques for the treatment of the aging face has given impulse to the search for alternative treatments. Four human studies have been published on the treatment of localized fat with the subcutaneous application of phosphatidylcholine [37–40]. The first study published included 30 patients with varying degrees of lower eyelid fat pads. The patients received one to four injections of phosphatidylcholine into the

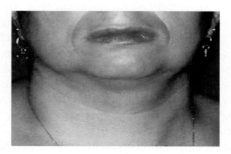

Fig. 3. Patient with fat accumulation after treatment with injections of phosphatidylcholine.

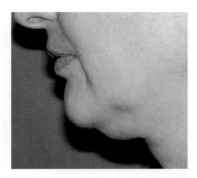

Fig. 4. Same patient before subcutaneous injections of phosphatidylcholine in the submento-nian region.

fat pads at intervals of 15 days. There was cosmetic improvement in all patients [37]. In another study published by the present authors, 213 patients, of whom 8 were HIV-positive, were treated with phosphatidyl-choline with the aim of reducing localized fat deposits. The patients were subjected to one to five subcutaneous applications at an average interval of 15 days. Thirteen patients from this study underwent laboratory evaluation, including blood tests, glycemia, lipid profile, and liver and renal function before treatment and 48 hours and 14 days after application, and there was no significant difference in the test results. Most patients reported a reduction of localized fat deposits in the areas treated, and this was confirmed with medical examination [38]. Yet another study reported the results of 50 patients who received applications of phosphatidylcholine for the treatment of localized fat, with reduction of deposits in all treated patients and without recurrence of treatment for a period of 2 years [39]. The most recently published clinical trial studied the efficacy and safety of injectable phosphatidylcholine for the treatment of eyelid fat pads. Ten

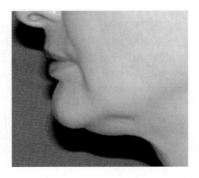

Fig. 5. Same patient after subcutaneous injections of phosphatidylcholine in the submentonian region.

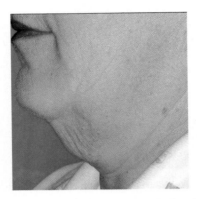

Fig. 6. Female patient before subcutaneous injections of phosphatidylcholine in the submentonian region.

patients were treated in three to five sessions. Improvement in fat herniation was reported in 80% and 70% of patients as graded by the physician and patients, respectively [40].

An animal model study was presented by Paschoal and colleagues [41]. They injected phosphatidylcholine in 6 healthy pigs and another group received placebo. Once a week, each pig received 10 subcutaneous injections of 0.5 mL phosphatidylcholine, 2 cm apart, into the flanks for 10 consecutive weeks. The total dose administered per pig, per week were 500 mg and the animals were submitted to physical and biochemical examination, over 6 months. Two days after the last injection, all the pigs became icteric (3+/4+), had prostration, and showed petechias, hematomas, bleeding from the mucous membranes and superficial ulcers at the extremities. Biochemical liver function alterations were observed in all pigs. The symptoms regressed in 5 of the 6 animals, following suspension of the treatment, but one of the pigs (from phosphatidylcholine group) died 2 days after the last injection due to cholestatic hepatitis. Probably these doses and frequency of injections can lead to hepatic overload, which may explain the results in the studied pigs. The pigs in the control group did not present complications. This is the first study reporting the effects of subcutaneous injection in animals, as used for cosmetic purposes. This study confirmed that further studies of phosphatidylcholine are needed to establish the safety of this drug prior to approval in humans, such as dose levels and frequency, and total doses as well as other possible side effects.

The side effects described in the previously cited studies included localized pain, infiltrative edema, erythema, localized heat, itching, and bruises at the treatment sites. These lasted for only a few days after the applications [37–39].

The present study shows similar results to those of previously published human studies on the use of phosphatidylcholine in the treatment of

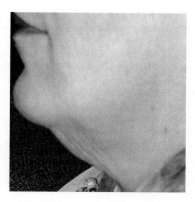

Fig. 7. Female patient after subcutaneous injections of phosphatidylcholine in the submentonian region.

localized fat and shows high levels of satisfaction in the treatment of areas of localized fat on the face in the studied sample in healthy and HIV-positive patients (Figs. 2–7). The local side effects reported by the patients in this study are also the same as those reported in previous publications, and no other variation or systemic side effect was found.

Summary

Despite the temporary side effects that cause a degree of discomfort, phosphatidylcholine injections can be used successfully in the treatment of localized and small fatty areas of the face, as it requires a few injections and less than one vial. Injection of phosphatidylcholine seems to be a better, safer, and more cost-effective treatment than liposuction in these specific cases. We point out that more studies should be performed to trace the safety profile and appropriate doses of phosphatidylcholine for the treatment of localized fat.

References

[1] Navder KP, Baraona E, Lieber SC. Polyenylphosphatidylcholine decreases alcoholic hyperlipemia without affecting the alcohol-induced rise of HDL-cholesterol. Life Sci 1997; 61(19):1907–14.
[2] Maranhao RC, Feres MC, Martins MT, et al. Plasma kinetics of a chylomicron-like emulsion in patients with coronary artery disease. Atherosclerosis 1996;27:126(1):15–25.
[3] Bialecka M. The effect of bioflavonoids and lecithin on the course of experimental atherosclerosis in rabbits. Ann Acad Med Stetin 1997;43:41–56.
[4] Brook JG, Linn S, Aviram M. Dietary soya lecithin decreases plasma triglyceride levels and inhibits collagen- and ADP-induced platelet aggregation. Biochem Med Metab Biol 1986; 35(1):31–9.
[5] Melchinskaya EN, Gromnatsky NI, Kirichenko LL. Hypolipidemic effects of alisat and lipostabil in patients with diabetes mellitus. Ter Arkh 2000;72(8):57–8.

[6] Ozerova IN, Paramonova IV, Akhmedzhanov NM, et al. Sinvastatin and lipostabil induce beneficial changes in high density lipoproteins phospholipid composition. Atherosclerosis 1999;144(Suppl 1):33.

[7] Polichetti E, Janisson A, La Porte PL, et al. Dietary polyenylphosphatidylcholine decreases cholesterolemia in hypercholesterolemic rabbits—role of the hepato-biliary axis. Life Sci 2000;67(21):2563–76.

[8] Takahashi Y, Mizunuma T, Kishino YJ. Effects of choline deficiency and phosphatidylcholine on fat absorption in rats. Nutr Sci Vitaminol 1982;28(2):139–47.

[9] Simonsson P, Nilsson A, Akesson B. Postprandial effects of dietary phosphatidylcholine on plasma lipoproteins in man. Am J Clin Nutr 1982;35(1):36–41.

[10] Maggiori S. Traitement mésotérapique des xanthelasmas à la phosphatidilcoline poluinsaturèe (EPL). V Congrès Internacional de Mésothérapie, Paris, 1988. Dermatologie. p. 364.

[11] Madeira MC. Anatomia da face: bases anátomo-funcionais para a prática odontológica. 3ª edição. São Paulo, Brazil: SAVIER; 2001.

[12] Freedberg IM. Fitzpatrick's dermatology in general medicine. 6th edition. New York: McGraw Hill; 2003.

[13] Kirkland JL, Tchkonia T, Pirtskhalava T, et al. Adipogenesis and aging: does aging make fat go MAD? Exp Gerontol 2002;37:757–67.

[14] Karagiannides I, Tchkonia T, Dobson DE, et al. Altered expression of C/EBP family members results in decreased adipogenesis with aging. Am J Physiol Regulatory Integrative Comp Physiol 2001;1280:R1772–80.

[15] White AJ. Mitochondrial toxicity and HIV therapy. Sex Transm Infect 2001;77:158–73.

[16] Pond CM. Long term changes in adipose tissue in human disease. Proc Nutr Soc 2001;60: 365–74.

[17] Flageul G, Illouz YG. Isolated cervico-facial liposuction applied to the treatment of aging. Ann Chir Plast Esthet 1996;41(6):620–30.

[18] Krauss MC, Kaminer MS. Liposuction. In: Nouri K, Leal-Khouri S, editors. Techniques in dermatologic surgery. London: Mosby; 2003. p. 315–22.

[19] Goodstein WA. Superficial liposculpture of the face and neck. Plast Reconstr Surg 1996; 98(6):988–96 [discussion: 997–8].

[20] Ziccardi VB. Adjunctive cervicofacial liposuction. Atlas Maxillofac Surg Clin North Am 2000;8(2):81–97.

[21] Gross CW, Becker DG, Lindsey WH, et al. The soft-tissue shaving procedure for removal of adipose tissue. A new, less traumatic approach than liposuction. Arch Otolaryngol Head Neck Surg 1995;121(10):1117–20.

[22] Grotting JC, Beckenstein MS. Cervicofacial rejuvenation using ultrasound-assisted lipectomy. Plast Reconstr Surg 2001;107(3):847–55.

[23] Navarro VF. Rhytidectomy assisted with ultrasound techniques: the ultra-lipo lift technique. Aesthetic Plast Surg 2001;25(3):175–80.

[24] Wilkinson TS. New perspectives in facial contouring using external ultrasonography. Clin Plast Surg 2001;28(4):703–18.

[25] Mommaerts MY, Abeloos JV, De Clerq CA, et al. Intraoral transmental suction lipectomy. Int J Oral Maxillofac Surg 2002;31(4):364–6.

[26] Langdon RC. Liposuction of neck and jowls: five-incision method combining machine-assisted and syringe aspiration. Dermatol Surg 2000;26:388–91.

[27] Gryskiewicz JM. Submental suction-assisted lipectomy without platysmaplasty: pushing the (skin) envelope to avoid a face lift for unsuitable candidates. Plast Reconstr Surg 2003; 112(5):1393–405 [discussion: 1406–7].

[28] Jasin ME. Submentoplasty as an isolated rejuvenative procedure for the neck. Arch Facial Plast Surg 2003;5(2):180–3.

[29] Butterwick KJ. Enhancement of the results of neck liposuction with the FAMI technique. J Drugs Dermatol 2003;2(5):487–93.

[30] Kamer FM, Pieper PG. Surgical treatment of the aging neck. Facial Plast Surg 2001;17(2): 123–8.

[31] Cook WR Jr. Cook "Weekend Alternative to the Facelift." Liposculpture of the face, neck, and jowls with laser dermal resurfacing and platysmal plication. Dermatol Clin 1999;17(4): 773–82.

[32] Cook WR Jr. Laser neck and jowl liposculpture including platysma laser resurfacing, dermal laser resurfacing, and vaporization of subcutaneous fat. Dermatol Surg 1997;23(12):1143–8.

[33] Phosphatidylcholine monograph. Alternative Medicine Review. April 2002. Available at: www.findarticles.com. Accessed March 3, 2004.

[34] The United States Pharmacopeia. The National Formulary, USP 27, NF 22. Rockville, MD: United States Pharmacopeial Convention. 2004.

[35] Andreo-Filho A, Oda CY, Scarpa MV, et al. Quantitative determination of phosphatidyl-choline by high performance liquid chromatography using silica column. Rev Cien Farm 1999;20(91):107–15.

[36] Rotunda AM, Suzuki BSH, Moy RL, et al. Detergent effects of sodium deoxycholate are a major feature of an injectable phosphatidylcholine formulation used for localized fat dissolution. Dermatol Surg 2004;30(7):1001–8.

[37] Rittes PG. The use of phosphatidylcholine for correction of lower lid bulging due to prominent fat pads. Dermatol Surg 2001;27(4):391–2.

[38] Hexsel D, Serra M, Mazzuco R, et al. Phosphatidylcholine in the treatment of localized fat. J Drugs Dermatol 2003;2(5):511–8.

[39] Rittes PG. The use of phosphatidylcholine for correction of localized fat deposits. Aesthetic Plast Surg 2003;27(4):315–8.

[40] Ablon G, Rotunda AM. Treatment of lower eyelid fat pads using phosphatidylcholine: clinical trial and review. Dermatol Surg 2004;30(3):422–7.

[41] Paschoal LH, Lourenço L, Ribeiro A, et al. Um alerta! Efeitos sistêmicos e teciduais da fosfatidilcolina em suínos. Faculdade de Medicina do ABC, Santo André - SP e Medicina Veterinária da UNIP- São Paulo-SP. [poster]. Presented at 16° Congresso de Cirurgia Dermatológica. Porto de Galinhas, PE. June, 2004.

ELSEVIER
SAUNDERS

Otolaryngol Clin N Am
38 (2005) 1131–1135

OTOLARYNGOLOGIC
CLINICS
OF NORTH AMERICA

Index

Note: Page numbers of article titles are in **boldface** type.

Changing Your Address?

Make sure your subscription changes too! When you notify us of your new address, you can help make our job easier by including an exact copy of your Clinics label number with your old address (see illustration below.) This number identifies you to our computer system and will speed the processing of your address change. Please be sure this label number accompanies your old address and your corrected address—you can send an old Clinics label with your number on it or just copy it exactly and send it to the address listed below.

We appreciate your help in our attempt to give you continuous coverage. Thank you.

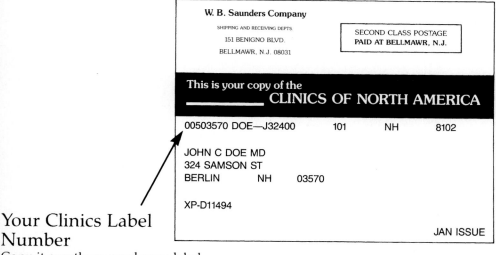

Your Clinics Label Number

Copy it exactly or send your label along with your address to:
W.B. Saunders Company, Customer Service
Orlando, FL 32887-4800
Call Toll Free 1-800-654-2452

Please allow four to six weeks for delivery of new subscriptions and for processing address changes.